Integrated Psychological Therapy (IPT)

Integrated Psychological Therapy (IPT)

for the Treatment of Neurocognition, Social Cognition, and Social Competency in Schizophrenia Patients

Volker Roder
University Hospital of Psychiatry, University of Bern, Switzerland

Daniel R. Müller
University Hospital of Psychiatry, University of Bern, Switzerland

Hans D. Brenner
Viña del Mar, Chile

William D. Spaulding
University of Nebraska, Lincoln, USA

In collaboration with
Anna Heuberger, MSc
University Hospital of Psychiatry, University of Bern, Switzerland

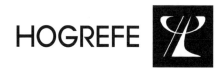

Library of Congress Cataloging in Publication

is available via the Library of Congress Marc Database under the
LC Control Number 2010930748.

Library and Archives Canada Cataloguing in Publication

Integrated psychological therapy (IPT) for the treatment of neurocognition, social
cognition, and social competency in schizophrenia patients / Volker Roder . . . [et al.].
— 1st ed.
Includes bibliographical references.
ISBN 978-0-88937-389-1
1. Schizophrenia—Treatment.   2. Cognitive therapy. 3. Schizophrenics—
Rehabilitation.   I. Roder, Volker
RC514.I585   2010   616.89'806   C2010-904337-5

Cover illustration © 2010 Artur Heras www.arturheras.com
© 2011 by Hogrefe Publishing

PUBLISHING OFFICES
USA: Hogrefe Publishing, 875 Massachusetts Avenue, 7th Floor,
                        Cambridge, MA 02139, Phone (866) 823-4726, Fax (617) 354-6875
                        E-mail customerservice@hogrefe-publishing.com
EUROPE: Hogrefe Publishing, Rohnsweg 25, 37085 Göttingen, Germany
                        Phone +49 551 49609-0, Fax +49 551 49609-88
                        E-mail publishing@hogrefe.com

SALES & DISTRIBUTION
USA: Hogrefe Publishing, Customer Services Department,
                        30 Amberwood Parkway, Ashland, OH 44805, Phone (800) 228-3749
                        Fax (419) 281-6883, E-mail customerservice@hogrefe.com
EUROPE: Hogrefe Publishing, Rohnsweg 25, 37085 Göttingen, Germany
                        Phone +49 551 49609-0, Fax +49 551 49609-88
                        E-mail publishing@hogrefe.com

OTHER OFFICES
CANADA: Hogrefe Publishing, 660 Eglinton Ave. East, Suite 119–514, Toronto,
                        Ontario M4G 2K2
SWITZERLAND: Hogrefe Publishing, Länggass-Strasse 76, CH-3000 Bern 9

Hogrefe Publishing. Incorporated and registered in the Commonwealth of Massachusetts,
USA, and in Göttingen, Lower Saxony, Germany.

Printed and bound in the USA
ISBN 978-0-88937-389-1

Foreword

It is a special privilege to be asked to write a foreword for this book, which is the fruit of over two decades of visionary and ground-breaking work in support of the recovery process in schizophrenia and, indeed, other psychotic disorders. I recall visiting Bern in the late 1980s, as a young academic psychiatrist, when this work was being formulated and pioneered, and feeling very excited that a scientific approach to the psychosocial care of patients was in development. Bern was one of the very few places in the world providing leadership in this field. It attracted a cohort of like-minded people and inspired many of them to pursue this type of approach in their own settings. At the time there were very few therapeutic tools in the toolkit to treat psychotic patients apart from basic nursing care and antipsychotic medications. We are now in a much better position, although still far too few patients around the world are given access to truly holistic recovery-oriented care from the onset of their illnesses. If this were to occur, the burden of these illnesses would be dramatically lessened.

Based originally on stress/vulnerability and cognitive neuroscience models, IPT has covered all of the domains that are affected in schizophrenia from neurocognition and social cognition through relationships and social functioning in the real world. It has been evolved and evaluated progressively over a long period of time and now has an impressive evidence base to support its more widespread dissemination. This comprehensive text is a vital tool in this endeavor. People with schizophrenia or other psychoses and their families have many reasons to be grateful to these pioneers, committed therapists, and researchers who have produced this body of expertise. This new volume provides a highly accessible resource for clinicians and I really hope IPT is taken up much more widely within clinical care settings across the world so that many more patients and families can benefit.

Patrick McGorry, MD, PhD
University of Melbourne, Australia

Preface

The importance of cognitive factors in the therapy and rehabilitation of schizophrenia patients has been recognized, examined, and is increasingly being accepted internationally in recent years. Cognitive factors have proved to have a decisive influence on how successfully patients can be (re)integrated in the community ("recovery perspective").

The initial development of Integrated Psychological Therapy (IPT) in the 1980s was truly pioneering, since it was one of the very first comprehensive and manualized treatment approaches for schizophrenia patients that combined neurocognitive, social cognitive, and social competence interventions. It was also truly innovative, in that – for example – it already contained interventions addressing "social cognition" years before that term had even been defined. The original IPT manual, published in 1988 in German, became a sort of therapy "classic." Subsequently, both the theoretical background and practical procedures used in IPT were continuously adapted within this framework to reflect the latest results of clinical and basic research. The ultimate goal of IPT is to provide our patients with the best possible chances of a good recovery.

A total of 35 studies on IPT, involving 1,529 patients from 12 different countries in Europe, North, Middle, and South America, as well as Asia, have now been published (see Chapter 7). IPT is, therefore, one of the most widely studied approaches around, and a broad range of clinical experience and empirical results have been gathered over the years. The American Psychological Association (APA) has also adopted IPT in its recommendations for treating schizophrenia patients ("Catalog of Clinical Training Opportunities: Best Practices for Recovery and Improved Outcomes for People with Serious Mental Illness": http://www.apa.org/practice/resources/grid/index.aspx; June 2010).

The IPT manual itself has been published in 13 languages and in multiple editions. The first manual appeared more than 20 years ago, and the latest version (the 6th revised German edition) was published in 2008. Because the first (and to date only) English edition was last published in 1994 – and our knowledge and understanding of schizophrenia have improved immensely since then – we felt it was time to publish a new version. We, therefore, completely rewrote most of the chapters for this book and expanded it greatly.

The book is divided into three main parts:
– **Part A: Theoretical Background and Treatment Approaches: An Overview** contains two chapters. Chapter 1 describes the theoretical background of cognitive behavioral treatments, for example, vulnerability-stress models, and shows how neurocognition and social cognition are highly relevant variables for functional out-

come and recovery. Chapter 2 provides an overview of the different cognitive-behavioral treatment approaches (cognitive remediation therapy and cognitive therapy, social competence approaches, psychoeducation and family therapy, and integrative approaches) as well as empirical evidence concerning their efficacy.

- **Part B: IPT – Indication, Therapy, Assessment, and Evaluation,** comprises five chapters and forms the core of the book. Here, clinicians learn step by step how to use the therapy techniques of the five IPT subprograms and how to select the appropriate therapy materials (which themselves are described at the back of the book). Numerous vignettes and examples from real therapy sessions are used to illustrate the techniques. We also provide practical advice for dealing with (difficult) group processes as well as individual dyadic situations. Furthermore, therapists can learn how to use IPT within multimodal therapy and rehabilitation efforts (case management). Chapter 3 describes the conditions needed to carry out the therapy program, while Chapter 4 gives an overview of the IPT approach and its five subprograms. Chapter 5 then shows how these five IPT subprograms can be implemented in practice. Chapter 6 looks at assessment and treatment planning. Finally, Chapter 7 discusses empirical results of studies involving IPT.
- **Part C: Further Development of IPT.** The cognitive part of IPT is now directly oriented toward the NIMH MATRICS variables (Measurement and Treatment Research to Improve Cognition in Schizophrenia) for patients who are better socially integrated and show fewer negative symptoms. The social competence part has been expanded in three specific areas: residential, vocational, and recreational rehabilitation. New therapy programs were developed and evaluated for these areas.

Last, but not least, we would like to thank all patients as well as numerous clinicians and researchers for their (critical) feedback about IPT. This feedback has contributed enormously to the continuous development of IPT and to making it what it is today: a proven, empirically supported, and practical approach to treating schizophrenia. Our thanks also go to Anna Heuberger, MSc, and Manuela Christen, MSc, research psychologists at the Psychiatric University Hospital in Bern, Switzerland, who provided us with tremendous support in drafting and writing the different chapters of this book. Finally, we would also like to thank Hogrefe Publishing, especially Robert Dimbleby, who initiated this new edition of the IPT.

Bern, Switzerland, Summer 2010
Volker Roder

About the Authors

Volker Roder, PhD
Professor of Clinical Psychology
University Hospital of Psychiatry
University of Bern
Bolligenstr. 111
CH-3000 Bern 60
Switzerland
E-mail: roder@sunrise.ch

Daniel R. Müller, PhD
Senior Lecturer of Psychology
University Hospital of Psychiatry
University of Bern
Bolligenstr. 111
CH-3000 Bern 60
Switzerland
E-mail: daniel.mueller@spk.unibe.ch

Hans D. Brenner, PhD, MD
Professor of Psychiatry
5 Norte 206, Dpt. 1201
Viña del Mar
Chile
E-mail: hansdbrenner@hotmail.com

William D. Spaulding, PhD
Professor of Clinical Psychology
Department of Psychology
University of Nebraska-Lincoln
317 Burnett Hall
Lincoln NE 68588-0308
USA
E-mail: WSpaulding@neb.rr.com

Table of Contents

Foreword by Patrick McGorry v
Preface vi
About the Authors viii

A. Theoretical Background and Treatment Approaches: An Overview

1 Theoretical Basis of Cognitive Behavioral Treatments 3
1.1 Systemic Vulnerability – Stress Models 3
    1.1.1 Zubin and Spring's Vulnerability Model 3
    1.1.2 Nuechterlein and Colleagues' Heuristic Vulnerability/Stress Model . 4
    1.1.3 Elaborations of Systemic Vulnerability Models 4
    1.1.4 Pervasiveness and Homeorhesis 10
1.2 Systemic Models in Clinical Application 12
    1.2.1 Cognitive Science and Technology 12
    1.2.2 Functional Outcome: A Main Objective of Rehabilitation 15
    1.2.3 Rehabilitation and the Recovery Movement 18
    1.2.4 Distribution, Mediation, and Moderation of Treatment Effects . . . 21
    1.2.5 An Integrated Model 22

2 Treatment Approaches and Empirical Results 25
2.1 Psychoeducation and Family Therapy 27
2.2 Cognitive Behavior Therapy Approaches for (Persistent)
Positive Symptoms 28
2.3 Social Competence Therapy 29
    2.3.1 Developmental Stages of Social Competence Therapy Approaches . 30
    2.3.2 Efficacy of Social Competence Therapy Approaches 31
2.4 Cognitive Remediation Therapy 32
    2.4.1 Neurocognitive Remediation Therapy 34
        Efficacy of Neurocognitive Remediation Therapy 37
    2.4.2 Social Cognitive Remediation Therapy 38
        Efficacy of Social Cognitive Remediation Therapy 42
    2.4.3 Integrated Therapy Approaches 43
        Efficacy of Integrated Therapy Approaches 46

B. IPT: Indication, Therapy, Assessment, and Evaluation

**3   Conditions for Carrying Out the Therapy Program:
Implementation and Indication**   49

3.1 Institutional Conditions   49
3.2 Patients   51
3.3 Group Makeup   53
3.4 Therapists   53
3.5 Differential Indication for Carrying Out IPT   54

4   The Therapy Program and Its Five Subprograms – An Overview . .   57

4.1 General Structure and Integration into a Multimodal
Treatment Concept   57
4.2 Cognitive Differentiation   60
4.3 Social Perception   63
4.4 Verbal Communication   65
4.5 Social Skills   67
4.6 Interpersonal Problem Solving   71

5   Implementation of the Five IPT Subprograms   75

5.1 General Considerations   75
5.2 Cognitive Differentiation   80
    5.2.1 Introducing the Subprogram   80
    5.2.2 Description of the Subprogram's Different Steps   81
5.3 Social Perception   89
    5.3.1 Introducing the Subprogram   89
    5.3.2 Description of the Subprogram's Different Steps   92
5.4 Verbal Communication   101
    5.4.1 Introducing the Subprogram   101
    5.4.2 Description of the Subprogram's Different Steps   103
5.5 Social Skills   112
    5.5.1 Introducing the Subprogram   112
    5.5.2 Description of the Subprogram's Different Steps   114
5.6 Interpersonal Problem Solving   123
    5.6.1 Introducing the Subprogram   123
    5.6.2 Description of the Subprogram's Different Steps   125
    5.6.3 Revised Therapeutic Procedures for Interpersonal Problem Solving   133
5.7 Group Processes Considerations   135

6   Assessment and Therapy Planning   141

6.1 Problem Analysis   142
    6.1.1 Behavior and Problem Analysis   142
    6.1.2 Sociocultural Background   146
    6.1.3 Classificatory Diagnostics   147
    6.1.4 History of Past Problems and Treatments   147

6.1.5 Treatment Plan 147
6.2 Assessment Instruments 148
6.2.1 Psychiatric Symptoms and Mental Status 148
6.2.2 Cognitive Functioning 150
6.2.3 Social Functioning 154
6.3 Self- and Expert-Rating System 155

7 Description and Discussion of Empirical Results 157
7.1 Quantitative Review of IPT Studies 159
7.2 Robust IPT Effects 160
7.3 Effects in Functional Levels and Symptom Reduction 160
7.4 IPT Subprograms: What Works? 161
7.5 Efficacy and Effectiveness of IPT 162

C. Further Development of IPT

8 Introduction 165
8.1 Cognitive Subprograms: INT – Integrated Neurocognitive Therapy . . . 166
8.1.1 Treatment Concept of INT 166
8.1.2 Evaluation of INT 168
8.2 Social Skills Subprograms: WAF* – Vocational, Residential, and
Recreational Skills 169
8.2.1 Treatment Concept of WAF 169
8.2.2 Evaluation of WAF 171

Appendix: Therapy Materials and Questionnaires (Worksheets) 173

Bibliography 229

---

* We use the German abbreviation for "**W**ohnen, **A**rbeit, **F**reizeit."

Part A
Theoretical Background and Treatment Approaches:
An Overview

1 Theoretical Basis of Cognitive Behavioral Treatments

1.1 Systemic Vulnerability – Stress Models

Theoretical models for understanding schizophrenia-spectrum disorders have evolved over many decades. By the end of the 1980s, the most widely accepted models included multiple causal or etiological factors. Schizophrenia is not attributed to any sole origin, but to the contributions of multiple biological, psychological, and social factors over the course of development. Similarly, these multiple contributions do not occur in simple, unidirectional ways; linear etiological models, in which causal processes cascade from a single origin to produce the disease, have been replaced by systemic models, in which causal processes interact with each other in circular, reciprocal ways.

Vulnerabilities are abnormalities or impairments in specific systemic processes. They do not directly cause the disease, but rather interact with other vulnerabilities and environmental challenges, or stress, to produce the disease state. Research on vulnerability to schizophrenia has focused on genetic factors and their endophenotypes (e.g., anatomical abnormalities, abnormal distribution of neurotransmitter receptors, neuro-cognitive impairments), although vulnerabilities could also be acquired, for example, deficits in self-regulation skills. Because of the dual role of enduring vulnerabilities and environmental factors, these models are generally known as vulnerability or diathesis-stress models (diathesis being essentially a synonym for vulnerability).

1.1.1 Zubin and Spring's Vulnerability Model

The vulnerability model of schizophrenia articulated by Zubin and Spring (1977) was a landmark in the evolution of modern systemic models. In addition to its conceptual innovation, the Zubin and Spring (1977) model gave a much improved account of the disparate empirical evidence from rigorous research. The key concept in the model was a distinction between vulnerability to schizophrenia – a relatively stable, long-lasting trait – and the instable, oscillating states (acute psychotic episodes) recognized as diagnostic features of schizophrenia (see Figure 1.1).

The original Zubin and Spring (1977) vulnerability model was revised and elaborated by various theorists over the following years. However, the key concept remained: pre-

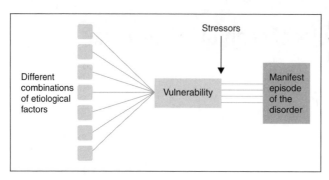

Figure 1.1: Zubin and Spring's vulnerability model (1977) as depicted by Brenner (1989)

morbid vulnerability associated with various causal factors. According to vulnerability models, a diagnosable episode of schizophrenia occurs only if a vulnerable individual is subjected to certain stressful demands. In individuals with more pronounced levels of vulnerability, minor demands can trigger an episode, whereas more severe stress may be required to trigger an episode in individuals with more moderate levels of vulnerability.

1.1.2 Nuechterlein and Colleagues' Heuristic Vulnerability/Stress Model

A more detailed and complex vulnerability model for schizophrenia was assembled by Nuechterlein and his colleagues (Nuechterlein & Dawson, 1984a; Nuechterlein, Dawson, & Green, 1994; see Figure 1.2). It was termed a *heuristic model* because its creators recognized that it identified only a subset of all possible vulnerabilities and causal pathways, but it did provide a reasonably complete description of the ways in which vulnerability factors might interact with other factors to produce the diagnosed disorder. In this model, a relatively stable vulnerable state is produced by biological factors, most importantly a dysfunction of dopamine neurotransmitter systems. Other features of the vulnerable state may include an instability and a hyperreactivity of the autonomic nervous system, cognitive deficits, and maladaptive social/behavioral traits. There may also be protective factors that may, at least partially, compensate for impairments caused by the vulnerabilities and/or mitigate the effects of stress, examples being high self-efficacy, good problem-solving skills, and a supportive family. Antipsychotic medication is a kind of protective factor that buffers a vulnerable central nervous system against neurophysiological dysregulation. The expression of diagnosable schizophrenia occurs when the net influence of all vulnerabilities overcomes the contributions of protective factors. Finally, the model of Nuechterlein and colleagues (1994) includes impairments of cognitive and autonomic functioning, which intermediate between stability and instability. These are the mechanisms by which the diagnosed disorder is expressed.

1.1.3 Elaborations of Systemic Vulnerability Models

Systemic vulnerability models of schizophrenia inspired the search for specific expressions in biological, psychological, and behavioral levels of functioning. A number of

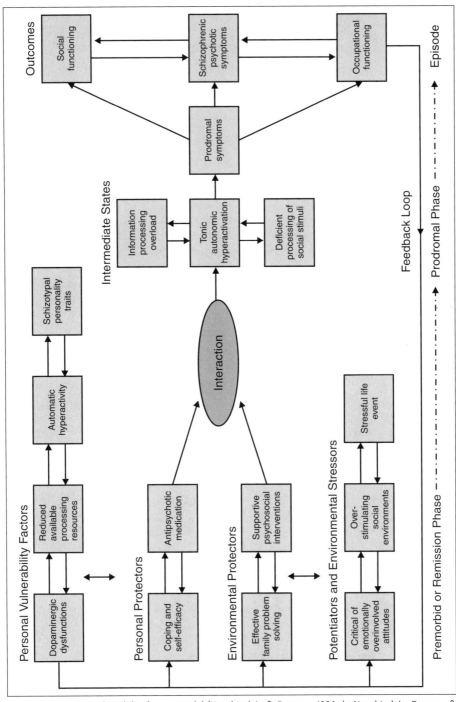

Figure 1.2: Heuristic vulnerability/stress model (Nuechterlein & Dawson, 1984a,b; Nuechterlein, Dawson, & Green, 1994)

such expressions were found, and several of them are described in this section. In some cases, these expressions may play a mechanistic role in etiology, such as causal links between a vulnerability genotype and a functional brain impairment. These mediating factors are receiving increasing attention in research on the endophenotypes of vulnerability. In other cases, the expressions may be measurable indications of vulnerability, but may play no role in the actual etiology of the disorder. These are generally termed *vulnerability markers*.

Genetic Factors

Genetic factors are still thought to be the primary source of biological vulnerabilities to schizophrenia. The concordance rate for monozygotic twins is estimated to be 50%–70% (Gottesman & Shields, 1982; Kendler et al., 1993; Sullivan, Kendler, & Neale, 2003). The remaining 30%–50% corroborate the vulnerability hypothesis that genetic factors interact with environmental factors to produce the disease (Mueser & McGurk, 2004; Portin & Alanen, 1997a,b; Tandon, Keshavan, & Nasrallah, 2008). A large number of specific genes are probably involved in vulnerability, and the specific mechanisms may range from structural flaws in dopamine system receptors to an immunological vulnerability to viral infection during gestation (van Os, Krabbendam, Myin-Germeys, & Delespaul, 2005).

Neurotransmitter Regulation

Dopamine remains a key neurophysiological factor in systemic models of schizophrenia, especially in the mesolimbic dopamine system (e.g., Broome et al., 2005; Kapur, Mizrahi, & Li, 2005). All antipsychotic medications act on the dopamine system, in particular on the D2 receptor (Garety, Bebbington, Fowler, Freeman, & Kuipers, 2007). Dopamine agonists, such as amphetamine, can precipitate psychosis in vulnerable individuals (Howes, Asselin, Murray, McGuire, & Grasby, 2006). Earlier hypotheses of an overabundance of dopamine have given way to hypotheses about the distribution and sensitivity of dopamine receptors. However, alternative models abound and the precise role of dopamine regulation as either a vulnerability marker or an endophenotype of schizophrenia is still not well understood. Generalized dopamine dysregulation clearly plays a key role in acute psychosis, and specific abnormalities in dopamine mechanisms may create a vulnerability to generalized dopamine dysregulation.

Brain Structure and Function

New medical imaging technologies, such as computer assisted tomography (CAT), positron emission tomography (PET), and magnetic resonance imaging (MRI), have stimulated much research on brain structure and function in schizophrenia (e.g., Blakemore & Frith, 2000; Buchanan & Carpenter, 1997; Kile, 2007). Initial studies failed to reveal differences in the brains of schizophrenia patients and normal controls, although this changed as imaging technology improved (Chua & McKenna, 1995). One of the most replicated findings is an enlargement of the lateral ventricles in schizophrenia patients, compared to normal controls (Crespo-Facorro et al., 2007; Kile, 2007; Lombardo-Ferrari, Kimura, Nita, & Elkis, 2006; Ohara, Sato, Tanabu, Yoshida, & Shibuya, 2006; Raz & Raz, 1990; Sharma et al., 1998; Van Horn & McManus, 1992). Nevertheless, ventricle enlargement is neither a necessary nor a sufficient factor in the development of schizophrenia (Stevens, 1997). Studies of identical twins discordant for schizophrenia suggest that ventricular enlargement is rather an indirect indication of subtle anatomical abnormalities in the limbic system (Suddath, Christison, Torrey, Casanova, & Weinberger, 1990), possibly due to developmental neurodysplasia.

Dynamic imaging, such as PET and functional MRI, tends to indicate reduced metabolic activity in the frontal lobes of schizophrenia patients compared to controls. This pattern is generally termed *hypofrontality* (for reviews see Blakemore & Frith, 2000; Ragland, Minzenberg, & Carter, 2007). Metabolic hypofrontality appears to be associated with impairments in neuropsychological functions in the frontal cortex, for example, working memory and executive functioning (Fu et al., 2005; MacDonald et al., 2005). This could form a link between the biological and cognitive levels of a specific type of vulnerability.

Specific brain structures implicated in schizophrenia include the dorsolateral, prefrontal, and temporal cortex, the various limbic system structures, the basal ganglia, parts of the thalamus, and the cerebellum (Andreasen, Paradiso, & O'Leary, 1998; Camchong, Dyckman, Chapman, Yanasak, & McDowell, 2006; Lee et al., 2006; Rüsch et al., 2007). The diversity of findings has inspired a more integrative perspective on brain impairments. For example, the cortical dysconnectivity syndrome model hypothesizes that normal interaction between multiple brain areas is impaired by synaptic processes common to those areas (James, James, Smith, & Javaloyes, 2004; Vogeley & Falkai, 1998; Wobrock et al., 2008). The failure is not situated in a specific brain structure or area, but in the transmission of information between them. Similarly, there is empirical evidence for fronto-temporal dissociation, or impaired transmission between frontal and temporal areas, in schizophrenia patients (Murray et al., 2008; Woodruff et al., 1997).

Cognition

Cognitive abnormalities have long been seen as core features of schizophrenia, arguably since Kraepelin (Green, 1998). Systemic vulnerability models stimulated new hypotheses about the etiological roles of these abnormalities – as markers, endophenotypes, and expressions of the disease. Soon after the first vulnerability models had appeared, cognitive abnormalities were found in children at risk (e.g., Asarnow, Steffy, MacCrimmon, & Cleghorn, 1978; Erlenmeyer-Kimling & Cornblatt, 1978) and in unaffected first-degree relatives (DeAmicis & Cromwell, 1979; Sitskoorn, Aleman, Ebich, Appels, & Kahn, 2004). In longitudinal studies, in support of the vulnerability hypothesis, impaired attention, and related information processing in children at risk for schizophrenia is related to eventual onset (Erlenmeyer-Kimling et al., 2000). Such abnormalities are also associated with impairments in social functioning in adulthood (Cornblatt, Lenzenweger, Dworkin, & Erlenmeyer-Kimling, 1992), suggesting more than a mere marker role in etiology.

As the cognitive research progressed, it became important to distinguish between trait-like and state-like abnormalities (Nuechterlein & Dawson, 1984b; Nuechterlein & Subotnik, 1998; Özgürdal et al., 2009; Wang, Chan, Yu, Shi, & Deng, 2008; Wykes & van der Gaag, 2001). Vulnerability factors tend to be more trait-like, present before as well as after onset, and relatively stable in severity (e.g., Aleman, Hijman, deHaan, & Kahn, 1999; Kurtz, 2005; Woods, Twamley, Dawson, Narvaez, & Jeste, 2007); state-like abnormalities tend to be associated with the acute psychotic state (e.g., Baxter & Liddle, 1998; Filbey et al., 2008; Nopoulos, Flashman, Flaum, Arndt, & Andreasen, 1994). Some abnormalities show characteristics of both, present at low levels before onset and between episodes, and becoming more severe after onset and/or during acute psychotic episodes. Many cognitive impairments appear to exert their effects over the course of the illness, producing poorer treatment adherence (Jeste, Patterson, Palmer, Dolder, & Jeste, 2003), functional behavioral impairments (Frith, 1992), higher risk of relapse (Chen et al., 2005), and a poorer overall prognosis (Green, Kern, Braf, & Mintz, 2000; McEvoy, 2008; Milev, Ho, Arndt, & Andreasen, 2005).

Another distinction of increasing importance is that between *neurocognition* and *social cognition* (Corrigan & Penn, 2001; Green, Penn et al., 2008; Penn, Corrigan, Bentall, & Racenstein, 1997; Penn et al., 2005). Most of the cognitive processes of interest in vulnerability research are relatively elemental, for example, reaction time, attention, and memory, derived from the laboratory methods of experimental psychopathology and clinical neuropsychology. These cognitive processes were used in a non-social context as neurobiological correlates (neurocognition). More recently, however, more complex levels of cognition have attracted the interest of schizophrenia researchers. The terms neurocognition and social cognition came to distinguish between these subdomains, although they are not necessarily distinct or nonoverlapping. Social cognition refers to how people think about themselves and others in the social world; simply put, it is people's thinking about people (Green, Olivier, Crawley, Penn, & Silverstein, 2005; Penn, Sanna, & Roberts, 2008). Interest in social cognition was inspired in part by the fact that, although more elemental measures appear linked to vulnerability factors, their actual mechanistic role in etiology has been difficult to establish. Green and Nuechterlein (1999) proposed a model including social cognition as a possible mediator between neurocognitive and behavioral functioning, and empirical evidence supports such a role (Addington, Saeedi, & Addington, 2006b; Bell, Tsang, Greig, & Bryson, 2008; Brekke & Nakagami, 2010; Brekke, Kay, Lee, & Green, 2005; Brüne, 2005; Pinkham & Penn, 2006; Pinkham, Penn, Perkins, & Lieberman, 2003; Roder & Schmidt, 2009; Schmidt, Mueller, & Roder, 2009; Sergi, Green et al., 2007; Sergi, Rassovsky, Nuechterlein, & Green, 2006; Sergi, Rassovsky et al., 2007; Vauth, Rüsch, Wirtz, & Corrigan, 2004). Also, since social cognition is more functionally proximal to the deficits in social behavior that are of primary clinical concern in schizophrenia, it is hoped that a better understanding of social cognition will lead more directly to improved clinical assessment and treatment methods (Addington et al., 2006b).

Specific social cognitive impairments under current study include theory of mind (a person's ability to infer the cognitive and emotional states of other people), social schema, social attribution, and social perception (Bellack, Morrison, & Mueser, 1989; Corcoran, Mercer, & Frith, 1995; Frith, 2004; Nienow, Docherty, Cohen, & Dinzeo, 2006; Penn et al., 1999; Pinkham, Penn, Perkins, Graham, & Siegel, 2007; Toomey, Wallace, Corrigan, Schuldberg, & Green, 1997; Zanello, Perrig, & Huguelet, 2006). Our understanding of this level of organismic functioning will probably expand considerably over the next few years. Many aspects of social cognition pertinent to severe mental illness have likely not yet been identified or measured. Also, the relationship between social cognition and neurocognition may not be purely hierarchical: There are differences between processing of social versus nonsocial information at fairly elemental levels, for example, between visual processing of the physical features of alphanumeric characters versus human faces.

Environmental Factors

Studies of the stress side of the vulnerability hypothesis were influenced by two distinct research paradigms: life events and expressed emotion. Life-events research typically involves an enumeration of specific stressful events that may either accumulate over time to interact with vulnerabilities or precipitate onset in a single stroke (Bebbington et al., 1993; Day, 1989; Dohrenwend, Shrout, Link, Skodol, & Stueve, 1995; Phillips, Francey, Edwards, & McMurray, 2007; Tennant, 1985). Both types of mechanisms appear to operate in the etiology of schizophrenia. After onset, both major stressors and minor "daily hassles" may influence the course of the disorder. Recently, the disproportionate representation of persons with histories of major trauma, childhood abuse, and childhood neglect among those with serious mental illness has given life-events research a new focus (Bebbington et al., 2004; Janssen et al., 2004; Read, van Os, Morrison, & Ross, 2005; Spauwen, Krabbendam, Lieb, Wittchen, & van Os, 2006). As with other life events, trauma appears to influence the course of the disorder over time as well as to precipitate the onset (Schenkel, Spaulding, DiLillo, & Silverstein, 2005).

Expressed emotion research has evolved from early findings that the emotional climate in a family has an impact on the stability of family members with schizophrenia (Leff & Vaughn, 1985). Stress in a high-expressed emotion family may be produced by family members' negative, critical attitudes – or by well-intended overinvolvement with the identified patient (Brown, Birley, & Wing, 1972; Butzlaff & Hooley, 1998; Hooley, 2007). Therapeutic techniques designed to reduce the expressed emotion in family networks demonstrated clear clinical efficacy in preventing relapse (Pilling et al., 2002).

Environmental stress relevant to vulnerability for schizophrenia may come from a variety of other sources. Stressors known to influence the incidence of schizophrenia include urban birth (McGrath, 2006), lack of social cohesion (Kirkbride et al., 2007), emigration (Smith et al., 2006), poverty (Cohen, 1993), and war (van Os & Selten, 1998). A model of vulnerability to schizophrenia (Walker & Diforio, 1997) proposes links between extreme environmental stress, fetal exposure to maternal cortisol (a hormone secreted in response to stress), developmental neurodysplasia, and vulnerability.

1.1.4 Pervasiveness and Homeorhesis

Another landmark in the evolution of systemic vulnerability models of schizophrenia was the concept of *pervasiveness* (Brenner, 1986; Spaulding, 1986). Inspired by vulnerability models, experimental psychopathology had produced a proliferation of laboratory paradigms that revealed abnormalities associated with schizophrenia (Cromwell & Spaulding, 1978). The processes measured by these paradigms were mostly cognitive, but they spanned a range of complexity, from elemental visual feature processing, to attention, to trait-like characteristics of social judgment and attribution. Borrowing from concepts originating in learning theory, these processes were ordered on a continuum ranging from relatively molecular to relatively molar levels of organization. Consistent with the information-processing models of cognition that predominated at that time, it was hypothesized that information is passed from more molecular processes to more molar processes in the course of apprehending the environment and responding to it. In the context of psychopathology, this means that impaired molecular processes pass corrupted information to more molar processes, thus distributing the effects upward throughout the cognitive system. Similarly, failures in the cognitive level of organismic functioning would be distributed to the behavioral and social levels. Schizophrenia came to be understood as a pervasive disorder, with significant impairments at every level of biological, psychological, behavioral, and social functioning.

As systemic theories became increasingly influential in psychology (e.g., Bronfenbrenner, 1979), the pervasiveness concept in schizophrenia research continued to evolve. Linear models of information processing, in which deficits are passed upward from molecular to molar levels, gave way to nonlinear models, wherein deficits are passed in both directions, within and between levels of functioning. The effects of vulnerabilities are reciprocal. For example, impaired attention can induce paranoid interpretations of social behavior, which in turn can compromise performance of social skills. Deficient social skills put greater demands on attention and create stress, which has neurophysiological consequences. The neurophysiological consequences of stress exacerbate attention deficits and paranoia, further impairing social skills. Impaired social skills also create a more stressful social environment, as family members struggle to respond. The functional deficits of schizophrenia came to be seen as the results of vicious circles between specific impairments (Brenner, Hodel, Roder, & Corrigan, 1992).

This insight into the reciprocal interactions of specific impairments or vulnerabilities intersected with the evolution of cognitive perspectives in psychology and psychopathology (as discussed in the previous section). The paradigms that had dominated experimental psychopathology and neuropsychology were under increasing attack as paradigms of "cold" cognition, meaning paradigms that analyze cognition in contrived laboratory conditions. The new concept of social cognition was developed in part to study "hot" cognition, meaning cognition with personal relevance and emotional significance as it actually occurs in natural settings. Systemic models that posit reciprocal interactions between cognition and other levels of organismic functioning and environmental events are better suited to understanding the role of "hot" social cognition in psychopathology (Penn et al., 2008). Integration of personally relevant material in laboratory assessments of social cognition is not yet common, but this may become an important development in the near future.

Systemic psychological models have implications for human development, and this applies to psychopathology as well. The familiar concept of homeostasis, referring to the static stability of a biological system, is now complemented by the concept of *homeorhesis*. A system in homeorhesis is homeostatic, in the sense that it is stable in the short term, but in the long term undergoes gradual changes. Humans are in homeorhesis because, while they maintain short-term homeostasis, they grow and change in various ways throughout the life course. Sometimes the change is desirable – as in the maturation of children – and sometimes less desirable, as in advanced aging. Eventually a deteriorating homeorhetic system may reach a point of collapse, in which homeostasis is disrupted, such as in death.

Schizophrenia can be understood as a condition of homeorhesis. In the short term, people with schizophrenia sustain a degree of homeostasis, preserving basic functioning despite some number of vulnerabilities that compromise the efficiency and long-term stability of their organismic system. However, the inefficiencies and the environmental stress they cause create a long-term tendency toward less efficiency and more stress. When extended over time, vicious circles become downward spirals, and at some point the spiral may accelerate enough to create a cascading system collapse, resulting not in death but in acute psychosis. Thus, advanced system theories and the concept of homeorhesis provide an expanded understanding of the actions of vulnerabilities over time.

The developmental dimension of system theory also sheds new light on how impairments become pervasive. An impaired component influences the rest of the system, not just at one point in time, but over time as human development progresses. For example, the cumulative effect of an attention deficit on social skills is not just during the moment of skill performance, but over the developmental period during which social skills are being acquired and refined. This insight was particularly important in light of the finding that crucial aspects of neuropsychological development extend through adolescence and early adulthood (e.g., Kolb & Nonneman, 1976). Since the onset of schizophrenia typically occurs in late adolescence or early adulthood, it disrupts some crucial developmental processes, leaving the person without specific cognitive abilities that normal adults take for granted.

The implications of advanced system theory define and guide an era of schizophrenia research that continues to this day. The implication that functional deficits are caused by impairments distributed throughout the system stimulated analysis across multiple levels of organismic functioning (e.g., Addington & Addington, 1999; Brekke et al., 2005; Green, 1996; McGurk & Mueser, 2004; Prouteau et al., 2005; Semkovska, Bedard, Godbout, Limoge, & Stip, 2004; Wykes & van der Gaag, 2001). These analyses provide empirical support for the systemic nature of schizophrenia.

1.2 Systemic Models in Clinical Application

One particularly important implication of biosystemic models is that treatment of schizophrenia should address multiple levels of functioning in a coordinated way. This was the key idea behind the development of Integrated Psychological Therapy (IPT). In the broadest sense it is also one of the key principles of psychiatric rehabilitation as such (Liberman, 2008; Spaulding, Sullivan, & Poland, 2003), and generally regarded as the comprehensive treatment approach of choice for severe mental illness, an approach in which modalities like IPT form core components. Outcome research on the effectiveness of treatments that address multiple levels of functioning provide empirical support for the hypothesis that a systemic approach to treatment meaningfully enhances recovery from schizophrenia (e.g., Cohen, Forbes, Mann, & Blanchard, 2006; Dickerson, Boronow, Ringel, & Parente, 1999; Hofer et al., 2005; Liddle, 2000; Milev et al., 2005; Reeder, Smedley, Butt, Bogner, & Wykes, 2006; Revheim et al., 2006; Roder, Mueller, Mueser, & Brenner, 2006; Spaulding, Reed, Sullivan, Richardson, & Weiler, 1999; Twamley, Savla, Zurhellen, & Heaton, 2008; Twamley, Woods et al., 2008; Velligan et al., 2000; Wykes, Reeder, Corner, Williams, & Eyeritt, 1999).

The remainder of this chapter discusses some key considerations in comprehensive application of biosystemic models in clinical assessment, treatment, and rehabilitation.

1.2.1 Cognitive Science and Technology

As discussed previously in this chapter, cognitive research has had a significant impact on the evolution of systemic vulnerability-stress models of schizophrenia. Accordingly, there has been a growing awareness of the need for new cognitive technology for clinical assessment and treatment (Spaulding, 1994).

A key empirical finding of the past 20 years of schizophrenia research was the ubiquity of neurocognitive impairments in people with schizophrenia. As many as 75%–85% of all schizophrenia patients have persistent deficits on neuropsychological performance measures, independent of patients' age (Bowie, Reichenberg, McClure, Leung, & Harvey, 2008; Gray & Roth, 2007). The average patient scores two standard deviations below healthy controls on neuropsychological tests, lying in the lowest 5%–10% of the general population (Keefe, 2007; Wilk et al., 2004). These findings corroborate a traditional view of schizophrenia, arguably dating back to Kraepelin (Green, 1997) but certainly to Bleuler (1911), namely, that cognitive impairments are distinctive and even defining features of the illness. In modern terminology, schizophrenia can be considered a *neurocognitive disorder* (Green, 1998). As discussed earlier in this chapter, social cognitive paradigms also promise to add much to our understanding of the cognitive impairments of schizophrenia (e.g., Bigelow et al., 2006; Horan et al., 2009; Kee et al., 2009; Sprong, Schothorst, Vos, Hox, & van Engeland, 2007).

Despite the prevalence and severity of cognitive impairment in schizophrenia, there is no single type or profile that characterizes the illness. Heterogeneity, in both the quality and severity of impairments, is the rule. A substantial minority of schizophrenia patients score in or above the average range on neuropsychological tests. There is sufficient variability that cognitive measures can predict within-group differences on other dimensions, for instance, treatment compliance and risk of relapse in first-episode patients (Chen et al., 2005) and longer-term outcome in more chronic patients (e.g., Brekke et al., 2005; Norman et al., 1999; Peer & Spaulding, 2007; Silverstein, Harrow, & Bryson, 1994; Silverstein, Mavrolefteros, & Close, 2002; Straube, 1993). This means that, for clinical purposes, assessment must be able to identify and characterize individual cognitive differences between people with schizophrenia – and treatment must be flexible enough to accommodate these differences.

The increasing recognition of the importance of cognitive factors in schizophrenia produced a proliferation of treatment approaches and assessment tools. Integrated Psychological Therapy (IPT) is representative of an array of treatment modalities that target neurocognitive and social cognitive impairments. The proliferation of assessment tools has, in fact, been so great that there are too many to ensure any comparability of findings across research studies. Concern about this has become great enough that a major effort to standardize cognitive assessment in schizophrenia research was undertaken by the U. S. National Institute of Mental Health (NIMH), the Measurement and Treatment Research to Improve Cognition in Schizophrenia (MATRICS). This initiative reflects widespread recognition (1) that cognitive factors are central to the understanding and treatment of schizophrenia, but (2) that the complexity of cognition and a proliferation of assessment tools threaten to inhibit scientific progress by generating large amounts of data that cannot be compared across studies or research groups. The solution to the problem was to assemble a single battery of cognitive measures, broad enough in scope to cover the major domains of cognition implicated in schizophrenia but small enough to be highly portable and suitable for a wide range of research applications (Green & Nuechterlein, 2004; Kern & Horan, 2010; Nuechterlein et al., 2004). A major motivation in the MATRICS initiative was to produce a battery well suited for research on psychopharmacological treatment of cognitive impairment. However, it was also expected that a standardized battery suitable for that purpose would also be suitable for a broad range of applications.

The MATRICS initiative involved a large number of schizophrenia researchers in a process of reaching consensus about the optimal contents of a cognitive assessment battery for schizophrenia research. The initial focus was on the neurocognitive domain, because the proliferation of assessment tools had been greatest in that domain, and there was a great desire to find psychopharmacological agents with benefits in that domain. After considerable deliberation, six independent subdomains of neurocognition relevant for schizophrenia disorders were identified on the basis of assessments used in research (Nuechterlein et al., 2004):

– **Speed of information processing:** This domain emphasizes the speed of performance including perceptual and motor components with which information is processed (e.g., cognitive flexibility, sensomotor speed).
– **Attention/Vigilance:** Selective attention works as a filter, with the function of selecting information prior to its further treatment according to its importance. Insufficient filtering of the mass of information and a lack of inhibition of irrelevant stim-

uli lead to an overflow of stimulation and a functional breakdown of thinking and feeling according to the context, respectively. The maintenance of attention over a longer period of time is referred to as vigilance.

– **Verbal and visual learning and memory:** Reception and long-term storage of verbal and nonverbal information. The verbal and visual memory – separately presented in the MATRICS-Initiative – is associated with secondary or long-term memory and also serves the purpose of distinguishing the latter from short-term memory.
– **Reasoning and problem solving:** In literature also subsumed as executive functions. It is helpful to distinguish between working memory and complex strategies of planning and decision-making.
– **Working memory:** Verbal and nonverbal (visual and spatial) working memory are classified as executive functions and form the prerequisite for complex cognitive processes like planning actions. Under an elevated level of stress or strain, schizophrenia patients experience an increasing limitation of working memory functions.

A major purpose of the MATRICS initiative was to choose specific neuropsychological tests for those neurocognitive domains. Late in the MATRICS development process, an increasing appreciation of social cognitive deficits separate from neurocognitive deficits (discussed in the previous section) led to the addition of a social cognitive domain.

The MATRICS project led to the commercial availability of a standardized test battery, consisting of 10 instruments covering the 7 measurement domains (Matrics Assessment, Inc., 2006). The subdomains and specific instruments in the consensus battery are shown in Table 1.1.

The MATRICS project is further developing the subdomain of social cognition, even as research in that area is rapidly expanding. A recent discussion of researchers associated with the MATRICS project yielded consensus on five relatively distinct types:

Table 1.1 The MATRICS Consensus Cognitive Battery (MCCB)

Subdomain	Instrument(s)
Speed of Processing	Brief assessment of cognition in schizophrenia (BACS) Symbol-coding Category Fluency: Animal naming
Attention/Vigilance	Continuous Performance Test: Identical pairs version (CPT-IP)
Verbal Learning	Hopkins Verbal Learning Test – Revised (HVLT-R)
Visual Learning	Brief Visuospatial Memory Test-Revised (BVMT-R)
Reasoning & Problem Solving	Neuropsychological Assessment Battery (NAB): Mazes
Working Memory	
(Verbal)	Wechsler Memory Scale – III (WMS-III): Spatial span
(Nonverbal)	Letter-number span
Social Cognition	Mayer-Salovey-Caruso Emotional Intelligence Test (MSCEIT^{TM}): Managing Emotions

– **Emotional Processing:** perceiving and using emotions. Emotion perception or affect recognition is one domain of emotion processing. Impairments include slower and less accurate recognition of emotional stimuli as well as deficient regulation of emotional responses. Impairments tend to be more severe when the emotional content of processed information is more intense.

– **Social Perception:** apprehension of key features of social situations and interactions. Impairments include deficient recognition of social cues and deficient processing of contextual information.

– **Theory of Mind (ToM):** the ability to apprehend the mental and emotional states, perspectives, and intentions of others. ToM also appears to be related to metacognition, the ability to apprehend, observe, and understand one's own cognitive activity.

– **Social Schemas:** also called social knowledge – bodies of declarative and procedural information that guide social behavior. Scripts are particular types of schemas that contain information on social behavior appropriate to specific situations or circumstances. Impairments may represent deficient informational structures or deficient access to or execution of the information they contain.

– **Social Attributions:** the causal explanations a person formulates in order to understand social events and behaviors. Impairments may involve disproportionate or perseverative use of external personal attributions (causes attributed to other people), external situational attributions (causes attributed to situational factors), or internal attributions (causes due to oneself). Attributional impairments may overlap with emotional processing, social perception, and ToM impairments. For instance, neutral facial expressions and social behaviors may stimulate attributions of angry emotional states, hostile intent, and aggression.

As research on social cognition in schizophrenia accelerates and expands, the need for systematic and standardized assessment of specific social cognitive domains will intensify. The near future will probably see further development of the social cognitive components of assessment batteries such as the MCCB (MATRICS Consensus Cognitive Battery).

1.2.2 Functional Outcome: A Main Objective of Rehabilitation

From our human perspective, the importance of our physiological and cognitive functions is that they support social functioning, which means participating in life, as a member of a family, a community, and a culture. By definition, severe mental illness compromises a person's social functioning. The specific ways in which mental illness affects social functioning, for example, through neurophysiological dysregulation, neurocognitive impairments, social cognitive problems, or emotional dysregulation, are highly diverse, even within severely disabled populations. People experience individually unique patterns of problems that span all levels of their organismic biosystem. Specific treatments target specific problems, but ultimately the value of any treatment is determined by the degree to which it contributes to improved social functioning.

This may seem like a truism, but historically psychiatry has a tendency to focus on the most proximal effects of treatment while neglecting the bigger picture of social functioning. This tendency is most pronounced in the pharmacological treatment of psychotic symptoms. Symptoms are the key criteria in diagnosis, and they are also the main targets of psychopharmacological treatment. However, people often maintain social functioning despite psychotic symptoms, and suppression of psychotic symptoms does not necessarily or automatically improve social functioning.

Since psychiatric rehabilitation was first formulated in the 1970s, attention to the big picture of social functioning has been one of its key principles. More recently, the importance of social functioning has become more broadly recognized. There is now general agreement that the outcome of treatment and other services for severe mental illness must ultimately be evaluated in terms of social functioning or functional outcome. Compared to other mental illnesses, the functional outcome of schizophrenia tends to be poor (Bellack, Mueser, Gingerich, & Agresta, 2004; Malla & Payne, 2005; Thornicroft et al., 2004; Wittorf, Wiedemann, Buchkremer, & Klingberg, 2008). This is reflected not only in the quality of life of the patient, but also in the distress of family and friends and the high cost of treatment and support services (Bellack et al., 2007; Roder, Mueller, Mueser et al., 2006; Wittorf et al., 2008).

Increased concern about functional outcome leads to issues of measurement. Much of the previous research on functional outcome has used inconsistent operational definitions – if at all (Bellack et al., 2007; Malla & Payne, 2005). Social functioning is arguably too broad a concept to be measured by a single definition. A methodologically useful strategy is to separate *social functioning, social competence*, and *social skills*. Social skills (also-called interpersonal skills) are the timely execution of the cognitive, verbal, and nonverbal behaviors necessary for effective interaction with others (Penn, Mueser, Doonan, & Nishith, 1995; Pinkham & Penn, 2006). Social competence means a broader ability to achieve goals by interacting with others (Bellack, 2004; Kopelowicz, Liberman, & Zarate, 2006). Social functioning means the exercise of skills and competence comprehensively to meet one's instrumental and affiliative needs (Mueser, Bellack, Morrison, & Wixted, 1990; Penn et al., 1995). Viewed in this way, social skills can be understood as supporting social competence at a more molecular level of the person's biosystem, whereas social competence supports social functioning at a more molar level. Social skills can be measured in laboratory or clinical settings, through use of roleplay-based tests of specific abilities (e.g., to apprehend the nature of a situation or conflict, to formulate an appropriate behavioral response, and then to execute the response). Social competence and social functioning are typically measured with checklist-type instruments that inventory a person's social activities, affiliations, achievements, problems, and quality of life (Bellack, 2004; Boden, Sundström, Lindström, & Lindström, 2009; Conley, Ascher-Svanum, Zhu, Faries, & Kinon, 2007; Green et al., 2000; Roder, Zorn, Mueller, & Brenner, 2001; Roder et al., 2002). Measured this way, social social skills are not correlated with psychiatric symptoms, but are highly correlated with social competence and social functioning (Bellack, Morrison, Wixted, & Mueser, 1990).

Ideally, functional outcome is assessed as the person's functioning in the "real world" (e.g., Bowie, Reichenberg, Patterson, Heaton, & Havey, 2006; Heinrichs, Ammari, Miles, & McDermid Vaz, 2008). However, "real world" functioning is difficult and expensive to measure in research studies – and prohibitively so within the practical

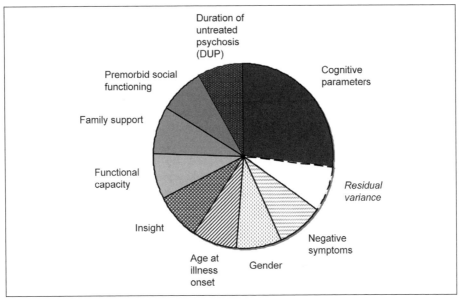

Figure 1.3: Heuristic model of possible sources of influence on functional outcome

constraints of some clinical settings, for instance, inpatient units (Bellack et al., 2007; Bustillo, Lauriello, Horan, & Keith, 2001; McKibbin, Brekke, Sires, Jeste, & Patterson, 2004). Yet social-skills training and related rehabilitation modalities can generate meaningful data in any setting. Demonstrations of improved social skills, leisure skills, disorder management skills, or occupational skills in restrictive clinical settings are not ipso facto positive functional outcomes; but they are valid indicators of progress toward greater social competence and social functioning (Green et al., 2000; Kurtz & Mueser, 2008). Development of instruments for measuring all relevant aspects of functional outcome has become a key methodological issue in mental health research and practice (Mausbach, Moore, Bowie, Cardenas, & Patterson, 2009).

Of course, social skills and social competence are not the only factors that compromise social functioning and, hence, functional outcome. Probable sources of influence on functional outcome are summarized in the heuristic model in Figure 1.3.

A large body of mostly cross-sectional study findings provide evidence that functional outcome is related to negative symptoms, neurocognition, and social cognition, but relatively independent of positive symptoms (e.g., Addington & Addington, 2008; Addington, Saeedi, & Addington, 2006a; Bowie et al., 2006; Brekke et al., 2005; Brüne, 2005; Brüne, Abdel-Hamid, Lehmkämper, & Sonntag, 2007; Cohen, Leung, Saperstein, & Blanchard, 2006; Conley et al., 2007; Couture, Penn, & Roberts, 2006; Dibben, Rice, Laws, & McKenna, 2009; Green & Nuechterlein, 1999; Green et al., 2000, 2004; Harvey, Koren, Reichenberg, & Bowie, 2006; Heinrichs et al., 2008; Kee, Green, Mintz, & Brekke, 2003; Leeson, Barnes, Hutton, Ron, & Joyce, 2009; Lysaker, Lancaster, Nees, & Davis, 2004; Matza et al., 2006; Milev et al., 2005; Nelson, Combs, Penn, & Basso, 2007; Pinkham & Penn, 2006; Sergi et al., 2006; Sergi, Green et al., 2007; Sergi, Rassovsky et al., 2007). Nevertheless, a few studies found associations between positive symptoms and functional outcome in longitudinal studies (e.g., Norman et al., 1999; Perlick, Rosenheck, Kaczynski, Bingham, & Collins, 2008; Racenstein, Harrow, Reed, Martin, & Penn, 2002; Wittorf et al., 2008). This inconsistency may simply reflect an inconsistent definition and measurement of functional outcome. Perhaps positive symptoms in a later stage of illness and after treatment are better predictors of functional outcome than those in acute phases (Boden et al., 2009; Helldin, Kane, Karilampi, Norlander, & Archer, 2007; Norman et al., 2002).

Cognitive impairments are generally thought to be rate-limiting factors in the acquisition of new skills and other key processes of rehabilitation (e.g., Bowen et al., 1994; Kern, Green, Mintz, & Liberman, 2003). As such, they are expected to be significant factors in functional outcome (Green, 1996). Other factors showing evidence of impact on functional outcome include duration of untreated psychosis (DUP) (Crumlish et al., 2009; Schimmelmann et al., 2008; White et al., 2009), premorbid social functioning (Bechard-Evans et al., 2007; Jeppesen et al., 2008; Malla et al., 2006; San, Ciudad, Alvarez, Bobes, & Gilaberte, 2007), family support (e.g., Bustillo et al., 2001; O'Brien et al., 2006), functional capacity or competence in the sense of practical thinking and skills demanded in real-life situations (e.g., Aubin, Stip, Gelinas, Rainvill, & Chapparo, 2009; Heinrichs et al., 2008; Heinrichs, Statucka, Goldberg, & McDermid Vaz, 2006; Twamley et al., 2002), insight into one's own psychotic symptoms, into their consequences, and into the need for treatment (e.g., Drake, 2008; Lysaker, Roe, & Yanos, 2007; Medalia, Thysen, & Freilich, 2008; Mutsatsa, Joyce, Hutton, & Barnes, 2006; Smith et al., 1999), age at onset (e.g., Kurtz & Mueser, 2008; Malla et al., 2006; Ochoa et al., 2006; Roder, Mueller, & Zorn, 2006; Thorup et al., 2007), as well as sex (Fiszdon, Choi, Goulet, & Bell, 2008; Moriarty et al., 2001; Thorup et al., 2007; Usall, Haro, Ochosa, Marquez, & Araya, 2002; Usall et al., 2007).

Despite the evidence for multiple contributions to functional outcome, it is doubtful that a prognosis can be reduced to a simple linear regression. Longitudinal studies tend to produce results different from those of cross-sectional studies. As with remission of symptoms, the prognostic significance of any factor may be moderated when it is present over the course of the disorder. Vulnerabilities interact with personal resources and protective factors in complex ways (e.g., Brekke et al., 2005). Even such factors as intrinsic interest and motivation may mediate prognostic significance, for instance, in the relationship between neurocognition and functional outcome (Barch & Carter, 2005; Nakagami, Xie, Hoe, & Brekke, 2008; Velligan, Kern, & Gold, 2006). Although multivariate studies can identify the statistical importance of various factors, recovery from mental illness is ultimately an individually unique process.

1.2.3 Rehabilitation and the Recovery Movement

In the 1970s the concept of psychiatric rehabilitation took shape as the principles of physical rehabilitation (rehabilitation of physical injuries and disabilities), which were translated into a mental-health context (e.g., Anthony, 1979). A key principle was that severe mental illness is understood as a set of disabilities to be overcome, rather than a disease to be cured. The term *recovery* economically captures the process of overcoming disabilities and thereby achieving a desirable functional outcome. Psychiatric rehabilitation came to be understood as the technological armamentarium or "toolbox" for recovery. Recovery is the "lived experience of rehabilitation" (Deegan, 1988). This reframing of psychiatric treatment definitively modifies the traditional role of "patient" and "practitioner." Instead of a practitioner "administering" treatment to a passive patient, rehabilitation consists of a person recovering with the assistance of the practitioner.

The concept of recovery in rehabilitation converged over the next decades with a social movement of consumers and advocates dissatisfied with traditional mental health services, especially for severe mental illness. Their activities came to be known as the recovery movement. Although it was essentially a social policy reform movement, it gained considerable momentum from various scientific findings. These included outcome studies showing unexpectedly high long-term recovery rates (Davidson, O'Connell, Tondora, Lawless, & Evans, 2005; Rabinowitz, Levine, Haim, & Häfner, 2007), epidemiological studies showing previously undetected differences in expression and morbidity across cultures, indicating moderation of the course by social factors (McGrath, 2005), and surveys showing that the unmet needs of people with severe mental illness extend beyond symptom control, for example, to access to daytime activities, company, reduction of psychological distress, information about their condition, and intimate relationships (Thornicroft et al., 2004). Consensus has developed throughout the consumer, professional, and scientific communities that recovery from mental illness must encompass far more than symptom remission (see Andreasen et al., 2005) to include all domains of daily living (e.g., cognitive and social functioning) as well as quality of life (Bellack, 2006; Brekke & Nakagami, 2010; Leucht & Lasser, 2006; Liberman & Kopelowicz, 2005; Liberman et al., 2008; Ralph & Corrigan, 2005; Roder et al., 2002; Rosen & Garety, 2005; van Os et al., 2006).

In the United States the recovery movement found an influential voice in a presidential commission on mental health reform. The commission's report (President's New Freedom Commission on Mental Health, 2004) included a devastating critique of traditional mental health services and practices as well as a call for the integration of the recovery concept into a new paradigm. By then, the concept of recovery had expanded to incorporate a variety of additional features and values, including a renewed sense of purpose, a sense of self beyond the role of "mental patient," acceptance of the limitations of illness and disability, involvement in meaningful activities, overcoming stigma, assuming control and responsibility for one's own treatment and recovery, managing symptoms, and participating in community life (Amering & Schmolke, 2007; Davidson et al., 2005; McEvoy, 2008). To some, valuing these aspects of outcome represented a radical departure, especially from the preoccupation with biological processes, medication, and symptom reduction that characterized the second half of the 20th century. Others (e.g., Anthony, 1993; Spaulding & Nolting, 2006) pointed out that expanded recovery values are consistent not only with the original principles of psychiatric rehabilitation, but also with traditional goals of psychotherapy. Criticisms of the "medical model" from the contemporary recovery perspective echo criticisms in the psychological treatment literature dating back to the 1960s (e.g., Ullman & Krasner, 1965, Introduction). In this perspective, the recovery movement is (among other things) a rediscovery of the relevance of psychological treatment approaches to severe mental illness.

As with other revolutionary ideas, recovery has come to mean different things to different people (e.g., Bellack, 2006; Davidson et al., 2005; Deegan, 1988; Frese, Stanley, Kress, & Vogel-Scibilia, 2001). From the original perspective of psychiatric rehabilitation, recovery consists of measurable dimensions of personal and social functioning. This may seem different from more subjective or experiential characterizations, especially personal accounts of people with severe mental illness. However, the empirical analysis of subjective experience has an honorable history in psychology and mental-health research, and is certainly not incompatible with psychiatric rehabilitation or recovery. Empirical analysis of the subjective aspects of recovery (e.g., Resnick, Fontana, Lehman, & Rosenheck, 2005) corroborates experiential accounts, identifying such dimensions as empowerment, hope, and optimism, knowledge, and life satisfaction. When psychiatric rehabilitation is informed by an integrated, biosystemic model of mental illness, the subjective aspects of recovery are easily included as important factors that inhabit the sociocognitive level of organismic functioning. There is no incompatibility between recognizing the importance of the subjective experience of recovery and pursuing a scientific agenda to measure, facilitate, and enhance that experience (Silverstein & Bellack, 2008).

Recovery is both a process and an outcome (Corrigan, 2006). The concept contributes importantly to what we mean by a positive functional outcome: a sense of control over one's life, satisfying relationships, and an acceptable quality of life. In the language of biosystemic models of mental illness, the sociocognitive processes associated with recovery are potentially important targets for treatment. Cognitive and cognitive-behavioral therapies can help people change attitudes and beliefs inconsistent with recovery and a good functional outcome, such as hopelessness and a sense of victimization. Of course, actual success in meaningful activities is an even more powerful way to change such attitudes, and rehabilitation can provide opportunities for such successes.

The recovery concept also calls our attention to sociocognitive processes that may be important moderators of treatment response and functional outcome. Motivation is one example (Velligan, Kern et al., 2006). Practitioners have traditionally observed that people with schizophrenia are often "unmotivated" to engage in treatment – a major barrier. Whether or how motivation is associated with the cognitive features of schizophrenia is unclear (Barch & Carter, 2005), but individual case analysis usually reveals that people are not *generally* unmotivated, but rather unmotivated to do what the practitioner wants. In the recovery perspective, a person is motivated to engage in treatment for distinct reasons:

1. The treatment "makes sense" to the person as a way of achieving desirable goals.
2. The treatment has intrinsic motivational properties, that is, it is interesting or satisfying or fun in its own right.

Treatment makes sense to the degree that people understand how it relates to their condition or problems. Understanding "the need for treatment" is associated with the concept of insight, which traditionally means understanding that one has a mental illness, that symptoms and related problems are caused by the illness, and that treatment can indeed help. The concept of insight as traditionally measured appears to be an important moderator of outcome (Drake, 2008; Lysaker et al., 2007; Medalia et al., 2008; Mutsatsa et al., 2006; Smith et al., 1999) and is in turn associated with depressive and negative symptoms (Karow et al., 2008; Mintz, Dobson, & Romney, 2003; Mutsata et al., 2006) and with cognitive impairment (Aleman, Agrawal, Morgan, & Davis, 2006; Drake & Lewis, 2003; Iqbal, Birchwood, Chadwick, & Trower, 2000; Lysaker, Bryson, Lancaster, Evans, & Bell, 2002; Mohamed, Fleming, Penn, & Spaulding, 1999; Mutsata et al., 2006). Insight problems are not limited to the illness and its symptoms. For example, patients' self-reports about their own cognitive deficits and resources as well as their objective performance in neuropsychological assessments are generally inaccurate (e.g., Medalia & Lim, 2004; Medalia & Thysen, 2008; Moritz, Ferahli, & Naber, 2004). The recovery perspective teaches that a careful analysis of a patient's "insight" is required to fully understand how and why the patient is or is not motivated for treatment.

Intrinsic motivation is clearly a powerful moderator of treatment effects (Roder, Mueller, & Zorn, 2006). Some treatment activities are more intrinsically motivating than others, although ultimately the intrinsic motivation of any task is an interaction between the nature of the task and the individual person's sociocognitive beliefs, attitudes, preferences, and values (Medalia & Lim, 2004; Medalia & Richardson, 2005; Nakagami et al., 2008). As a consequence, assessment and enhancement of intrinsic motivation became the goals of psychological intervention in schizophrenia (e.g., Medalia, Revheim, & Casey, 2001).

1.2.4 Distribution, Mediation, and Moderation of Treatment Effects

The multiple, reciprocal interactions in biosystemic models of schizophrenia create a conundrum in clinical application. Although we know that vulnerabilities such as dopamine dysregulation or neurocognitive impairments, or social-skill deficits exert significant influence on the overall course of the disorder, it has been surprisingly difficult to identify *causal relationships* between these vulnerabilities and specific failures in personal or social functioning. Instead, multiple vulnerabilities interact with other personal characteristics and environmental circumstances to produce the unique clinical presentation of a person with schizophrenia. Identifying the causal processes that underlie a specific person's clinical presentation may require extremely complex mathematical models, perhaps comparable to meteorological models that predict the paths of certain types of storms over specific terrains – if they can be identified at all (Heinrichs, 2001).

Traditionally, the principles of Western allopathic medicine lead us to think about both, disease and treatment, as the products of linear sequences or cascades. Disease starts at molecular levels of functioning and cascades to more molar levels. For example, microbes produce toxins that cause cell death, which produces tissue damage, which brings about organ failure, which leads to organ system failure, which disrupts organismic homeostasis, which ends in death. Accordingly, treatment is designed to prevent the cascade, preferably at the lowest possible level, that is, by killing the microbe. Treatment directed more downstream in the cascade – without addressing its origin – is merely palliative. But if schizophrenia is a state of deteriorating homeorhesis there is no single cause and no linear cascade. There is, therefore, no single target for an allopathic "magic bullet." What then should be the targets of treatment?

Current research does identify general relationships between processes at different levels of analysis, for example, between cognitive impairments, emotional dysregulation, psychotic symptoms, and metacognition (apprehension of one's own cognitive functioning: Garety et al., 2007; Wykes & Reeder, 2005). The neurocognitive domain itself has a hierarchical structure, ranging from basic attentional processes to executive functions (McGurk & Mueser, 2004). Empirical findings suggest a link between cognitive deficits and negative symptoms (e.g., Allen, Strauss, Donohue, & van Kammen, 2007; Cohen,Leung et al., 2006; Greenwood, Landau, & Wykes, 2005; Harvey, Koren et al., 2006; Sergi, Rassovsky et al., 2007). Social capacity, the ability to engage in everyday tasks and activities, is a mediating factor between cognitive and everyday functioning (Bellack, 2004; Bellack et al., 2007; Heaton et al., 2004). Cognition, positive and negative symptoms, and functional outcome can be incorporated in a model of pharmacological efficacy (Green & Nuechterlein, 1999). Analyses using advanced mathematical modeling techniques support the existence of complex, interacting causal pathways of treatment effects between processes across levels of functioning (e.g., Bell, Tsang et al., 2008; Brekke et al., 2005; Peer, Rothmann, Penrod, Penn, & Spaulding, 2004; Roder & Schmidt, 2009; Schmidt et al., 2009; Sergi et al., 2006; Vauth et al., 2004). So far, taken together the evidence suggests that the benefits of any treatment directed at any level of functioning may potentially be distributed throughout the organismic system. Whether any particular intervention produces a measurable increment in functional outcome is an empirical question. However, the interconnectedness of processes impaired in schizophrenia suggests that the overall impact of treatment on functional outcome is maximized not by a magic bullet, but by the total number of beneficial interventions that can be applied across all levels of functioning. This has been one of the guiding principles in the development of IPT.

1.2.5 An Integrated Model

All the foregoing considerations lead to an expansion of the integrated model originally constructed by Green and Nuechterlein (1999). The expanded model is shown in Figure 1.4. The model suggests that functional outcome ("coping with life successfully") is determined by a multiplicity of organismic factors, including neurocognitive and sociocognitive impairments in the various domains described by the MATRICS model as well as positive and negative symptoms, all interacting with the sociocognitive factors associated with the recovery perspective. Psychological interventions can address all these factors at their respective levels. This leads pragmatically to various treatment options, especially for cognitive-behavioral approaches, which will be discussed in the next chapter.

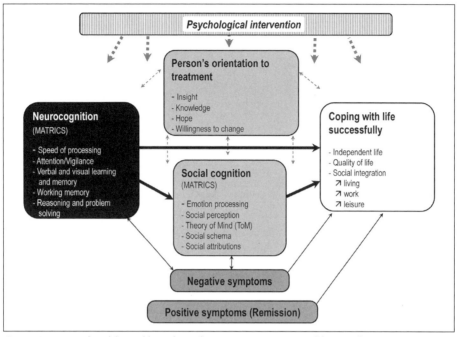

Figure 1.4 Integrated model: Possible mediators between neurocognition and functional outcome

2 Treatment Approaches and Empirical Results

Unlike conventional antipsychotic medication, the newer atypical neuroleptics seem to have a potentially better profile of some side effects, and their efficacy is probably greater (e.g., Davis, Chen, & Glick, 2003; Harvey & Keefe, 2001; Woodward, Purdon, Meltzer, & Zald, 2007). However, these assumptions are being controversially discussed. The results of the CATIE study (Clinical Antipsychotic Trial of Intervention Effectiveness) were unable to support either a superiority of atypical neuroleptics over conventional drugs (Keefe, Bilder et al., 2007; Keefe, Sweeney et al., 2007; Lieberman et al., 2005) or a greater cost efficacy of atypical neuroleptics (Rosenheck, Leslie, & Doshi, 2008; Rosenheck et al., 2006). The latter finding corresponds with the results of the British CUTLASS (Cost Utility of the Latest Antipsychotic Drugs in Schizophrenia Study; Davies et al., 2007; Jones et al., 2006). A more differential approach to the spectrum efficacy of atypical neuroleptics showed only a very small effect on cognitive disorders – and only moderate effects on negative symptoms, psychosocial functioning, and employment outcome (Bowie & Harvey, 2005; Harvey, Patterson, Potter, Zhong, & Brecher, 2006; Hori et al., 2006; Keefe, Bilder et al., 2007; Resnick et al., 2008; Sergi, Green et al. 2007; Swartz et al., 2007). Consequently, purely pharmacological treatment can only reach some of the therapeutic goals required for recovery.

Against the background of integrative models (e.g., the mediator model shown in Figure 1.4), it seems plausible that therapeutic approaches that focus on cognitive and social deficits caused by the disorder are most effective within a multidimensional treatment approach. Essentially, four main approaches of cognitive behavioral interventions can be distinguished:
1. Psychoeducation and Family Therapy
2. Cognitive Behavior Therapy for (Persistent) Positive Symptoms
3. Social Competence Therapy
4. Cognitive Remediation Therapy

The Integrated Psychological Therapy Program (IPT) connects the two treatment approaches of Cognitive Remediation Therapy and Social Competence Therapy. Note that, aside from cognitive behavioral approaches, other therapeutic methods might be effective in the treatment of schizophrenia (e.g., psychodynamic therapy); to date, however, there is no well-founded evidence for a clinical effect. This lack of evidence can be shown exemplarily with two meta-analyses: One of the meta-analyses dealing with psychodynamic short-term therapy for specific disorders failed to include any controlled schizophrenia study (Leichsenring, Rabung, & Leibing, 2004). Another meta-analysis evaluated the efficacy of Supportive Therapy (ST). Thereby, ST was defined as an intervention for individuals to maintain current functioning or to assist preexisting abilities as opposed to educating, training, or changing the person's way of coping. This analysis did not find any additive effects of ST compared to standard care – and found weaker effects of ST compared to other therapeutic approaches, mainly cognitive behavioral therapy approaches (Buckley & Pettit, 2007). On the other hand, the four cognitive behavioral therapy approaches mentioned above fulfill the criteria established for evidence-based psychotherapeutic intervention. The Cochran Collaboration (www.cochrane.org), for instance, hierarchically arranged the criteria of external validity: On the basis of expert judgments, the lowest level of validity contains nonexperimental designs (e.g., no control group included; field study), followed by quasiexperimental (e.g., unrandomized patient allocation to compared treatment conditions), and finally the methodologically valuable randomized-control trials (RTC). RTC are the studies with the highest criterion and can be summarized and quantitatively analyzed in a meta-analysis. Accordingly, an overview of the past 30 years showed an exponential increase in the number of schizophrenia-related meta-analyses. A total of 237 meta-analyses have been published, 58 concerning genetics, 38 cognition, 30 pharmacology, and 19 psychosocial treatment (Nasrallah, 2008). Systematically summarizing the evaluation of empirical results elevates the replicability and generalizability of the results from individual studies. A standardized effect measure is required in order to statistically integrate such findings. The measure of effects used in meta-analyses is the effect size (*ES*). Below, we list the most important methodological steps of a meta-analysis, in order to help in the understanding and interpretation of *ES* discussed in this chapter and Chapter 7:

– Literature research and selection of studies (e.g., RCT, diagnosis, description of the intervention, availability of statistical values).
– Calculation of *ES* from statistical values (*t*-value, *F*-value, χ^2, etc.) following the formula $ES = 2(F/df)^{1/2}$; or taking the difference of the mean raw values of the condition of comparison in relation to the variance of the formula $ES = (M_{\text{experimental group}} - M_{\text{control group}})/SD$. *ES* = 1.0, therefore, means that the difference between the experimental groups and the control condition is at one standard deviation (*SD*) of the population.
– Weighting the *ES* of the primary studies with their inverse variance.
– Test of homogeneity of the *ES* to summarize the outcome variables from the individual studies and analysis of moderators for heterogeneous effects: categorizing *ES* (e.g., sex, duration of therapy, medication).
– Test of significance of the mean *ES*, for example, by means of the 95% confidence interval (CI; lower bound > 0).
– Judging the effects independent of their level of significance. *ES* can be small (*ES* = .2), moderate (*ES* = .5), or large (*ES* = .8) (Cohen, 1988).

The fact that evidence-based cognitive behavioral therapeutic approaches dominate over other approaches is also evident in the elaboration of treatment guidelines (e.g., the Schizophrenia Patients Outcomes Research Team (PORT) [Lehman & Steinwachs, 2003]; Catalog of Clinical Training Opportunities: best practices for recovery and improved outcomes for people with serious mental illness, APA task force [www.apa.org/practice/grid.html]). The rationale of these therapeutic approaches, their typical contents, their respective empirically founded spectrum of efficacy using examples from current meta-analyses, as well as related open questions, is summarized below. Psychoeducation and Family Therapy approaches will be summarized in Chapter 2.1, Cognitive Behavior Therapy approaches for (Persistent) Positive Symptoms in Chapter 2.2, Social Competence Therapy approaches in Chapter 2.3, and Cognitive Remediation Therapy approaches will be illustrated separately in Chapter 2.4.1 through 2.4.3 under the terms Neurocognitive Remediation, Social Cognitive Remediation, and Integrated Therapy approaches.

2.1 Psychoeducation and Family Therapy

These approaches have a long tradition and are widely used in the treatment of schizophrenia patients. In an international study carried out in Germany, Austria, and Switzerland, for instance, 72% of all institutions indicated that they offered psychoeducation for schizophrenia inpatients. Within these offerings, 66% of interventions are directed toward the patients, 33% toward patients and their relatives, and only about 1% only toward just the relatives (Rummel-Kluge, Pitschel-Walz, Bäuml, & Kissling, 2006). The aim of these interventions is to augment the possibilities for coping with the disorder and reduce the resulting burden on the patients and/or their relatives. Different forms of treatment are used: single families (Falloon, Boyd, & McGill, 1984; Hogarty & Anderson, 1986; Leff, Kuipers, Berkowitz, Eberlein-Vries, & Sturgeon, 1982; Tarrier et al. 1988), groups of relatives together with the patients (McFarlane et al., 1995) and without the patients (Bäuml, Kissling, Meurer, Wais, & Lauter, 1991; Leff et al., 1989), as well as bifocal therapies with patients and relatives in separate group sessions (Buchkremer, Klingberg, Holle, Schulze Mönking, & Hornung, 1997; Roder, Zorn et al., 2008). In past years, so-called peer-to-peer psychoeducation concepts have come to be accepted as well. These concepts are based on training patients and/or their relatives, who in turn act as group moderators in psychoeducative groups. After receiving training, they instruct other patients, and train family members to take over the tasks of moderator in other groups of relatives (e.g., Rummel, Hansen, Helbig, Pitschel-Walz, & Kissling, 2005; Rummel, Pitschel-Walz, & Kissling, 2005).

Even though the general frameworks for carrying out therapy approaches concerning the disorder and the resulting burden vary greatly, most of them have three central therapeutic elements in common: psychoeducation, coping with signs of early symptoms, and training in communication skills.

These approaches typically start with psychoeducation, that is, explaining the current knowledge about the disorder as well as the treatment options, based on a vulnerability-stress coping model. Information concerning the effects of drugs is crucial in this context, as one aim is to increase the patients' compliance with the medical treatment. Subsequent to the elements of educative therapy, the issue of identification and coping with signs of early detection, symptoms and stress is usually broached, with the aim of augmenting the patients' as well as their relatives' strategies and resources for coping. Finally, communication training can be carried out to improve the patients' possibilities of interacting with their social environment. Two recent meta-analyses examined the efficacy of these approaches by including only randomized controlled studies (RCT) (Lincoln, 2006; Pfammatter, Junghan, & Brenner, 2006). The mean outcome implied a significant reduction of relapse rates at 6–12-month follow-up ($ES >$ 0.42). However, the results of these meta-analyses were not consistent concerning functional outcome at posttreatment ($ES = -0.03$ to 0.38), symptom reduction at follow-up ($ES = 0.19$ to 0.40), and rehospitalization rates at follow-up lasting longer than 12 months ($ES = 0.21$ to 0.51). Additionally, an increase in the relatives' knowledge about the disorder after treatment was observed ($ES = 0.39$ to 0.48). Interventions that included the families were more effective in relapse prevention during follow-up ($ES = 0.48$) than interventions addressed only toward patients ($ES = 0.18$) (Lincoln et al., 2007). Finally, despite the lack of data there is no strong evidence for an improvement of patients' medication compliance. To prevent relapses and to improve understanding of schizophrenia, psychoeducation and family interventions are the approaches of choice.

2.2 Cognitive Behavior Therapy Approaches for (Persistent) Positive Symptoms

Various work groups from England (e.g., Chadwick, Birchwood, & Trower, 1996; Fowler, Garety, & Kuipers, 1995; Kingdon & Turkington, 2005; Tarrier, 1992), North America (e.g., Beck & Rector, 2000; Rector, Seeman, & Segal, 2003), Scandinavia (e.g., Perris, 1989), German-speaking countries (Lincoln, 2006; Vauth & Stieglitz, 2007), and Australia (e.g., Jackson et al., 1998; Kingsep, Nathan, & Castle, 2003) have developed cognitive behavioral intervention approaches over the past 10 years. The majority of these approaches are offered in an individual setting, although in some studies, especially from the United States, group settings may also be found (overview in Wykes, Steel, Everitt, & Tarrier, 2008). The primary aim of most approaches is to reduce positive symptoms; some approaches additionally aim for the reduction of negative symptoms and social anxiety, as well as an increased level of functioning (Wykes et al., 2008). The cognitive treatment of the irrational patterns of explanation that form the basis of delusions and hallucinations is central to these therapeutic approaches. These irrational patterns of explanation can be modified by the cognitive therapy techniques of Beck (1970) and Ellis (1957) (e.g., Socratic dialog, behavioral experiments for reality check, reattribution). Additionally, the approaches often contain psychoeducative elements, imparting the current state of knowledge about the causes of the disease, as well as training in appropriate coping strategies.

Several recent and differentiated meta-analyses have summarized the efficacy of such approaches (e.g., Lincoln et al., 2008; Pfammatter et al., 2006; Wykes et al., 2008; Zimmermann, Favrod, Trieu, & Pomini, 2005). The meta-analyses of Zimmermann and colleagues, as well as that of Wykes and colleagues, included studies that were not randomized, although in the latter this influence on the results was controlled for. In general, a significant reduction of the general psychopathology at the posttreatment measurement (ES = .25 to .45) as well as positive symptoms (ES = .21 to .47) was found. However, these effects were stronger in postacute patients (ES = .48) compared to chronic patients (ES = .26) (Zimmermann et al., 2005). The significant reduction of positive symptoms remained during a follow-up of 8.6 months (ES = 0.35) (Lincoln et al., 2008).

Significant effects during the therapy phase were also found for negative symptoms (ES = 0.44), functioning (ES = 0.39), and mood (ES = 0.36) (Wykes et al., 2008). Furthermore, there was no statistical evidence of any difference in target symptoms between individual therapy (ES = 0.42) and group therapy (ES = 0.39). However, the methodological rigor of the ratings seems to play an important role with respect to the outcome: Nonblind ratings tended to have 50–100% higher effects than blind ratings (Wykes et al., 2008; Zimmermann et al., 2005). Moreover, the results were related to the type of control condition: The comparison of CBT with active control groups did not imply a significant reduction of general psychopathology and positive symptoms during therapy, although a comparison of CBT with treatment as usual (TAU) revealed significant effects favoring CBT (Lincoln et al., 2008). Finally, to date there is little evidence that cognitive behavior therapy for (persistent) symptoms also increases the underlying cognitive functions. Nevertheless, these approaches seem to be the treatment of choice for reducing general psychopathology and positive symptoms in many schizophrenia patients.

2.3 Social Competence Therapy

From a rehabilitative perspective, (re)establishing social and community functioning are considered to be among the hallmarks of schizophrenia therapy (*Diagnostic and Statistical Manual of Mental Disorders*, American Psychiatric Association) as well as social and community reintegration. Social competence, which is defined as the ability to achieve personally relevant goals through interacting with others in situations such as work, residence, recreation, and medical care, is essential for social and community functioning and quality of life. Social competence, thus, comprises (1) social cognition (especially social and emotion perception) on the basis of established neurocognitive functioning to decode contextual social input, to effectively process social information, and to plan a behavioral response as well as social problem solving; and (2) the behavioral response to act adequately in a specific context with appropriate verbal and nonverbal behavior and expression of emotions. In contrast, social skills represent the constituent behavior that depends on perceiving skills, processing skills, and sending skills, which enable the individual to be successful in everyday life as reflected by social competence. Social skills are predominantly based on learning principles and experiences (Bellack, 2004; Kopelowicz et al., 2006).

We decided to use the term *social competence therapy* instead of the commonly used term social skills therapy. Social competence reflects self-efficacy and real-world success in everyday life through favorable experiences.

Thus, social competence therapy approaches have a long tradition and were developed on the basis of learning principles. These cognitive behavioral therapy approaches can be categorized in three chronological developmental stages (Roder et al., 2000; Roder, Zorn et al., 2001).

2.3.1 Developmental Stages of Social Competence Therapy Approaches

Stage 1

Token-programs were the first step toward augmenting social skills in schizophrenia patients. They are based on Skinner's model of operant conditioning from the 1960s and 1970s (Cohen, Florin, Grusche, Meyer-Osterkamp, & Sell, 1973). Activation and a positive influence of token programs on very specific areas of social behavior is evident (McMonagle & Sultana, 2000; Paul & Lentz, 1977). Because recent developments have led to more efficient methods – and also for ethical reasons – nowadays these approaches are justifiable only with patients presenting very pronounced negative symptoms and resistance to other treatment approaches.

Stage 2

These treatment approaches were developed in the 1970s and 1980s. Based on the paradigms of model learning and roleplay, augmentation of "molecular skills" (eye-contact, currency of speech, gesture, etc.) as well as complex "molar skills" (thanking someone, asking for favors, etc.) is targeted (Roder, Brenner, & Kienzle, 2008; Smith, Bellack, & Lieberman, 1996). These approaches are usually carried out in a step-by-step procedure (e.g., Bellack, Mueser, Gingerich, & Agresta, 1997, 2004). Additional core elements of such group approaches are individual problem analysis, communication of the therapy rationale, planning the therapy, practical instructions, stepwise structuring of the target behavior, positive reinforcement, and corrective feedback, and – in order to enable the transfer to everyday life – in vivo exercises and homework.

Stage 3

The third phase of development took place in the USA in the 1980s and 1990s and included rehabilitation themes relevant to schizophrenia patients (e.g., symptom management, coping with medicaments, body hygiene, and clothing [Liberman et al., 1986, 1993; Mueser, Wallace, & Liberman, 1995]). Also, a problem-solving model formed the basis of the definition of these "therapy modules." After the turn of the millennium, additional focus on aftercare completed these modules. Case managers in the community exercised the skills learned during therapy with the patients in aftercare, in order to support a vertical generalization and a transfer to everyday life. Furthermore, the therapeutic methods dealing with social skills became an integral part of outpatient management (Glynn et al., 2002; Liberman, Kopelowicz, Venture, & Gutkind, 2002). This third stage of therapy approaches to augment social skills formed the basis for the development of new specific therapy programs in the fields of living, work, and leisure (WAF*) for schizophrenia patients (Mueller & Roder, 2005; Roder et al., 2000, 2002; Roder, Brenner et al., 2001; Roder, Zorn et al., 2001; Roder, Zorn et al., 2008; Roder, Mueller, & Zorn, 2006). These therapy approaches evolved from the further development of the subprograms "Social Skills" and "Interpersonal Problem Solving" of Integrated Psychological Therapy (IPT). Along with the technique of role-playing problem solving, a wide range of cognitive behavioral therapy methods was included in these therapy approaches (see Chapter 8).

2.3.2 Efficacy of Social Competence Therapy Approaches

Two recent meta-analyses quantitatively reviewed the results of social competence therapy approaches evaluated in randomized controlled trials (RCT) (Kurtz & Mueser, 2008; Pfammatter et al., 2006). The results of these meta-analyses are summarized in Table 2.1.

Although the two meta-analyses partially used a different terminology and a different categorization system, the results are very similar: As postulated by the model purporting a continuum from proximal (direct therapy targets) to distal outcomes (not directly targeted in therapy reflecting generalization) (Kurtz & Mueser, 2008), the effect sizes (*ES*) of the measurements were higher for more proximal outcomes. As expected, the largest effects after therapy were found in content mastery exams (*ES* =

Table 2.1 Recent meta-analyses and efficacy of social competence therapy approaches

Authors	Outcome variable	Weighted effect size
Pfammatter et al. 2006	Skill acquisition	0.77
K = 19 RCT	Skill acquisition (follow-up)	0.52
	Assertiveness	0.43
	Social functioning	0.39
	Social functioning (follow-up)	0.32
	General psychopathology	0.23
Kurtz & Mueser 2008	Content mastery exams	1.20
K = 22 RCT	Social skills and daily living skills	0.52
	Social functioning	0.52
	Negative symptoms	0.40
	Other psychiatric symptoms	0.15
	Relapse/rehospitalization (follow-up)	0.23

K = number of studies; RCT = randomized-controlled trial. *Note:* only variables with K ≥ 3 are included.

* We use the German abbreviations (**W**ohnen, **A**rbeit, **F**reizeit)

1.20), the lowest in psychopathology ($ES \geq 0.15$). However, the *ES* addressing social skills, social functioning, and negative symptoms also reach significance ($ES \geq 0.39$). Only the small *ES* of psychiatric symptoms is slightly heterogeneous across the two analyses and is not significant (Kurtz & Mueser, 2008). Not all of the effects are homogeneous over the included studies; some moderator variables could be identified (Kurtz & Mueser, 2008). For example, stronger effects in social skills were found in studies with younger samples, inpatients, and treatment as usual (TAU) as the control condition. The reduction of negative symptoms was affected by patients' age and the methodological rigor of the design: Younger age and a lower quality of studies predicted greater reduction of negative symptoms. Finally, the improvements in social skills ($ES = 0.52$) and social functioning ($ES = 0.32$) were maintained during follow-up (Pfammatter et al., 2006), and a small but significant reduction in the relapse of patients who participated in a social competence therapy was observed compared to those in the control condition ($ES = 0.23$) (Kurtz & Mueser, 2008).

Neither of the meta-analyses reflected the impact on the outcome of different contents and aims associated with the described developmental stages of the social competence therapy approaches included. Furthermore, there is a general lack of data addressing the efficacy of social competence therapy approaches in neurocognition and social cognition, which underlie social competence (see Chapter 8). However, the follow-up results (Pfammatter et al., 2006) indicate a vertical generalization of the effects after treatment, which is in contrast to the assumption of insufficient generalization and transfer effects discussed over the past decade. Against the background of the recovery concept, (re)establishing social skills and social competence and supporting the social integration of schizophrenia patients represent a main topic of modern psychiatric rehabilitation. To date, Social Competence Therapy is the only available and successfully evaluated treatment that directly intervenes on this level. During the evaluation of IPT and its further developments, we found evidence that the effectiveness of Social Competence Therapy could be optimized by combining it with Cognitive Remediation Therapy (see Chapter 7).

2.4 Cognitive Remediation Therapy

Cognitive impairments are considered a core component of schizophrenia. There is growing evidence for the association of various cognitive deficits (see the MATRICS dimensions discussed in Chapter 1) with functional outcome and, therefore, with reduced success in "classical" psychosocial rehabilitation in schizophrenia patients (Keefe & Fenton, 2007). Most schizophrenia patients show cognitive impairments compared to healthy controls as well as to people with affective disorders in any state of the illness. These impairments are already present during childhood and adolescence, in the premorbid phase, during the first episode, and in chronic patients. However, neither the diagnostic criteria nor the subtypology of schizophrenia of the present edition of the *Diagnostic and Statistical Manual of Mental Disorders* (DSM-IV-TR) includes cognitive impairment as a criterion for schizophrenia. The definition and inclusion of a specific cognitive criterion into the DSM-V was recently proposed and discussed by experts (Keefe, 2008; see Forum in *World Psychiatry*, 7, February 2008). Against this background, it seems evident that the improvement of cognitive functions represents a main treatment target.

Cognitive disturbances largely remain after symptom remission and, therefore, continue to act as a feature of the disorder, which is essentially independent of the positive symptoms (see Chapter 1). This is yet another indicator for the differential effect of neuroleptics: While neuroleptics have a clear effect on psychotic symptoms, their impact on cognitive deficits is moderate (Keefe, Bilder et al., 2007; Keefe, Sweeney et al., 2007). The results of the CATIE study (Clinical Antipsychotic Trial of Intervention Effectiveness [Keefe, Bilder et al., 2007; Keefe, Sweeney et al., 2007; Lieberman et al., 2005]), especially, suggest that the currently available neuroleptics are unable to produce an efficient improvement in cognitive functioning, making additional interventions necessary (Green, 2007). The close link between deficits in cognitive capacity and the success of rehabilitative interventions, namely, improvements in social behavior, work, and living standards, implies that a decrease in cognitive deficits might lead to a direct improvement of social functioning. These implications are the main reason for the increasing interest in cognitive deficits specific to schizophrenia – and the most important premise of their therapeutic focus. Cognitive Remediation Therapy aims at a systematic enhancement of cognitive processes through a rehearsal learning approach of specific cognitive achievements. A compensatory approach consisting of behavioral therapeutic and didactic learning strategies is also employed. These exercises include repeated practice of cognitive achievement either on the computer or as paper-and-pencil exercises. Building up compensatory strategies involves teaching strategies to cope with problems associated with own deficits (e.g., chunking of information), but also environmental engineering (e.g., the use of external aids to memory and organizational support such as notepads or to-do lists). Rehearsing cognitive exercises and communicating compensatory strategies is supported by several therapeutic techniques: positive reinforcement of immediate, correct proposals for solutions (shaping), presentation of cues (prompting), direct and corrective feedback (coaching), instructions, learning rules, internal repetition of exercises (cognitive rehearsal), systematic problem solving, adaptation of the difficulty of tasks to the actual capacities of the patient (scaffolding), and the technique of errorless learning.

A number of cognitive remediation approaches have been clinically evaluated over the past years. Several reviews have summarized the evaluation of these approaches (Krabbendam & Aleman, 2003; Kurtz, 2003; Mueller, Pfammatter, Roder, & Brenner, 2006; Twamley, Jeste, & Bellack, 2003; Velligan, Kern et al., 2006; Wykes & Reeder, 2005). These reviews consider psychological therapy approaches to enhance neurocognition and integrated approaches including interventions on neurocognition and social cognition, among others. However, interventions focusing exclusively on social cognition are missing in these reviews. Consequently, Cognitive Remediation Therapy can be categorized into Neurocognitive Remediation Therapy, Social Cognitive Remediation Therapy, and Integrated Therapy approaches. These are discussed separately in the following sections.

2.4.1 Neurocognitive Remediation Therapy

Neurocognitive Remediation Therapy has a long tradition, especially in connection with war veterans and brain-injured patients (summary in Twamley et al., 2003). The first neurocognitive interventions for treating schizophrenia patients were developed 30 years ago. Most of these approaches aimed at improving neurocognitive functions by means of laboratory tasks, for instance, with repeated practice including enhanced instructions using the Wisconsin Card Sorting Test (WCST, Heaton, 1981; computerized version: Loong, 1989). The WCST measures higher executive functions. The results of WCST studies were summarized in a meta-analysis by Kurtz et al. (2001). Approaches such as lab-based interventions for the improvement of executive functions are not very clinically oriented, since they are based on the measurement of functioning in one neurocognitive domain being dependent on a person's momentary state. However, over the past 20 years, broad-based and clinically oriented neurocognitive therapy approaches have undergone increasing development. These approaches are summarized in Table 2.2. The subprogram Cognitive Differentiation of the Integrated Psychological Therapy (IPT) (Brenner et al., 1980; Roder, Kienzle, & Studer, 1988; Roder, Brenner et al., 2008) is among the first neurocognitive remediation therapy approaches to be empirically founded and evidence based. This therapy approach is discussed in the section concerning integrated therapy approaches.

The American Psychological Association Task Force on Serious Mental Illness and Severe Emotional Disturbance (APA/CAPP) included several of these neurocognitive approaches in its *Catalog of Clinical Training Opportunities: Best Practice for Recovery and Improved Outcomes for People with Serious Mental Illness* (www.apa.org/practice/grid.html), which represents state-of-the-art interventions. Approaches to the improvement of specific neurocognitive functions can be categorized, according to their intervention goals, into therapies of executive functions, memory, and attention.

Cognitive Remediation Therapy (CRT) was originally developed in Australia (Delahunty & Morice, 1993) and then adopted for use in the United Kingdom by Wykes and colleagues (1999, 2003; Rose & Wykes, 2008; Wykes & Reeder, 2005). CRT originally used paper-and-pencil exercises in an individual setting. It targets executive functioning and consists of three modules: cognitive flexibility, working memory, and planning. In recent years the focus was expanded to metacognitive functions that underlie certain symptoms. CRT procedure places a strong emphasis on teaching methods and uses errorless learning principles adapted to each participant's own pace.

Other training procedures for memory and attention are strongly based on the use of computer programs (e.g., Benedict et al., 1994; Medalia, Revheim, & Casey, 2000). These interventions successfully improve the specifically targeted neurocognitive functions but generally fail to promote generalization effects. They have also been criticized for their lack of an explicit reference to any underlying theoretical models (Wykes & van der Gaag, 2001).

One exception is Attention Process Training (APT), originally designed to remediate attention deficits in individuals with brain injury (Sohlberg & Mateer, 1987) and then adopted for cognitive rehabilitation of schizophrenia patients (Kurtz et al., 2001; Lopez-Luengo & Vasquez, 2003; Silverstein et al., 2005). APT provides an individual-

Table 2.2 Examples of nonintegrated neurocognitive remediation approaches

Neurocognitive remediation approach	Type of intervention	Author
1. Training of specific neurocognitive functions		
1a. *Training of executive functions*		
Cognitive Remediation Therapy CRT*	restitution & strategy learning; originally noncomputerized	Delahunty & Morice, 1993; Wykes, Reeder, Corner, Williams, & Eyeritt, 1999; Wykes et al., 2003
1b. *Memory training*		
Memory remediation	restitution; computerized	e.g., Medalia, Revheim, & Casey, 2000
1c. *Attention training*		
Attention Process Training APT*	restitution; noncomputerized	Sohlberg & Mateer, 1987
Attention training	restitution; computerized	e.g., Benedict et al., 1994
Attention Shaping*	restitution; noncomputerized	Silverstein et al., 1999
2. Broad-based neurocognitive remediation		
Computer-based trainings	restitution; computerized	e.g., Bellucci et al., 2002; Kurtz, Seltzer, Shagan, Thime, & Wexler, 2007; Lindenmayer et al., 2008; McGurk, Mueser, Feldman, Wolfe, & Pascaris, 2007; McGurk, Mueser, & Pascaris, 2005; Sartory, Zorn, Groetzinger, & Windgassen, 2005; Vauth et al., 2005
Cognitive Training CT	Compensatory & environmental strategy learning; noncomputerized group setting	Twamley, Savla, Zurhellen, & Heaton, 2008
3. Compensatory approaches		
Cognitive Adaption Training CAT*	Compensatory & environmental strategies for home and work	Velligan & Bow-Thomas, 2000; Velligan, Kern, & Gold, 2006; Velligan et al., 2000, 2002
Errorless learning approach*	Short-time training and teaching method; Individual or group format	Kern, Green, Mintz, & Liberman, 2003; Kern, Liberman, Kopelowicz, Mintz, & Green, 2002; Kern et al., 2005; Kern, Liberman et al., 2009

*State-of-the-art interventions, APA Training Grid 2007.

ized, highly structured multilevel intervention. It consists of hierarchically organized tasks that train different components of attention. ATP follows a building-block approach: Skills acquired in earlier stages serve as prerequisites for skills to be developed during later training stages. ATP material includes auditory attention tapes and combines auditory and visual activities.

Attention Shaping is another attention training approach (Silverstein, Menditto, & Stuve, 2001; Silverstein et al., 1999, 2005). Against the background of research findings suggesting that sustained attention deficits have a rate-limiting effect on cognitive rehabilitation, APT was designed for treatment-refractory schizophrenia patients. Shaping is an operant conditioning technique and involves the differential reinforcement of successive approximations toward an intended behavior. Behavior approximating the intended behavior is reinforced (e.g., by the use of tokens) and nondesired behavior is not (Velligan, Kern et al., 2006). Attention-shaping procedures have also been combined with APT (Silverstein et al., 2005).

Published studies used various licensed computer programs: CogPack (Olbrich, 1996, 1998, 1999; www.markersoftware.com), Ben-Yishay's Orientation Remediation Module (Ben-Yishay, Piasetsky, & Rattok, 1985), Captain's Log Software (Sandford & Browne, 1988), and CogRehab (Bracy, 1995). The following software programs have all been used in treatment evaluation studies with schizophrenia patients: Captain's Log Software (Bellucci, Glaberman, & Haslam, 2002), CogRehab (Kurtz et al., 2007), Ben-Yishay's Orientation Remediation Module (Hogarty et al., 2004), and Cogpack (Lindenmayer et al., 2008; McGurk et al., 2005; McGurk, Mueser et al., 2007; Sartory et al., 2005; Vauth, Dietl, Stieglitz, & Olbrich, 2000; Vauth et al., 2005). In some studies CogPack was combined with work rehabilitation (McGurk et al., 2005; McGurk, Mueser et al., 2007; Vauth et al., 2005) or with discussion group sessions to support the transfer of the cognitive skills to daily activities (Lindenmayer et al., 2008). In general, these remediation approaches contain repeated practice methods (restitution) based on errorless learning principles, and usually they do not promote group interaction and group dynamics.

In contrast, Twamley and colleagues' (Twamley, Savla et al., 2008). Cognitive Training (CT) is a group-based, noncomputerized, and manualized approach with a focus on teaching and practicing compensatory and environmental strategies. The repeated practice is intended to familiarize clients with these strategies. The interventions include tasks concerning prospective memory, attention/vigilance, learning and memory, and executive functions as well as their relationship to daily life. The tasks were adapted from various sources such as social skills training (Bellack et al., 1997) or Cognitive Remediation Therapy (CRT, Wykes et al., 1999). The interventions were designed to be practical, not very technical, and yet appealing to clients. CT tries to bridge the gap between traditional restitution approaches and compensatory approaches within neurocognitive remediation.

In contrast to the neurocognitive remediation approaches discussed above, compensatory approaches place their primary emphasis on bypassing neurocognitive impairments in order to improve broader aspects of functioning (Kern, Glynn, Horan, & Marder, 2009; Velligan, Mueller et al., 2006). Therefore, the focus lies on two intervention topics: recruiting relatively intact neurocognitive processes or using environmental supports and adapting intended behavior.

An important compensatory approach is errorless learning (Kern et al., 2002, 2003, 2005), which is an integrated part of other cognitive remediation approaches. The key principle underlying this approach is the elimination of errors in the learning process and the automation of responses. Tasks are broken down into individual components,

with the simplest component being trained first, followed by more complex components. Errorless learning is a short-term training and teaching approach conducted in
small groups. Kern and colleagues applied errorless learning procedure in lab-based
studies, although recently they have extended their efforts to community settings (Kern,
Liberman et al., 2009).

Another compensatory approach is the manual-based Cognitive Adaptation Training
(CAT) (Maples & Velligan, 2008; Velligan & Bow-Thomas, 2000; Velligan et al., 2000,
2002; Velligan, Mueller et al., 2006). Many schizophrenia patients suffer from impairments in executive functioning, which lead to problems of initiating and inhibiting
appropriate behavior. CAT uses at-home environmental support and structure (e.g.,
checklists, alarm signs for medication, reorganizing placement of belongings) to facilitate independent living. Using behavioral principles, one sets up environments to cue
specific behavior, discourage distraction, and maintain goal-oriented activity. Additionally, adaptations can be customized for neurocognitive limitations, e.g., in attention
and memory (Velligan, Kern et al., 2006). Individual treatment involving home visits
is based on comprehensive behavioral, neuropsychological, functional, and environmental assessments at intake.

Efficacy of Neurocognitive Remediation Therapy

Some years ago, it was argued that this type of cognitive behavioral intervention was being
evaluated in very few RCTs and was consequently found to have accumulated little empirical evidence concerning its efficacy. Only recently did two meta-analyses quantitatively
review the results of 19 and 26 RCTs, respectively, addressing cognitive remediation as the
experimental condition (McGurk, Twamley et al., 2007; Pfammatter et al., 2006). The
results of these meta-analyses are summarized in Table 2.3.

Both meta-analyses found significant treatment effects in the neurocognitive domains of attention and executive functioning as well as social functioning and symptom
reduction. The only exception within neurocognitive functions was visual learning and
memory, where no effects were found (McGurk, Twamley et al., 2007). Overall, neurocognitive remediation works quite well on the proximal outcome. The effect sizes
(ES) in neurocognition were positively associated with a longer duration of therapy at
posttreatment and could be maintained over a follow-up to 8 months ($ES = 0.66$) (Mc-
Gurk, Twamley et al., 2007). Additionally, small to moderate generalization effects on
functioning and symptoms were identified (McGurk, Twamley et al., 2007; Pfammatter
et al., 2006). The combination of restitution and strategy learning methods led to significantly larger effects ($ES = .62$) compared to the use of restitution techniques alone
($ES = 0.24$) (McGurk, Twamley et al., 2007). These results are in line with the results
of an earlier meta-analysis (Krabbendam & Aleman, 2003). Both meta-analyses (Table
2.3) found among the highest ES in social cognition, though this surprising result is
strongly affected by the inclusion of studies evaluating integrated therapy approaches,
which also comprise social cognition as an intervention topic. At least in the analysis
of McGurk and colleagues (McGurk, Twamley et al., 2007), studies of integrated therapies were the only ones assessing social cognition.

A: Background

Table 2.3 Recent meta-analyses and efficacy of cognitive remediation approaches

Author	Outcome variable	Weighted effect size
Pfammatter, Junghan, & Brenner, 2006 K = 19 RCTs	Attention	0.32
	Memory	0.36
	Executive functioning	0.28
	Social cognition	0.40
	Social functioning	0.49
	General psychopathology	0.20
	Negative symptoms	0.24
McGurk, Twamley, Sitzer, McHugo, & Mueser, 2007 K = 26 RCTs	Global cognition	0.41
	Attention/vigilance	0.41
	Speed of processing	0.48
	Verbal working memory	0.52
	Verbal learning and memory	0.39
	Visual learning and memory	0.09
	Reasoning/problem solving	0.47
	Social cognitions	0.54
	Symptoms	0.28
	Functioning	0.35

K = number of studies; RCT = randomized controlled trial.

Finally, there is a lack of studies addressing compensatory approaches as well as social cognitive remediation approaches within the two meta-analyses. The few studies that do evaluate compensatory approaches (errorless learning, CAT) consistently show significant effects in proximal outcome (target behaviors), although they did not measure secondary outcomes corresponding to neurocognitive functioning (Kern, Glynn et al., 2009; Velligan, Mueller et al., 2006). On the other hand, studies on social cognitive remediation generally also assess the outcome in neurocognition in addition to the outcome in social cognition. To our knowledge, however, no meta-analysis addressing social cognitive remediation has been conducted to date.

2.4.2 Social Cognitive Remediation Therapy

A literature search in the Medline database using the terms "schizophrenia" or "psychosis" and "social cognition" showed that the latter term was first used in relation with schizophrenia disorders in 1993 (Corrigan & Green, 1993). There has been a continuous increase of publications dealing with the construct of social cognition in schizophrenia patients in the last 10 years. This tendency runs parallel to the knowledge that the different dimensions of social cognition in schizophrenia patients (described in Chapter 1) are first and foremost distinguished from basic neurocognition, functional outcome, and symptoms. Second, they appear to function as a moderator between neurocognitive functions and functional outcome. Third, they explain an additional proportion of variance of the functional outcome through their unique relationship. As a result, the social cognitive dimensions have become an increasingly important intervention goal in cognitive-behavioral therapy approaches.

We should note that several therapy approaches included certain social cognitive dimensions as intervention goals before the term "social cognition" was defined in the 1990s. The Integrated Psychological Therapy program (IPT) exemplifies this: Its first evaluation study was published as far back as 1980 (Brenner et al., 1980); the first therapy manual in German being released in 1988 (Roder, Brenner, Kienzle, & Hodel, 1988). The development and research on IPT, therefore, offers some pioneering achievements.

Recently, there have been several reviews published on social cognitive remediation approaches (Corrigan & Penn, 2001; Couture et al., 2006; Horan, Kern, & Green, 2008; Kern, Glynn et al., 2009; Penn et al., 2008; Roder, Zorn et al., 2008). It is important to distinguish between lab-based interventions to prove the concept, which last only 1–3 sessions; and goal-oriented psychological treatment for sustainable improvement of individual or multiple social cognitive functions. Horan and colleagues (2008) identified seven proof-of-concept studies (Combs, Tosheva, Wanner, & Basso, 2006; Corrigan, Hirschbeck, & Wolfe, 1995; Kayser, Sarfati, Besche, & Hardy-Baylé, 2006; Penn & Combs, 2000; Russell, Chu, & Phillips, 2006; Sarfati, Passerieux, & Hardy-Baylé, 2000; Silver, Goodman, Knoll, & Isakov, 2004), the majority of which targeted facial emotion perception. Of course, these research studies are of limited interest to clinicians since they are of too short duration; they include rather small samples and measure only cues identical with training content in well-controlled lab-based situations. However, the positive results of these studies provide strong evidence for the possibility of manipulating and increasing social cognition in schizophrenia patients during goal-oriented psychological therapy.

In the meantime, a growing body of social cognitive remediation approaches has been developed in the United States, Switzerland, Germany, The Netherlands, Italy, and South Korea. The majority of these studies target one single social cognitive dimension defined as the "primary target." Others include a broad-based focus on a combination of various social cognitive dimensions. Table 2.4 gives an overview of social cognitive remediation approaches. Broad, integrated therapy approaches combining intervention on social cognition with other treatment targets are discussed in the next section.

Nonintegrated social cognitive remediation approaches are relatively new psychological interventions. They were all developed within the last 8 years, the only exception being the innovative Emotional Management Therapy (EMT) (Hodel & Brenner, 1996). The research group in Bern, Switzerland, who had conceptualized IPT some years earlier, also developed EMT. In general, this type of intervention can be categorized into (1) approaches targeting one single primary social cognitive dimension or (2) broad-based approaches addressing various social cognitive functions.

The Training of Social Perception and Perception of Emotions (van der Gaag et al., 2002) is an individually administered remediation program. Skills in social perception and perception of emotions are the primary treatment goal; the included training to enhance memory, attention, and executive functions are defined as necessary basic

Table 2.4 Examples of nonintegrated social cognitive remediation approaches

Social cognitive remediation approach	Type of intervention	Author
1. Approaches addressing specific social cognitive functions		
1.a. Emotion and social perception		
Training of Social & Emotion Perception	Individually administered; various verbal, visual, and auditive stimuli	van der Gaag, Kern, van den Bosch, & Liberman, 2002
Training of Affect Recognition TAR	Pairs of patients, using pictures of expressed emotions; PC-tasks and desk work	Frommann, Streit, & Wölwer, 2003; Wölwer et al., 2005
1.b. Additionally addressed to coping and emotional intelligence		
Emotional Management Therapy EMT	Group therapy, using pictures of expressed emotions in the social context; role-plays to train coping strategies	Hodel & Brenner, 1996; Hodel, Kern, & Brenner, 2004
Training of Emotional Intelligence TEI	Group therapy, using education sheets, pictures of expressed emotions, euthymic training	Vauth, Rüsch, Wirtz, & Corrigan, 2004; Vauth & Stieglitz, 2008
1.c. Theory of mind (ToM)		
Instrumental Enrichment Program IEP	Group therapy, using pictures of expressed emotions, cartoons, paintings, and role-plays	Rancone et al., 2004
Social Cognition Enhancement Training SCET	Group therapy, using 4-column cartoons	Choi & Kwon, 2006
2. Broad-based approaches addressing several social cognitive functions		
Social Cognition and Interaction Training SCIT	Group therapy, using video clips, slides, and handouts; written and visual stimuli (brief social vignettes, pictured facial affects)	Combs, Adams et al., 2007; Penn, Roberts, Combs, & Sterne, 2007; Penn et al., 2005; Roberts, Penn, & Combs, 2006
Metacognitive Skills Training MCT	Group therapy, using slides and handouts, written and visual stimuli (pictured facial affects, comic)	Moritz & Woodward, 2007a,b; Moritz, Woodward, Stevens, Hauschildt, & Metacognition Study Group, 2009
Social Cognition Skills Training SCST	Group therapy, using photos, audio and video clips, brief social vignettes	Horan, Kern et al., 2009

skills for perceptual social cognitive functions. Training of Affect Recognition (TAR) (Wölwer et al., 2005) has become quite popular since its complete integration into a recently developed new treatment approach of the UCLA (SCST, Horan et al., 2008, see below). TAR is administered to pairs of patients at a time. The founders of TAR like to describe the training as a molecular treatment approach since it is reduced to enhancing affect recognition. TAR starts with facial affects associated with (basic) emotions and gradually progresses to more complex facial expressions, eventually aiming for the patients to understand emotions based on nonverbal gestures and social context. Both treatments, Training of Social and Emotion Perception and TAR, involve restitution and compensation strategies following errorless learning principles.

Two further approaches expand the treatment target of emotion perception by adding coping strategies and the concept of emotional intelligence. The development of Emotional Management Therapy (EMT) (Hodel & Brenner, 1996; Hodel et al., 2004) was based on IPT. EMT addresses the perception of one's own and others' emotional expression as well as its functional consequences on social adjustment and psychopathology. Patients' limited stress tolerance, denoting the negative influence of their psychopathology, and their poor social adjustment can be improved by efficient coping strategies, which are accomplished through role-plays and in vivo exercises. In a further advancement, a brief stress inoculation program for immediate relaxation was added to the standard EMT program (Hodel, Brenner, Merlo, & Teuber, 1998). The intervention goal of the Training of Emotional Intelligence (TEI) (Vauth et al., 2001; Vauth & Stieglitz, 2008) is social intelligence, a topic currently being discussed in the literature. This represents an important intervention goal for schizophrenia patients. However, the Mayer-Salovey-Caruso Emotional Intelligence Test (MSCEIT) is the only existing assessment of social cognition included in the MATRICS Consensus (cognitive) Test Battery (see Chapter 6). Based on the models and conceptualization of emotional intelligence by Salovay, Mayer, and Caruso (Mayer, Salovey, & Caruso, 2000; Salovay & Mayer, 2000), TEI focuses on three domains: emotional perception, emotional understanding, and emotional management. Similar to EMT, TEI improves coping with negative emotions like depression, anxiety, anger, shame, and blame. Additionally, TEI tries to reestablish joy and pleasure (positive feelings) associated with individual interests to increase leisure time activities.

The following two approaches provide an example of possible interventions dealing with deficits in Theory of Mind (ToM): The Instrumental Enrichment Program (IEP) was originally developed for people with learning disabilities (Feuerstein, 1980) and was subsequently adapted for the treatment of schizophrenia patients with deficits in ToM (Rancone et al., 2004). The IEP is based on mediated learning, which means it is predicated on a metacognitive learning strategy focusing on the learning process rather than on the product of learning. The IEP addresses patients' erroneous beliefs and thinking strategies. Therapists work as mediators, their task being to lead discussions with the goal of supporting patients' capacity to mentally anticipate interpersonal actions. The IEP includes exercises that aim to improve the perception of emotions, social intelligence, and role-played social situations dealing with ToM issues. Social Cognition Enhancement Training (SCET) (Choi & Kwon, 2006) aims at improving the ToM functions of context appraisal and perspective-taking abilities. The major training materials used are four-column content cartoons. For each of the cartoons presented, the patients are encouraged to spot social cues, to arrange the four pictures based on contextual information, and to provide coherent explanations for the chosen arrangement of the social situation.

The following three approaches are examples of broad-based social cognitive remediation: Social Cognition and Interaction Training (SCIT) developed by Penn and Colleagues (Combs, Adams et al., 2007; Horan, Kern et al., 2009; Horan, Nuechterlein et al., 2009; Penn et al., 2005, 2007; Roberts et al., 2006) is directed toward several social cognitive functions and aims to transfer the improved social cognitive skills into patients' real lives. SCIT consists of three phases: (1) emotion perception linked to facial expression, (2) attribution bias and ToM in figured-out situations, and (3) integration and generalization of the learned social skills by applying them to realistic social situations. Recently, Penn and colleagues made an effort to evaluate the effectiveness and feasibility of SCIT in various settings. It was applied to schizophrenia inpatients (Penn et al., 2005), to schizophrenia outpatients (Roberts & Penn, 2009), and to forensic inpatients with psychotic disorders (Combs, Adams et al., 2007).

Metacognitive Skills Training (MCT) (Moritz & Woodward, 2007a, 2007b; Moritz et al., 2009) is a metacognitive remediation approach based on two components: knowledge translation and a demonstration of the negative consequences of cognitive biases. In a series of incremental steps, MCT treats the metacognitive bias underlying psychotic symptoms (e.g., attribution, jumping to conclusions, bias against disconfirmatory overconfidence in errors, ToM). The conceptualization of MCT lies somewhere between social cognitive remediation and cognitive behavior therapy (CBT) for psychotic symptoms. While CBT directly approaches target positive symptoms, MCT represents a sort of "back-door" approach, focusing on the thoughts underlying a psychosis. On the other hand, MCT is closely related to social cognitive remediation since it targets social cognitive domains like emotions and social perception as well as ToM and attribution style. The goal of MCT is to improve patients' thinking by minimizing cognitive errors.

Finally, Social Cognition Skills Training (SCST) from the UCLA research group of Michael Green (Horan, Kern et al., 2009) recently developed a social cognition intervention approach including tasks from SCID and TAR. SCST primarily targets emotion and social perception as well as social attribution and ToM. The training incorporates the following skill-building strategies widely used in other treatment approaches discussed above: breaking down social cognitive processes into their basic skill components, initially teaching and exercising skills at the most basic level and gradually increasing the complexity of skill acquisition, and, finally, automating these skills through repetition and practice (Horan, Kern et al., 2009).

Efficacy of Social Cognitive Remediation Therapy

The most detailed review on social cognitive remediation approaches available (Horan et al., 2008) showed that certain evaluation studies found evidence for proximal benefits in schizophrenia patients participating in specific and broad-based social cognitive interventions. However, to date, no meta-analysis quantitatively summarizing the outcome of the reviewed approaches to treat social cognitive deficits in schizophrenia patients has been published. Therefore, we only have a small amount of data indicating whether or not social cognitive remediation supports functional outcome. However, the preliminary results of a meta-analysis (Mueller, Roder, & Heuberger, 2009), including 21 randomized-controlled trials to evaluate social cognitive remediation and combined treatment approaches, shows some promising results: Over an average duration of 5.8 months a significant global therapy effect was demonstrated (average effect size of all calculated variables). The global therapy effect was maintained during a follow-up period of an average of 9.5 months. Superior effects of social cognitive remediation compared to controls were found in proximal as well as in distal outcome variables. Setting, control groups, and type of intervention were identified as moderators. This study provides strong evidence for social cognitive remediation and combined treatment (including social cognitive remediation) having a broad effect on various areas of functioning and symptoms relevant to schizophrenia.

2.4.3 Integrated Therapy Approaches

Some combined treatment approaches are available today. These approaches aim at enhancing neurocognitive and social cognitive functioning in schizophrenia patients. Furthermore, their cognitive remediation aspect has been expanded and in some approaches combined with other therapeutic and rehabilitative goals such as social functioning, work, and education. This integrates specific cognitive and noncognitive interventions and therapy goals into one broad-based treatment concept. Generally, these approaches are used in group-based settings, partially supplemented by individual sessions. The best-evaluated and most promising integrated cognitive therapy approaches are summarized in Table 2.5.

The Integrated Psychological Therapy Program (IPT) was the first systematically structured, comprehensive, and manualized integrated therapy approach for schizophrenia patients. It combines neurocognitive and social cognitive interventions with a social and interpersonal problem-solving skills approach.

The conceptualization of Cognitive Enhancement Therapy (CET) (Hogarty & Flesher, 1999a, 1999b; Hogarty et al., 2004, 2006) was influenced considerably by IPT. CET is a holistic, developmental approach that aims at the rehabilitation of social cognitive and neurocognitive deficits among patients with schizophrenia. The underlying model of CET postulates that impaired social cognition is a result of neurodevelopmental disturbances. Furthermore, it is postulated that a presumed neuroplasticity reserve can respond to enriched cognitive experiences. CET strives to achieve four major goals. First and foremost, it attempts to facilitate the attainment of social cognitive milestones that are appropriate for healthy adults. Among these milestones are the attainment of a "gistfulness" in social exchange, effortful and active processing of social content, cognitive flexibility, a tolerance for ambiguity and uncertainty, and personal comfort with abstraction. The second aim is to incite patients to display appropriate behavior

Table 2.5 Examples of Integrated Therapy approaches including cognitive remediation

Integrated therapy approach	Type of intervention addressing neuro-cognition	Intervention topic additional to neurocognition	Author
Integrated Psychological Therapy IPT*	Restitution and strategy learning, noncomputerized, group therapy	Social cognition and social competence	Brenner et al., 1994; Roder, Brenner, Kienzle, & Hodel, 1988
Cognitive Enhancement Therapy CET*	Restitution and strategy learning, computerized, group therapy	Social cognition	Hogarty, & Flesher, 1999a,b; Hogarty, Greenwald, & Eack, 2006; Hogarty et al., 2004
Neurocognitive Enhancement Therapy NET*	Restitution and strategy learning, computerized, group therapy	Social cognition and work rehabilitation	Bell, Bryson, Greig, Corcoran, & Wexler, 2001; Bell, Zito, Greig, & Wexler, 2008
Neuropsychological Educational Approach to Rehabilitation NEAR*	Restitution and strategy learning, computerized, group therapy	Educational approach addressing intrinsic motivation	Medalia & Freilich, 2008; Medalia & Richardson, 2005; Medalia, Revheim, & Casey, 2002; Medalia, Revheim, & Herlands, 2002
Integrated Neurocognitive Therapy INT	Restitution and strategy learning, partly computerized, group therapy	Social cognition (all MATRICS dimensions)	Mueller & Roder, 2010; Roder & Mueller, 2006

*State-of-the-art interventions, APA Training Grid 2007.

in social contexts, which requires proper appraisal of the context as well as the ability to take another person's perspective. The third goal is to create a personally relevant understanding of schizophrenia by providing patients with psychoeducation. Patients may be more inclined to actively participate in planning and maintaining a treatment strategy that is specifically designed to meet their own cognitive difficulties, strengths, and rehabilitative goals. Finally, CET also addresses patients' neuropsychological impairments, albeit in an interactive process rather than with formal didactic exercises. Neurocognitive deficits are addressed by administering computer-based training, using progressive exercises drawn from Ben-Yishay and colleagues' (1985) attention software and Bracy's (1995) memory and problem-solving software. Computer sessions are conducted in pairs of patients with the therapist's supervision. In addition, patients receive social cognitive group exercises, containing activities such as categorization exercises; formation of gistful, condensed messages; solving real-life social dilemmas; abstraction of themes from the editorial pages of *USA Today*; appraisal of affect and social contexts; initiating and maintaining conversations; writing plays; and the center stage exercises (e.g., introducing oneself or a friend) adapted from Ben-Yishay and colleagues' (1985) curriculum.

Neurocognitive Enhancement Therapy (NET) is a comprehensive approach to cognitive remediation developed by Bell and colleagues (Bell, Zito, Greig, & Wexler,

2008; Bell et al., 2001) with a particular focus on work rehabilitation. In the cognitive part, NET is closely related to CET. It is based on models of neuroplasticity highlighting the need for intense and repetitive practice in order to influence neurocognitive impairments. The program consists of three main components: computer-based cognitive training, a social information processing group, and a work feedback group. Cognitive exercises are based on a modified version of the multimedia CogReHab software, originally designed for individuals with traumatic brain injury and other neurological impairments (Bracy, 1995). Tasks are designed so that they are initially relatively simple in order to enable patients to accomplish them. The level of difficulty then gradually increases according to errorless learning principles. Patients are usually paid for doing cognitive exercises. The group session for social information processing takes place weekly and resembles an exercise from the traumatic brain injury program (Ben-Yishay et al., 1985): One patient prepares an oral presentation with the assistance of a staff member and then introduces it to the group. Group members are required to ask questions and provide specific feedback. The third component addresses work feedback, which includes ratings of job-related attention, memory, and executive function, and is provided biweekly, by using the Cognitive Functional Assessment Scale. Based on these feedbacks, patients are also encouraged to develop new goals.

The comprehensive, evidence-based, manualized Neuropsychological Educational Approach to Cognitive Remediation (NEAR) (Medalia & Freilich, 2008; Medalia, Revheim, & Herlands, 2002) constitutes a synthesis of knowledge derived from educational psychology, behavior and learning theories, rehabilitation psychology, and neuropsychology. NEAR postulates that cognitive remediation is in its essence a learning activity in which educational principles, promoting intrinsic motivation and task engagement, are taken into account. Patients are encouraged to reflect on their personal learning styles, since many of them have encountered repeated failure in learning situations during adolescence because of their cognitive and social deficits. In order to promote a positive learning experience that elicits intrinsic motivation to learn and use their cognitive skills, the NEAR exercises are designed to be highly engaging, enjoyable, and rewarding. Tasks are, therefore, presented in a contextualized, personalized, multisensory manner that also allows the learner to exert a certain level of control over nonessential aspects (Medalia, Revheim, & Casey, 2002). Independence, self-efficacy, and persistence toward learning tasks are fostered. Unlike other cognitive remediation approaches, NEAR generally favors a top-down approach to remediation where tasks incorporate several skills simultaneously (Medalia & Richardson, 2005). Training is usually conducted with a group of 6 to 10 patients who each work at their own pace on tasks chosen to address their particular needs. Usually, patients perform computer-based cognitive tasks in 2 of 3 sessions and then in a third session attend a group meeting where social skills are practiced and the real-world relevance of the individually performed exercises is discussed. Tasks are taken from commercially available educational software packages that not only address various neuropsychological functions, but are also designed to be engaging, enjoyable, and intrinsically motivating.

Integrated Neurocognitive Therapy (INT) (Mueller & Roder, 2010; Roder & Mueller, 2006) is an advancement of the cognitive part of IPT. As a proximal goal, INT intends to restitute and compensate neurocognitive and social cognitive (dys)functions by systematically targeting all 11 dimensions defined by the MATRICS initiative. These domains are subsumed into four modules. INT is a resource-oriented intervention that considers the functional impact of cognitive functioning on patients' daily life. A task in each targeted cognitive function associated with patients' own experience aims at increasing participants' insight into their individual cognitive resources and deficits – and at supporting intrinsic motivation. Following the IPT technology, INT systematically supports group processes and dynamics, partially in PC-based exercises. In a large, ongoing multisite evaluation study, the restitution part of neurocognitive enhancement used the CogPack computer-software program (Olbrich, 1996) distributed by Marker Software. A more detailed description of the INT procedure is given in Chapter 8.

Efficacy of Integrated Therapy Approaches

With the exception of the newly developed INT, which is currently being evaluated in a study, the other integrated therapy approaches represent interventions with a broad empirical basis. The results are encouraging inasmuch as improvements were found not only in proximal cognitive performance, but also in the more distal areas of psychosocial functioning and psychopathology. IPT, CET, NET, and NEAR are all included in the *Catalog of Clinical Training Opportunities: Best Practice for Recovery and Improved Outcomes for People with Serious Mental Illness* published by the American Psychological Association (APA/CAPP) Task Force on Serious Mental Illness and Severe Emotional Disturbance (see Table 2.5). Evaluation studies of high quality addressing these approaches were also largely included in the discussed meta-analyses on neurocognitive and social cognitive remediation (McGurk, Twamley et al., 2007; Mueller et al., 2009; Pfammatter et al., 2006). Integration in adjunctive rehabilitation programs appears to have an advantage over programs that include only cognitive remediation (McGurk, Twamley et al., 2007). Furthermore, strong empirical evidence of integrated therapy came from IPT research: An analysis of IPT intervention indicated that the intervention combining neurocognition and social cognition had superior effects in proximal and distal outcomes compared to neurocognitive intervention alone (Mueller & Roder, 2008). Only a treatment with IPT including all subprograms had long-lasting and progressively increasing effects after therapy. The use of single subprograms did not show these effects (Roder, Mueller, Mueser et al., 2006). The improvement of functional outcome is a key goal of recovery, and it is often defined as the ultimate goal of any therapeutic treatment (Mueller & Roder, 2007; Spaulding & Nolting, 2006) as well as of cognitive remediation. Integrated therapy seems to be a powerful and promising method to reach this goal within a multimodal rehabilitation process.

Part B
IPT: Indication, Therapy, Assessment, and Evaluation

3 Conditions for Carrying Out the Therapy Program: Implementation and Indication

3.1 Institutional Conditions

This chapter deals with the various ways of implementing the therapy program in institutions, for example, in a psychiatric clinic.

Inpatient Services

Across Wards

Patients from different wards normally meet twice a week in a specified room of the hospital for therapy sessions. Good coordination between the team treating the patients on the ward and the (external) therapists carrying out the therapy program has proven to be extremely important. This is, of course, time consuming for the therapist, and it requires considerable cooperation on the part of the ward teams. Within the therapy group, there is not much room to discuss matters of group dynamics, for instance, how the behavior of patient A affects patient B and vice versa. This is why such matters should remain the task of the ward team. If the therapists do not belong to the ward team, it can be difficult to support patients' behavior modifications during therapy outside the sessions, in the sense of generalizing them. For example, the therapists do not have the opportunity to observe, and thus to reinforce and encourage, a patient's improved alertness and concentration in real-life situations in the ward. The same is true for other areas, such as social behavior.

Additional difficulty in carrying out the therapy program across wards concerns the patients' motivation for taking part in the therapy as well as the group's cohesion. A possible consequence would be that patients do not regularly attend the sessions. Furthermore, mutual trust between the group members may take longer to develop and will need to be built up by the therapist very slowly.

Within a Ward

For the reasons mentioned above, it has proven to be more advantageous to integrate the therapy program into the overall concept of a ward. The therapists are then part of the ward team, and the team of therapists can carry out therapy planning centrally. Consistency of staff and time is an absolute prerequisite for the successful rehabilitation of schizophrenia patients; the therapy program becomes an integral part of a broad ward concept.

In a Specialized Ward

The ideal arrangement is a ward of about 10 to 15 beds, specialized for schizophrenia patients. In such a ward, a multimodal concept of treatment, based on the present state of schizophrenia research, should be applied (Roder & Kienzle, 1986). Both the therapists and the patients should participate in planning the therapy, based on a broad behavior and problem assessment. Thus, one theme guides all of the therapy, with all participants heading in the same therapeutic direction. In addition to social therapy, occupational therapy, movement therapy, and family management, the therapy program itself forms the principal part of the work in the ward. Each patient has his or her own individual program, in which demands are successively increased until he/she is able, for example, to live in a more or less protected external living community. The ward should be organized according to the principles of learning theory and behavior therapy, characterized by a clearly defined therapeutic concept.

Most therapeutic activities, such as the therapy program, cooking and cleaning groups, and movement therapy, are carried out in small groups of 4 to 5 patients. This, on the one hand, counteracts the patients' typical tendency toward withdrawal behavior (caution: overstimulation). On the other hand, small groups promote strong relationships, for example, by allowing patients to live together outside the hospital in an apartment house. Observations made during therapy sessions can also be compared to behavior in everyday situations on the ward. This often results in important implications for further therapy planning. Under these circumstances, it is also easier to approach particular deficits of individual patients (e.g., social behavior) in individual sessions or within the scope of ward life.

Outpatient Services / Day Care

The therapy program has also proved advantageous with daycare patients and outpatients. Previous experience shows that such therapy groups tend to concentrate on the final two subprograms (Social Skills and Interpersonal Problem Solving). Additionally, exercises from the first three subprograms (Cognitive Differentiation, Social Perception, Verbal Communication) can be included. These patients' cognitive level of functioning is not so low that cognitive skills would need to be learned before beginning with the problem-solving and social-skills training. Furthermore, outpatients are usually so intensely concerned with their everyday problems (e.g., partner and work problems) that they first need to deal therapeutically with these problems. To this end, it is practical to use the "instruments" offered by the more advanced subprograms of IPT.

Mixed Group Settings with In- and Outpatients

The IPT program has also been conducted in groups with in- and outpatients. This is a challenging intervention for experienced and well-trained therapists, since they have to find a balance between different demands (e.g., needs and abilities) in heterogeneous groups. Against the background of systematic support of group processes and dynamics, inpatients may benefit from the skills of outpatients. Outpatients have already learned how to cope with negative experiences they had during an acute phase in the hospital. One outpatient participating in a mixed group summarized these aspects as follows: "First, it was really hard to come back to the hospital to participate in the group. But then I realized that I could improve my (cognitive) skills by training. And most important: It was the first time I had the feeling that I really had overcome my negative experiences concerning the acute phase in the hospital."

3.2 Patients

A wide variety of different groups of patients have provided their experiences with the Integrated Psychological Therapy program. The groups ranged from severely chronic and long-term hospitalized patients to postacute patients in the initial remission phase (see Chapter 7). These experiences suggest differentiating between medium-chronic and severely chronic patients. A criterion of chronicity is present if the illness has lasted for more than 1 year without remission. To differentiate between medium and severe chronicity, one possible criterion is whether the illness has existed for more than 5 years. According to results from various longitudinal studies, changes for the better often occur after about 5 years.

Severely Chronic Schizophrenia Patients

A patient who has been hospitalized for more than 7 years is considered severely chronic. The greatest difficulty in working therapeutically with severely chronic patients lies in their initial lack of motivation. Severely chronic patients are often afraid of any change in their habitual rhythm of life, especially when it comes to participating in regular group activities. If patients have been hospitalized for such a long period of time, their behavior and thinking usually also change in ways that are difficult to modify. A motivation phase in a dyadic setting (therapist – patient) prior to the beginning of the therapy group seems to be necessary as well as advantageous. During this phase, the therapist can identify things the patient is interested in (usually very few) and, thus, try to establish compliance. After creating a stable relationship, which can take weeks or even months, it is usually possible to convince the patient to participate in a therapy group. In the beginning, the term "therapy" should be avoided, and expressions like "practice group" or "discussion group" should be used instead. Again it can take months of individual sessions to convince the patient of the usefulness and importance of the therapy group. Moreover, once the group sessions have begun, it is important to start off at a slow pace, with two weekly sessions of 30 minutes each, for instance. During this first period of group sessions, the patients need to have a lot of positive experiences during the sessions (positive feedback) in order to build up group cohesion and trust.

The therapists need to have great patience, since it can take a long time for the patient to attain a greater measure of independence or even to become capable of moving into an external community. Accordingly, with severely chronic patients, the different subprograms will also take longer (see Chapter 4). Well-known exercises need to be repeated continually in order to maintain the therapeutic effects over a longer period of time. The patients' fear and insecurity toward new exercises can be overcome by the recurrent repetition of well-known exercises. Finally, the duration of the sessions is increased to 60 minutes each (later perhaps to 90 minutes each). Such groups make very great demands on the therapists in terms of perseverance, frustration tolerance (relapses), and the ability to provide continuous and intense care as well as warmth. Normally treatment duration is 1 to 2 years.

Medium-Chronic Schizophrenia Patients

The comments above are also valid for medium-chronic schizophrenia patients (overall hospitalization of 1 to 6 years), although to a somewhat lesser degree. For example, it depends considerably on the patient's level of hospitalism whether and to what extent a motivation phase is necessary before commencing therapy sessions. In many cases, the psychological-psychiatric examination carried out in order to determine indication and group makeup (see Chapter 6) is sufficient to establish contact with the therapist and provide the necessary motivation and compliance. This intimate interview and assessment is often less stressful and upsetting than an unstructured conversation.

The duration of therapy is anywhere between 6 months and 1 year. Usually, sessions are held twice a week for 60 minutes each. The subprograms can be carried out more rapidly than with severely chronic schizophrenia patients; in particular, the continuous repetitions of earlier exercises are not necessary.

Postacute Schizophrenia Patients

Compared to the severely or medium-chronic schizophrenia patients, a group of post-acute schizophrenia patients need a therapy that is considerably shorter. As soon as the acute episode has abated, the patients can be admitted to a therapy group. Since patients with acute episodes are usually hospitalized for about 4 to 6 weeks, there are normally only 2 to 4 weeks left for the patient to participate in the inpatient therapy program after remission. This is, of course, not enough time to carry out the entire program.

Instead, the therapists need to make choices based on the deficits present. Generally speaking, a combination of perceptive/cognitive exercises with exercises on problem solving has proven to be of value. The therapy sessions are held 2 to 4 times a week for 60 to 90 minutes each. Special attention should be paid to stimulating the patients optimally. Particularly right after an acute episode, patients typically experience exacerbations from emotional overstimulation. After releasing the patients from the clinic, one can best help them with an IPT outpatient therapy group (see section 5.1 above).

3.3 Group Makeup

Groups of 4 to 8 patients have proven optimal, except with very "difficult" patients, where smaller groups are more convenient. Particular attention should be paid when putting together groups of medium and severely chronic patients: Groups should be roughly homogeneous with respect to intelligence as well as deficits in information processing. A heterogeneous group constellation is also advantageous with respect to age (between 20 and 50) and sex. The group members' IQ should range between 80 and 110. The first parts of the therapy program (Cognitive Differentiation, Social Perception, and, in part, Verbal Communication) are less suitable for patients with above-average intelligence: Because the exercises are kept quite "simple" in these sections, more intelligent patients do not see their purpose or importance. The Social Skills and Interpersonal Problem-Solving subprograms, however, can be employed very well with intelligent patients as well. On the other hand, patients with an IQ that lies considerably below average are often quickly overtaxed by these subprograms.

Only patients with the primary diagnosis of "schizophrenia" should be included in the therapy group. Patients with brain-organic diseases, severe psychogenic disorders, etc., should not be included. Taken individually, some of the exercises may be appropriate for nonschizophrenia patients as well (e.g., Cognitive Differentiation for brain-damaged patients) and can be applied for them. But the order and content of the subprograms as well as the behavior of the therapists have been conceived of esspecially for schizophrenia patients and are based on the results of empiric schizophrenia research.

Patients with an insufficient mastery of the English language should not take part in such a group, because of the linguistic nature of many of the exercises. In the past, it has proven difficult to keep patients in the group who have difficulties properly understanding and communicating in English. Positive symptoms should not play too prominent a role; the therapy program shows the best results in patients with negative symptoms.

3.4 Therapists

Finally, a few comments on the qualification of the therapists and the demands put upon them. The therapists should have detailed knowledge of two fields: On the one hand, they need to be very familiar with the structured therapy methods of the five subprograms; on the other hand, they need to have a profound knowledge of group processes and group dynamics.

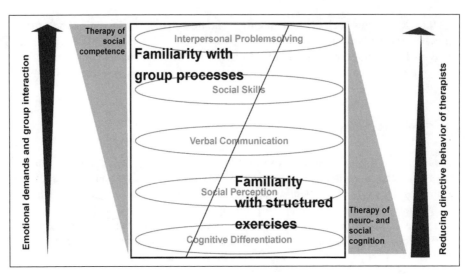

Figure 3.1: IPT: Training of therapists

This book gives many suggestions of therapy methods. Their implementation, however, without further practical training is not recommended. The nature of group processes is addressed only briefly in this volume and cannot be applied without further training.

As shown in Figure 3.1, the therapists' knowledge about the structured therapy methods is of crucial importance with the first subprograms (Cognitive Differentiation, Social Perception and, in part, Verbal Communication). Initial knowledge of group dynamics and group processes is less emphasized here. During the later subprograms (in part Verbal Communication, Social Skills, Interpersonal Problem Solving), these relations are inverted, and the directive therapeutic behavior simultaneously decreases.

It is important to point out that even in the last subprogram the structured therapeutic approach, which is so important for schizophrenia patients, still plays a very decisive role in the group therapy.

3.5 Differential Indication for Carrying Out IPT

Experience in working with IPT and various studies (Hodel & Brenner, 1988; Roder, 1988) have demonstrated that cognitive intervention does not necessarily have to precede social and problem-solving skills training (The Modified Pervasiveness Theory [see Brenner, 1987; Brenner, Böker, Hodel, & Wyss, 1989] as briefly outlined at the beginning of this chapter). In other words, the five IPT subprograms do not necessarily have to be implemented sequentially. Rather, the sequence of administration should be determined by the information derived from the assessments discussed in Chapter 6. The assessment devices specifically designed for this purpose (Roder, Zorn et al., 2008, see Chapter 6.3), are of particular importance here.

Cognitive interventions are particularly useful with patients who manifest at least

Table 3.1 Indications of IPT – overview

1) **Cognitive Therapy**
   Cognitive Differentiation
   Social Perception
   Verbal Communication (Part I)
   – Severe cognitive deficits
   – Intense social fears
   – Negative symptoms
   – Little motivation for engaging in therapy
   – Long-term duration of illness
2) **Social Competence Therapy**
   Verbal Communication (Part II)
   Social Skills
   Interpersonal Problem Solving
   – Inability to cope with social situations appropriately
   – Relatively young age
   – Motivated for therapy
   – Revolving door patients

one of the following criteria: severe cognitive deficits, intense social fears, negative symptoms, little motivation for therapy, or long-term duration of illness. The high organizational structure and the minor emotional loading of the initial activities enable proper development of a therapeutic atmosphere and allow the patients to engage in social interactions (see Table 3.1).

Patients who do not suffer from severe cognitive impairment are advised to skip the first part of the program and begin directly with the second part of the IPT program. These patients typically show the following characteristics: They are unable to cope with social situations appropriately; they are relatively young; they are motivated for therapy; and they have had several (shorter) periods of inpatient treatment ("revolving-door patient"). This group of patients often lives or works outside the confines of the hospital and primarily has difficulty dealing with the demands of daily life in the community (i.e., problems at work or at home, or questions pertaining to homecare). That is why their treatment should focus on building and enhancing their social and independent living skills. In addition, various activities that are normally executed during the cognitive interventions can also be conducted in the second part of the program. Of course, patients who master the first part of the program may proceed to the second part.

4 The Therapy Program and Its Five Subprograms: An Overview

4.1 General Structure and Integration into a Multimodal Treatment Concept

The theoretical framework and the empirical data discussed in the previous chapters provide a compelling case that a multimodal approach to treating people with schizophrenia can be effective not only for managing symptoms, but also for improving personal and social functioning ("recovery perspective"). The functional outcomes produced by such an approach are essential to the values and goals of recovery. A comprehensive treatment program must make use of multiple therapeutic modalities, both pharmacological and psychosocial. This requires an interdisciplinary team of practitioners with the relevant knowledge and skills – of which the recovering person is also a key member, systematically pursuing an integrated treatment, rehabilitation, and recovery plan. The plan must be individually tailored to the patient's needs, preferences, and recovery goals.

The conception of IPT originally took into account the findings from the 1970s and 1980s in the fields of psychology and psychiatry. Particular emphasis was placed on experimental psychological and psychopathological research. Since the publication of the first German language IPT manual more than 20 years ago (Roder, Brenner et al., 1988), developments have continued, informed by new research on schizophrenia, clinical experience, feedback from patients and therapists, and worldwide outcome studies (Müller & Roder, 2010; Roder, Mueller, Mueser et al., 2006). As IPT evolved it kept up with increasing demands for multimodal treatment and rehabilitation, functional outcomes, and a recovery orientation. Today's IPT is designed to be a core component of modern comprehensive psychiatric rehabilitation.

IPT consists of five subprograms, aiming for the treatment of neurocognitive and social cognitive disturbances typical of schizophrenia and for specific deficiencies in overall social functioning. IPT was initially designed long before social cognitions were broadly accepted as important subjects of intervention in the mid-1990s. The development of standardized cognitive assessment batteries, the MATRICS initiative, occurred even later, in 2004 and 2005. Readers familiar with earlier IPT editions will note an evolution in the concepts, terminology, and technology, especially in the cognitive domain. This parallels the broader evolution of cognitive science and psychopa-

Table 4.1 The 5 subprograms of IPT

- Cognitive Differentiation
- Social Perception
- Verbal Communication
- Social Skills
- Interpersonal Problem Solving

thology described in Chapter 1 of this edition. These developments generally reflect an expansion, more than a revision, of IPT's original theoretical framework. The importance of a biosystemic vulnerability-stress view of schizophrenia and the need for a treatment that addresses multiple levels of organismic functioning are even more empirically supported today than they were when IPT was first designed.

As discussed in Chapter 2, this theoretical framework has also had an impact on other therapeutic approaches. The five subprograms of IPT are (see Table 4.1): The first subprogram (Cognitive Differentiation) primarily targets basic impairments in neurocognition (e.g., attention, verbal memory, cognitive flexibility, concept formation). The second subprogram (Social Perception) addresses deficits in social cognition (e.g., social and emotional perception). The fourth and fifth subprograms (Social Skills, Interpersonal Problem Solving) focus on developing patients' social competence through practice of interpersonal skills (e.g., role-plays) and group-based problem-solving exercises. The third subprogram (Verbal Communication) serves as a bridge between the first two and last two subprograms by focusing on neurocognitive skills, which have a direct impact on interpersonal communication, such as verbal fluency and executive functioning. The goal of each individual subprogram depends on the respective patient's deficits and strengths as well as the functional outcomes representing the main focus of treatment.

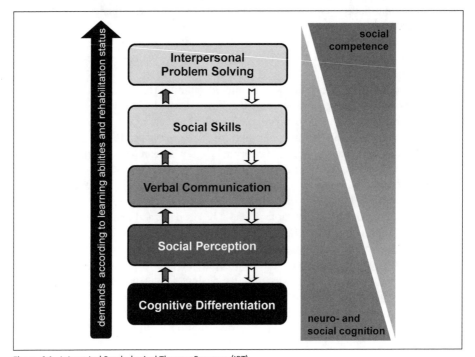

Figure 4.1: Integrated Psychological Therapy Program (IPT)

IPT is based on the assumption that basic deficits in neurocognitive functioning have a pervasive effect on higher levels of behavioral organization, including social skills as well as social and independent functioning (see the concept of pervasiveness and the integrative model in Chapter 1). Hence, basic neurocognitive and social cognitive functions need to be developed *before* more complex interactional modes of behavior can be fostered. Successful psychosocial rehabilitation requires remediation of both the underlying neurocognitive impairments and related social cognitive deficits as well as building social, self-care, and vocational skills. IPT strives to integrate cognitive and psychosocial rehabilitation in a systematic way with the goal of improving social competence in order to cope with life successfully (see Figure 4.1).

Each subprogram is designed to gradually increase demands on the individual and the group over the course of therapy. Group participants steadily progress from simple and obvious tasks to more difficult and complex ones. In the course of the program, these demands increase both within the tasks and in the overall therapy framework. The activities are initially very structured and task-oriented, progressively changing to more open group interaction. At the beginning, the therapeutic method is very directive and becomes less so toward the end, placing increasing emphasis on participants' own initiative and responsibility (see Chapter 5). It is important to advance slowly through small and clearly defined steps and to spend an adequate amount of time on each learning task. This avoids putting the group under too much pressure, which would be counterproductive.

Developing the ability to manage emotion and affect is assigned a particularly important role in each subprogram. People suffering from schizophrenia often experience increased impairment when under emotional stress. The initial exercises in each subprogram are, therefore, designed to be affectively neutral. As therapy progresses, more emotionally evocative material is gradually introduced. In the later stages of therapy, a greater emphasis is placed on coping with emotional stress.

In summary, three basic rules guide progress through the subprograms:
- Start with easy tasks and proceed to more complex and difficult tasks later on.
- Start with a high level of structure and reduce it in the course of therapy.
- Avoid emotional, stress-provocative material and interventions at the beginning of each exercise.

Generalization and Transfer of Therapy

Generalization (performance of new skills in different settings) and transfer of therapy (application of new skills to different problems) is a central concern in all forms of psychosocial treatment, including IPT. Outcome studies of earlier versions of IPT provide evidence that under IPT treatment effects are generalized and transfer of training occurs (see Chapter 7). It is important for the therapist to explicitly enhance and encourage these processes. As IPT evolved, activities specifically designed to do this were added. In each of the five IPT subprograms, especially in the subprograms addressing social skills and social competence, the patients' experiences and needs in everyday life need to be taken into consideration during therapy in order to support the transfer of the outcome into practice. Questions like "Do you see this problem in your everyday life?" or "Have any of you ever used this coping strategy in daily life?" are key components in the repertoire of an IPT therapist.

4.2 Cognitive Differentiation

Structure

The Cognitive Differentiation subprogram aims primarily to improve neurocognitive functioning by means of a variety of exercises. The exercises are organized into three steps.

> **Step 1:** Card-Sorting Exercises
> **Step 2:** Verbal Concept Exercises
>   – Conceptual Hierarchies Exercise
>   – Synonyms Exercise
>   – Antonyms Exercise
>   – Word Definitions Exercise
>   – Word Clue Exercise
>   – Context-Dependent Words Exercise
> **Step 3:** Search Strategies Exercise

The group normally progresses from Step 1 to Step 3 in the sequence described above. Step 1 is a good way of initially approaching severely chronic schizophrenia patients. Since the group members do not have to communicate very much with each other while doing the card-sorting exercise, they do not have to relate to people unfamiliar to them, which for some is quite difficult in itself.

Step 1: Card-Sorting Exercises*

Each group member gets a certain number of cards, which are printed with designs that differ in shape, number, days of the week, and color. Each participant is asked to pick out a particular kind of card, for example, all red cards with a two-digit number, from his/her pile and lay them out separately. Each participant's neighbor then checks to see if the exercise has been done correctly.

---

* The cards can be ordered from the first author.

Step 2: Verbal Concept Exercises

There are different exercises for conceptual hierarchies, synonyms, antonyms, word definitions, and context-dependent words, which can be carried out with word cards according to context and exercise:

– *Conceptual Hierarchies Exercise:* Participants are shown a word or phrase (e.g., cooking) and asked to name related words as they come to mind. Later all the words mentioned are organized into hypernyms and hyponyms (e.g., "cooking" is a hypernym of "roasting," and a hyponym of "housework").
– *Synonyms Exercise:* Group members name words with the same meaning as a particular word (e.g., work). They then make up sentences using these words and decide whether there are any differences in meaning or whether they mean the same.
– *Antonyms Exercise:* The procedure is analogous to the synonyms exercise, only with antonyms.
– *Word Definitions Exercise:* The group members are asked to explain a word (e.g., door) to the cotherapist. They try to determine important aspects that enable them to describe the word (example: What is it made of? Where is it? What is it used for?).
– *Word Clue Exercise:* Group member A is handed a card with two words printed on it, one of which is underlined (example: ballpoint pen – *fountain pen*), and requested to read both words aloud without revealing which one is underlined. Then he/she is asked to think of a word that enables the other group members to identify the underlined word (example: fountain).
– *Context-Dependent Words Exercise:* The group members explain and discuss the different meanings of a word (e.g., bulb: tulip bulb – light bulb).

Step 3: Search Strategies Exercise

Group member A and the cotherapist team up and choose an object in the room. The name of the object is written down for future reference, but this information is not shared with the other group members. The group's task is to determine which object the team was thinking of through a series of questions that can be answered only by "yes" or "no." The group members practice asking questions, gradually proceeding from very concrete questions to more conceptual ones. Their use of conceptual questions is encouraged. The initial focus on the immediate geographical surroundings from which objects can be chosen is progressively enlarged (e.g., ward, hospital grounds, city).

A detailed description of each exercise is presented in Chapter 5. The material used for therapy can be found in the Appendix (Worksheets 1–3).

It is important to note that that the initial exercises consist of material low in emotional loading. The reasons for this are discussed in Sections 4.1 and 5.1. Once the group masters a particular exercise with factually oriented material, more emotionally loaded material is introduced.

A combination of the card-sorting exercises and the search strategies exercise can be carried out with "high-functioning patients": Each of the IPT patients receives six cards, which are laid out so that every group member can see each of them. The co-therapist or a group member then memorizes one of the cards (six cards × number of group members) and writes down a short card description on a piece of paper (help in orientation and proof for the others). The other participants' task is to find out by asking specific "yes" or "no" questions which card has been selected. Of course, the contents of the questions represent the card categories (e.g., "Does the card contain the color blue?" – "Does the number have two digits?"). In a second step the group's task is to develop strategies for reducing the number of questions needed to find the solution. This task involves basic neurocognitive functions (attention, verbal, visual, and spatial memory), higher executive functions (problem solving) as well as social cognition within the group context.

Objectives

The main objective of the Cognitive Differentiation subprogram is to strengthen the neurocognitive factors that support more integrated social functioning. This also establishes a foundation for the more advanced subprograms that incorporate increasingly complex cognitive and behavioral abilities.

The Cognitive Differentiation subprogram utilizes a variety of principles derived from the psychotherapy, learning, neuropsychology, and psychopathology literature, including the principles of errorless learning (e.g., Kern et al., 2002). The main focus, however, is on using the dynamic interpersonal processes of the group to enhance engagement in the exercises. Ideally, participants whose cognitive functioning is relatively more intact share their resources with those experiencing greater difficulties. This creates opportunities for observational and imitative learning, diffuses performance demands, reduces stress, and strengthens participants' interpersonal orientation. Because of the heterogeneous nature of neurocognitive impairments in schizophrenia, the participants who have the most difficulty tend to show divergent performances in different exercises, although most patients do have some difficulty across the domains of attention, concentration, discrimination of relevant from irrelevant information, abstraction, concept formation, and conceptual search strategies. It is important for the therapist to evaluate individual strengths and weakness as the group proceeds through the exercises, facilitating interactions between participants as opportunity permits.

Similarly, the group process exercises the cognitive abilities involved in apprehending and processing other people's perspectives and intentions (discussed in Chapter 1 as theory of mind and related abilities). This is a recurrent theme throughout IPT, and its importance in interpersonal functioning becomes more obvious in later subprograms. At the neurocognitive level, such abilities are founded on an appreciation that even basic processes such as concept formation can produce different results in different people. The key therapeutic strategy for developing this appreciation is for the therapist to help the group work toward a consensus on the outcome of the exercises, and if consensus cannot be reached, to demonstrate that one can at least understand other people's perspectives even without agreeing with them.

4.3 Social Perception

Structure

The Social Perception subprogram is designed to improve the apprehension and interpretation of social situations. The subprogram involves a series of slides* depicting social situations (descriptions on Worksheets 4–7). Some of the slides also involve facial expressions or gestures (nonverbal communication). The slides, ordered according to their level of difficulty, vary in visual complexity (number of presented stimuli) and emotional loading. At the beginning of therapy, slides rated with a low degree of complexity and emotional loading are used, and the level of difficulty gradually increases as group members improve in the task. The group progresses through the slides, performing three steps on each as described below.

> **Step 1:** Gathering Information
> **Step 2:** Interpretation and Discussion
> **Step 3:** Assigning a Title

Step 1: Gathering Information

The group members are asked to describe a slide as accurately and in as much detail as possible. Describing a picture in such detail makes the patients learn to attend to the entire picture and prevents them from ignoring relevant details.

At this stage the slide should not be interpreted. Following this carefully structured procedure, in which the number of stimuli is gradually increased, reduces the risk of participants overreacting or getting upset. Gathering information and learning how to accurately describe situations is a fundamental and important objective in this subprogram, building the basis for further progress. For the interpretation and discussion of the slides, group members use the visual information gathered as arguments for their respective interpretations of the social situations as well as the suggested emotions. During this phase of training the focus should be on two main questions:
– "What can you see in the picture?"
– "Can you describe it to me in greater detail?"

Step 2: Interpretation and Discussion

Group members are asked to state their views on possible interpretations of the situation depicted on the slide. As described above, every opinion needs justification by reference to the actual visual information gathered in the first step. All group members engage in thoughtful reflection and consideration, and then discuss the different possi-

---

*   The slides are available on CD-ROM and can be ordered from the first author.

ble interpretations. They learn how to judge the correctness and the likeliness of each interpretation. By comparing and substantiating various interpretations, the participants learn to resolve cognitive dissonance rather than just adopting group consensus. In addition, they learn to decode facial affects and emotional gestures – and they learn to understand how and why a social situation can be interpreted in various ways. Thus, the ultimate goal of this phase of the training is to help the participants to understand their own and others' interpretations of social situations. In this phase the group mainly focuses on the following three questions:
– "What is the meaning of this picture?"
– "How can you justify your interpretation?"
– "What do the other group members think of this interpretation?"

Step 3: Assigning a Title

After gathering information and interpreting the pictures, the therapist asks the group members to choose a title for the picture. The title should be short and meaningful, reflecting the most important aspects of the social situation depicted on the slide (summarizing contents of the slide). The appropriateness of the suggested title enables the therapist to verify whether the key aspects of a situation have indeed been properly perceived and understood. If a group member has not succeeded in generating an appropriate interpretation, the process should be repeated.

With higher-functioning participants, a fourth step ("reframing") can be added. Once a title has been accepted by the group, the therapist says, "Now let's take a fresh look at this picture. Usually when we observe situations like this, it's possible to give them different interpretations. The title we gave to this picture shows one interpretation. Let's see if we can make up a completely different title by changing some of our interpretations." The therapist then gives an example of a key feature of the physical stimulus that allows a different interpretation. In the less complex pictures, this might be interpretation of a facial expression (e.g., "it could be surprise – or it could be a reaction to a joke"), gesture (e.g., "he could be pointing something out – or counting"), or situation ("she could be getting ready for bed – or to go out"). In the more complex pictures, this might be an interpretation of roles or relationships ("it could be his brother – or it could be a friend") or entire situations ("it could be an outdoor concert – or a picnic"). The therapist then describes how a different title, reflecting a different story about the picture, can be composed without contradicting the physical features of the picture. The participants are then engaged in a discussion of how other interpretive changes could create different stories and titles. As with the title step, the therapist constantly encourages the participants to understand each other's perceptions and to note how a single picture can be interpreted differently by different people – or by just one person changing his or her interpretations. The therapist must be prepared to provide much help and direction with this task, as many people (not just people with mental illness) find it extremely difficult to change their initial interpretations. This difficulty is best addressed by helping the person identify specific physical features suggesting simple interpretations (e.g., "there are two people here, and they could either be brothers or friends"), writing them on the blackboard if necessary and changing the initial story and title incrementally with each new interpretation.

Objectives

The ultimate objective of the Social Perception subprogram is to improve participants' ability to apprehend and understand social situations. This is accomplished by strengthening specific components of that ability, including accurate visual perception, correct interpretation of emotional cues and nonverbal communication, application of appropriate schemata and scripts, and logical but flexible interpretation. Specific problems that interrupt that ability are identified and corrected, including incomplete or fragmented visual processing, perceptual biases, and rigid or perseverative use of stereotypic schemata. As the subprogram progresses, participants' ability to process complexity and emotional loading is increasingly challenged, gradually approximating the levels of real-world situations. This also challenges the participants' stamina. Although the exercise is intrinsically interesting and motivating for most people, it requires a degree of information processing and interpersonal interaction that some quickly find exhausting. The therapist should be alert to this dimension of the group dynamics.

4.4 Verbal Communication

Structure

From the theoretical considerations on language and thought disorder in schizophrenia it follows that the Verbal Communication subprogram needs to focus on three basic communication skills:
- *Listening:* respecting and attending to other people's contributions to a conversation.
- *Understanding:* correctly perceiving and interpreting the content of the transmitted information.
- *Responding:* formulating and sending an appropriate response.

The group members practice these basic skills in five consecutive steps (Worksheets 8–10):

Step 1:	Literal Repetition Exercise
Step 2:	Paraphrasing Exercise
Step 3:	W-Questions
Step 4:	Asking Questions About a Topic
Step 5:	Focused Communication Exercise

The group progressively works through these five steps. The tasks assigned gradually become more difficult, as demands increase in the course of therapy. For the initial phases, the therapy material is highly structured and task-oriented, becoming less so as the therapy progresses. The purpose of this incremental procedure is to help participants to acquire more differentiated communication skills, which can eventually be applied to real-life interaction. The steps proceed as follows:

Step 1: Literal Repetition Exercise

A group member is handed a card with a sentence printed on it and is asked to read it to the group aloud. Another member of the group repeats this sentence literally. All group members check if the exercise is being done correctly.

Step 2: Paraphrasing Exercise

This exercise resembles Step 1, the sole difference being that on each card only one or two words are presented. One group member is handed a card and asked to make up his or her own sentence with the word (or words). The other group members are then asked to reproduce this sentence in their own words, while retaining its meaning.

Step 3: W-Questions Exercise

The group or the therapist introduces a topic of discussion (e.g., ward, hobby) and writes it down on the blackboard. The group compiles a list of words related to that topic. These words are written down on cards, analogous to Step 2. Each group member is asked to choose one of the word cards as well as a question word starting with "w" (where, when, who, why, etc.), to combine them in a question, and to pose this question to another group member. The group then monitors whether the question is related to the discussion topic and whether the answer refers to the question asked.

Step 4: Asking Questions About a Topic

The group poses questions about a certain topic to one or two members (e.g., newspaper article). Group members are again asked to monitor the process of communication, based on the observation criteria used in Step 3. Additionally, aspects from Step 5, which are central to evaluating the communication, may already be used.

Step 5: Focused Communication Exercise

Once more, the group is provided with a topic of discussion. The topic can be adopted from newspaper articles, short stories, proverbs or figures of speech, slides, or other topics of interest for the group members. The most important aspect of this activity is the evaluation of communication skills. Group members act as observers, and the therapist or the cotherapist serve as evaluators. The evaluation should take place on two levels. To evaluate the quality of the content, the following questions should be asked: "How well were the contributions understood?" (i.e., how well did the participants respond to what was said?) "How high was the quality of what was expressed?" (i.e., was the discussion superficial or deep and extensive?) "Did the conversation wander off to unrelated or irrelevant matters?" An evaluation of the nonverbal aspects of communication should be conducted as well (e.g., eye contact, fluency, loudness, tone of voice, etc.).

Objectives

The objectives of the Verbal Communication subprogram are based on the disturbed nature of schizophrenia patients' language and the three basic communication skills described earlier in this chapter. In the context of the incremental progression of IPT, the Verbal Communication subprogram is designed to serve as a bridge between the two first subprograms focusing on cognition and the two last subprograms addressing social functioning. Conceptually, this subprogram addresses the vicious circles of cognitive and social impairments described in Chapter 1. The subprogram challenges patients to use learned cognitive skills in interpersonal communication.

It is especially important to progress consecutively through the five steps of this subprogram. Repeated difficulty in one step may indicate a need to go back to the previous step and consolidate the skills exercised there. Persistent problems may require an individual therapy format in addition to the IPT group. As the subprogram nears completion in the fifth step, the therapist should take note of participants' interpersonal communication outside the confines of IPT, such as in ward or community meetings, other therapies and rehabilitation activities, casual social interactions, and family meetings. Generalization and transfer of training should be assessed in these other settings, and observed difficulties brought back to the IPT sessions for further work within the corresponding subprogram step. The criterion of successful skill acquisition in this subprogram is clear and appropriate verbal communication in naturalistic settings outside the IPT sessions.

4.5 Social Skills

Structure

In the Social Skills subprogram, the focus of IPT shifts from specific cognitive processes and verbal abilities to behavioral skills that employ those abilities in socially meaningful ways. This subprogram employs a range of techniques from classical behavior therapy (e.g., assertiveness training) adapted to the needs and abilities of people with schizophrenia. These techniques include didactic instruction, modeling and imitative learning, role-playing, feedback, and social reinforcement (Kelly & Lamparski, 1985). Also in keeping with classical techniques, problems and situations from the participants' daily lives provide material for therapy, including routine interpersonal interactions, working and dealing with coworkers, dealing with bosses and other authorities, housekeeping, and leisure activities. The subprogram draws upon the cognitive abilities addressed in the previous subprograms, especially in setting up the role-plays. In that sense, the subprogram has two distinct purposes: (1) to develop skills to successfully manage specific real-life situations, and (2) to develop cognitive and behavioral skills that will generalize to a variety of real-life problems. The steps in this subprogram progress as follows:

Step 1: Setting up the Role-Play
- Introducing the Role-Play
- Defining the Interaction Goal
- Preparing a Dialog
- Assigning a Title
- Discussing Anticipated Difficulties
- Assigning Observation Tasks
- Rating the Perceived Level of Difficulty

Step 2: Enacting the Role-Play
- Demonstration Role-Play by the Cotherapists
- Feedback Discussion
- Reenactment of Role-Play by Group Members
- Feedback Discussion
- In vivo Exercises

Step 1: Setting up the Role-Play

The therapist begins the session (usually after checking the homework) by explaining the new role-play to be practiced. The practice situation should be explained as simply, clearly, and concretely as possible. By asking questions, the therapist ensures that the task is understood, and that the group members are actually paying attention and are actively participating in the activity. Getting the group members involved in preparing the role-plays prevents the therapist from giving boring monologs and encourages the group members to become aware of potential problems involved in the assigned role-play. In other words, the group members are encouraged to identify the demands they are confronted with in a particular situation. This technique also motivates the group to define a common goal.

The given situations are constructed in a way that requires social interaction to reach the goal of the role-play, with dialogs being the center of focus. This is why the preparation of the dialog is the step subsequent to defining a goal. This phase of the procedure is particularly important since group members tend to manifest generalized avoidance tendencies at this point as a means of discontinuing therapy. Group members who are afraid of social interaction are particularly prone to emerging avoidance tendencies. Writing the role-play on the blackboard can help them feel more secure, both cognitively and emotionally. The group members are then asked to assign an appropriate title to the role-play. Asking the group to reach a consensus on an appropriate title enables the therapists to verify whether the group members have understood and retained the basic points and the interaction goals to be achieved.

The next step involves a discussion of anticipated difficulties, which serves to decrease fears and related anxieties. Each group member is then assigned to observe one of the mentioned aspects of behavior. In doing so, the group members realize that their fears and problems are being taken seriously, and that this procedure further allows each group member to take an active role during this phase of therapy.

The last step before initiating the role-play is to ask the group members to rate the perceived level of difficulty of the role-play using a scale from 1 (*very easy*) to 6 (*very difficult*).

Step 2: Enacting the Role-Play

First of all, a small stage area with realistic props is prepared. Then the two cotherapists enact the role-play the group has developed to provide a model for the group members. The cotherapists are instructed not to give a perfect performance. Participants benefit more if their models are not perfect.

Once this performance is over, the feedback phase begins. First, the "active cotherapist" comments on the role-play, then the group members acting as observers comment on specific aspects of the role-play. The "passive cotherapist" and the primary therapist should make sure all their feedback is of positive nature.

After the cotherapists' role-play, the other group members start participating in the plays. The participant who originally found the exercise to be particularly easy (i.e., had rated it low in difficulty) begins. This patient takes the role of the "active cotherapist," and the cotherapist keeps his or her role of the "passive cotherapist." Only at a later point in therapy will both roles be entrusted to group members. Feedback is given each time a group member enacts a role (analogous to the modeling enactment phase described above).

Therapists employ various techniques to assist group members (e.g., prompting, coaching). Positive reinforcement is, however, the most effective measure. Criticism (e.g., by other patients) should not have a counterproductive effect. Suggestions for changes in behavior should be constructive and concrete for behavior modification. The primary therapist should point out that role-playing skills can be improved with practice, particularly if group members should have to participate in more than one reenactment of the same role-play. Once the group has become adept at role-playing, they may benefit from examining a videotape of their performance. To assist group members in generalizing the Social Skills they are learning, each therapy session ends with the assignment of a homework exercise (in vivo transfer).

B4: Program Overview

B4: Program Overview

Objectives

The objective of this subprogram can be understood as reversing the processes that cause people to lose their social competence – or their failure to acquire it. In the context of the biosystemic model discussed in Chapter 1, social competence involves relatively molecular levels (cognitive and neurocognitive functioning) as well as more molar levels (skill performance, social role performance). In the context of vulnerability-stress models of schizophrenia, some deficiencies are developmental vulnerabilities present before the onset of illness, while others are the result of institutionalization and other dimensions of chronicity. Vulnerabilities prevent the acquisition of social competence, while postonset processes such as conditioned avoidance, psychotic disorganization, and impoverished institutional environments contribute to the neglect and subsequent loss of acquired competence at both the molar and molecular levels. The objective of therapy must, therefore, be (1) to exercise the molecular components that support social competence (attention, eye contact, appropriate voice volume, facial expressions, and nonverbal communication, e.g., gestures, and verbal communication), and (2) to exercise integrated use of the molecular component skills in molar behavioral responses to realistic situations.

Role-playing is the core of this subprogram because, on the one hand, it can be designed and controlled to emphasize use of particular molecular cognitive and behavioral skills, while at the same time it can be tailored to demand an integrated performance of molar social competence in situations that have personal meaning and importance to the participants. As with any other skill, the key to mastery is practice with feedback. Role-playing provides the structure for practice in a situation that maximizes constructive feedback (the IPT group), and allows for as much repetition as is needed for mastery.

Finally, social competence has important cognitive consequences as well as prerequisites. Positive feedback in role-plays, and positive outcomes of in vivo homework assignments, generate the experience of success and empowerment in people who seldom have those experiences. This contributes to the cognitive schema described by Bandura (1977) as self-efficacy, the expectation of success and reward as a consequence of one's own behavior. Loss of self-efficacy contributes heavily to the "negative symptom quality" of lost social competence. The patient no longer expects to be effective, no longer expects reward, and therefore no longer thinks about pursuing goals and objectives. As enhanced social competence generalizes – and the transfer of training brings new skills to ongoing problems – the patient's experience of success creates a higher level of self-efficacy as well as a return of the motivations and interests that had been lost over the chronic course of the disorder. Often, strengthened appropriate social behavior replaces the odd, inappropriate, or bizarre behavior associated with chronic schizophrenia.

4.6 Interpersonal Problem Solving

Structure

Interpersonal Problem Solving is the final step of the therapy program. The reason for its being the last step is not so much because it necessarily has to follow the preceding ones, but because the procedures of this subprogram are relatively complicated and, therefore, put rather high demands on the participants. Furthermore, it is an excellent means of preparing the group members to make important life decisions, such as choosing a discharge destination or an occupational pursuit. This phase of therapy is an independent building block of IPT (Worksheets 14–18), but it can also be combined with a variety of related behavior therapy techniques (e.g., Tarrier, Wells, & Haddock, 1998). Problem-solving strategies should be applied to real-life situations (in vivo) whenever possible.

Although Interpersonal Problem Solving is a highly structured technique, it also requires considerable flexibility and "thinking on one's feet" on the part of the therapist. Substantial experience with this approach is, therefore, especially valuable. The Interpersonal Problem Solving subprogram comprises the following 7 steps, which need to be conducted in sequence:

- Problem Identification and Analysis
- Problem Description
- Generating Alternative Solutions
- Evaluating Alternative Solutions
- Deciding on a Solution
- Implementing the Chosen Solution
- Subsequent Feedback

Problem Identification and Analysis

This represents the initial step of Interpersonal Problem Solving. The therapist chooses a problem area to be addressed with the group after having carefully assessed and defined it (Analysis of the Problem Area). He/she interviews the group members as well as their friends, relatives, and other people involved in the therapeutic process. By means of these interviews the therapist gathers information that will be helpful for obtaining greater insight into the patient's problem. The problem area to start working with is usually chosen according to its urgency as well as according to its probability of finding a solution, which also implies that it should be low in complexity and emotional loading, especially if the patients are not very familiar with the problem area. The principle of gradually increasing the level of emotional stress to cope with is acted upon analogously to the subprograms discussed earlier in this chapter.

Since individuals with a schizophrenia disorder tend to be severely impaired in their ability to identify and understand a problem, problem identification should focus on demands dictated by the process of rehabilitation rather than on tangible everyday problems which patients are more likely to pinpoint on their own accord.

B4: Program Overview

Problem Description

That the afflicted persons suffer from a severely limited and impaired capacity to identify problems points to the importance of this next step of Interpersonal Problem Solving training: the cognitive description of a problem. This step encompasses several goals, such as correcting idiosyncratic attitudes, learning to distinguish fact from fiction, and how to break down complex problems into integral, well-defined parts of the overall problem, identifying the behavioral aspects of a problem, and fostering pragmatic attitudes in order to enable a modification of the behavior. The therapist tries to help the group agree on what *is* and what *should be* in terms of the problem to be treated.

Generating Alternative Solutions

Once the group has successfully described the problem, it can proceed with working out possible alternative solutions. In this phase of the therapy, the therapist makes use of the brainstorming technique (Osborn, 1963). In other words, the group is encouraged to come up with as many solutions as possible. The therapist reinforces all the suggestions made and notes them (e.g., writes them on the blackboard). At this point, it is important for the therapist not to assess or judge the suggestions made.

Evaluating Alternative Solutions

Once various alternatives have been found, their advantages and disadvantages are weighed by assigning plus or minus points to each suggestion. The total number of points for each alternative can be calculated. This rating scale enables the group to develop an objective and neutral method of assessment. The therapist should accept emotionally biased judgments or assessments but not reinforce them. In most cases, challenging or attempting to correct cognitive distortions (e.g., as described by Beck, Rush, Shaw, & Emery, 1979) is not useful in this context.

Deciding on a Solution

The group selects an appropriate solution together, according to the previous objectifying/rationalizing procedure. However, each individual patient needs to decide which solution best fulfills his/her own needs. The therapist's job is to decide to what extent he/she should influence the decision-making process. It is important to make this decision individually, for each patient.

Implementing the Chosen Solution

Once a solution has been selected, the most difficult step of therapy follows, namely, the translation of the chosen solution into action. Specific homework assignments may be used to structure in vivo application, as in the previous subprogram. If the patient has access to other resources – for instance, lives in a residential rehabilitation program – those resources should be recruited for the task. Most importantly, in setting up the translation into action, the therapist should keep in mind that the benefits of the translation are heavily determined by the value of an effective solution in the patient's own experience.

Subsequent Feedback

It is important for the participants to report their experiences with the designated solution in subsequent IPT sessions. Each attempt at constructive problem solving should be encouraged beforehand and reinforced afterward. Not achieving the desired outcome should not be interpreted as a failure or a reason for resignation. Rather, the reason for failure should be objectively analyzed: Did it not work because it was the wrong solution? Or was the solution ineffectively implemented? Or was the problem not properly identified or described in the first place? The therapist should guide this analysis with a combination of Socratic questioning and objective, factual feedback. Working on a "problem" can require several IPT sessions. Keeping good notes and preparing for the sessions can save a great deal of time by preventing needless "rehashing." These are additional reasons that the therapist's depth of experience is especially advantageous.

Objectives

People with schizophrenia often experience great difficulty solving the routine problems of everyday life. This observation is reflected in Bleuler's historic identification of "ambivalence" as one of the principal "5 A's" of schizophrenia. This difficulty extends to decisions required in the course of psychiatric rehabilitation and recovery, which is why treatment sometimes generates counterproductive feelings of diffuse inadequacy.

In order to reduce the impact of failing in everyday life during the rehabilitation process, it is important for the patient to acquire objective and problem-oriented attitudes and reasonable ways of solving problems within the therapeutic setting. Thus, the main objective of the Interpersonal Problem Solving subprogram is to learn to make realistic interpretations of a problem and entertain feasible solutions, while managing the emotional stress that inevitably accompanies that activity.

Implicitly, other related cognitive goals should further be addressed in this subprogram. These include:
- **Improving the Ability to Identify a Problem:** The patients should learn to generalize the problem identification concept acquired in therapy to situations in their everyday life. This should include identifying needed skills and barriers to utilizing those skills.
- **Developing a Rational Attitude Toward Problems:** The patients should learn to define problems in objective, pragmatic terms, while perceiving their own specific

behavior as potentially an integral part of each problem situation. They should also learn to break a problem down into specific parts in order to facilitate analysis.

- **Developing a Solution-Oriented Attitude Toward Problems:** The patients should be encouraged to expect that there are solutions to be found for many problems. It is important for the patients to be able to find solutions to problems not identified in therapy.
- **Fostering a Way of Thinking that Anticipates the Consequences of a Solution and Takes Them into Account**: The patients are encouraged to deal with problems calmly, objectively, and analytically, rather than impulsively and emotionally. Identifying the consequences of emotionally driven actions is an important check on suffering those consequences.
- **Increasing the Chance of Real Problem-Solving Behavior:** The patients should be empowered to seek constructive solutions to the problems and demands they face in their natural environments.

As the Interpersonal Problem Solving subprogram progresses, the therapist should keep both the cognitive prerequisites and the cognitive consequences of effective problem solving in mind. The cognitive prerequisites are those processes addressed by the previous subprograms, most proximally those of Social Perception. Deficiencies at this level of functioning make interpersonal problem solving exceedingly difficult. The cognitive consequences of effective problem solving can be summarized as a greater degree of self-efficacy. This and related schemas, for instance, self-respect and self-esteem, are in and of themselves key components of functional outcome, in the perspective of recovery. In addition, these schemas are key antidotes to the sense of despair, hopelessness, and powerlessness that characterizes the negative symptom picture of chronic schizophrenia. Reversal of these cognitive factors changes the vicious cycles of cognitive and behavioral failure into complementary aspects of the recovery process, resulting in the comprehensive positive outcomes envisioned by biosystemic models, psychiatric rehabilitation, and the recovery movement.

5 Implementation of the Five IPT Subprograms

This chapter describes the implementation of the therapy program. The first section summarizes the general considerations of the therapy program (e.g., group size, tasks for therapist and cotherapists, ways of guiding discussions, etc.). The five subsequent sections provide detailed descriptions of the individual subprograms including brief dialogs taken from therapy sessions. Dialog examples serve solely for the purpose of familiarizing the therapist with the specific procedures. It is, therefore, important to keep in mind that they are only examples and are not applicable in all situations. Furthermore, because the examples are taken from real-life situations, the reinforcement strategies, length, and language may not always seem appropriate and should, therefore, be assessed critically. In contrast to "ideally" constructed examples, these real-life examples help a therapist to understand the problems he/she is faced with. The final section presents group processes.

5.1 General Considerations

Group Size

The group size should be between five and eight participants: Too many participants can prevent the therapists from focusing enough on each group member individually, making it more difficult to keep all group members focused and involved in the activities; and if the group is too small, the demands on the group members may become excessive, making it difficult to generate a variety of responses in therapy activities. In addition, a small group is always in danger of disintegrating when even one or two group members fail to attend or drop out completely.

Frequency of Therapy

In general, therapy sessions should be held twice a week. Determining factors that need to be taken into consideration are external circumstances, the time each patient can spare for group therapy, tolerance to stress, as well as degree of chronicity (see also Chapter 7).

Duration of Therapy Sessions

The sessions take between 30 and 90 minutes depending on the subprogram. Initial sessions of the Cognitive Differentiation subprogram should be limited to 30 or 40 minutes, whereas Social Perception and Verbal Communication subprogram sessions generally last 60 minutes. Finally, the Social Skills and Interpersonal Problem Solving subprograms usually require 90-minute sessions mainly because of the time-consuming nature of role-plays, which represent an integral part of these subprograms. With some group members it may be necessary to provide one or more short breaks in the 90-minute sessions to facilitate attention and concentration. Alternatively, the content of a 90-minute session can be divided into two sessions. The therapist should always define the duration of a session for a fixed time interval (e.g., 60-min sessions twice a week for the next 6 weeks) and inform the participants in a motivational way.

Duration of the Different Subprograms

It is difficult to define the general duration of each subprogram or the whole therapy program. The duration depends mainly on the severity and the chronicity of the disorder as well as on the patients' motivation. Accordingly, the number of sessions required to complete a particular subprogram varies depending on the group members' abilities to master therapy activities.

To foster the group members' motivation by bringing more variety into the sessions, in the course of the first three subprograms (Cognitive Differentiation, Social Perception, and Verbal Communication) activities from two separate subprograms may be conducted during the same session (e.g., carrying out a Cognitive Differentiation activity at the end of a Social Perception session). However, the first 3 to 10 sessions of each subprogram should be limited to only activities from that subprogram. If group members find it difficult to master the therapy activities of the Cognitive Differentiation subprogram, the first 10 to 20 sessions should even be limited to only activities of that subprogram. Because of the time-consuming nature of role-plays, the last two subprograms, Social Skills and Interpersonal Problem Solving, are generally limited to only one subprogram per session. During the Social Skills and Interpersonal Problem Solving subprograms, however, it is recommended that sessions focusing on earlier activities be inserted periodically in order to increase retention of cognitive skills learned in earlier subprograms ("booster sessions").

Explanation and Justification of the Therapy Program

A clear understanding of how the therapy relates to accomplishing personal goals increases the patients' motivation to attend and participate in the therapy sessions. Individually discussing self-expressed difficulties may further augment this motivation. In our studies, we used the Frankfurt Complaint Questionnaire (FCQ, Süllwold, 1977), a self-report questionnaire dealing with subjectively experienced cognitive difficulties, to increase group members' involvement in the therapy. The FCQ is not an instrument for differential diagnoses, but should merely be considered useful from a motivational point of view: If the questionnaire reveals cognitive difficulties in group members, discussing how the therapy addresses the experienced difficulties provides a way for them to understand how the therapy can help them to meet their own goals of reducing cognitive difficulties. However, some patients do not acknowledge subjectively experienced cognitive difficulties, despite obvious indicators. This implies that the patient is either not ready to discuss these disorders or does not perceive the disturbances himself. In this case, other means of motivating participation are necessary. Alternatively to the FCQ, the ESI (Eppendorfer Schizophrenia Inventory, Mass, 2001) can be used to motivate patients to participate in a group. The ESI is an instrument for differential diagnostics, dealing with difficulties typical for schizophrenia patients. Other assessment instruments may also be useful within this context (compare Chapter 6).

The basic principle and goals of the therapy are presented at the beginning of the therapy and are repeated only if the group as a whole expresses the need for clarification and explanation. However, the therapist(s) should not feel pressured to explain the purpose of each activity. In most cases it should be sufficient to elaborate the objectives if the group explicitly requests this. Individual discussions of purpose and objectives of the therapy outside the group may be useful for some group members who have particular difficulty retaining this information.

Preparation and Evaluation Meetings

Each therapy session needs to be planned and discussed in advance by the therapists (10 to 20 minutes). Special attention should be directed toward difficulties experienced in the previous session. After a therapy session, it is important for the therapist(s) to have another meeting in order to discuss the following points:
– Were any of the group members overburdened by the activities?
– Were they motivated?
– Which resources and deficits did they show?
– Which points need to be practiced in particular?
– Is there a need to expand certain issues over several sessions?
– Was there anything conspicuous regarding the group processes?
– What are our own feelings?

To help in structuring this evaluation meeting, the therapist can consult Worksheet 20 "Behavior in the Therapy Group (BT)" (in the Appendix).

Role-Plays

Therapists who have no experience with this therapy program will find role-plays before therapy sessions to be very useful. Role-playing provides therapists with the opportunity to draw important inferences about their own behavior, to explore the possibilities of the didactic use of the materials, and to experience the group process. Involving the supervisor of the therapist who is experienced in the different subprograms as well as the therapy program is recommended.

Team of Therapists

Continuity is important; it is therefore recommended that the same therapist(s) carry out the entire therapy. During each of the sessions, one therapist should be designated as primary therapist and the other therapist(s) fulfill the function of cotherapist(s). Therapists can, of course, swap their roles during a session. For example, after the first half of the session, the primary therapist can switch roles with one of the cotherapists. However, this change of roles needs to be clearly communicated to the group members in advance. The primary therapist could say, for instance: "Mr. Jones will now lead the group." Only one change of therapist roles is recommended during any single therapy session. If the group members are especially low-functioning, role alternation should not take place at all. The first three subprograms require one primary therapist and one cotherapist. Adding a second cotherapist is suggested for the last two subprograms to facilitate role-plays.

Primary Therapist

The main role of the primary therapist is to guide and structure the group sessions and to support as well as to encourage the group members. Group members are motivated to improve their performance through positive reinforcement, thereby reducing fear, discouragement, and disappointment, which may interfere with their performance. Negative feedback should be avoided; instead, the therapist should always point out and emphasize the positive aspects of feedback. Reinforcement should be informative rather than emotional or morally judgmental (i.e., right or wrong). For example, it is better to say: "Yes, you have just repeated the sentence absolutely correctly" rather than "Great" or "Wonderful." Emotional reinforcement may be perceived as not being genuine. The therapist should acknowledge the constructive contributions of all group members, for example, by responding in an informative and reinforcing way, or by acknowledging the contribution and nodding in agreement. Acceptance of self and others is facilitated by the therapist(s)' acknowledgment and acceptance of differing viewpoints by the group members. Instructions by the primary therapist should be directive but not authoritarian, and negative criticism is to be avoided.

Cotherapists

The function of the cotherapist(s) is formally equal to the patients' role. They should, however, restrain themselves concerning content (contributions).

Their special tasks are:
- To be always ready to take over the role of the primary therapist in a difficult situation, but to wait for a prearranged signal from the primary therapist before actually doing so.
- To serve as role models for group members. For example, the primary therapist may ask the cotherapist to demonstrate a new exercise or to assist with a role-play.
- To influence group processes in the sense of encouraging and supporting weaker group members or to express solidarity with them.
- They also serve as supervisors, monitoring group processes. Since the cotherapist(s) do not lead the group, they are in a better position to observe the group process and offer valuable information in postsession discussions, which in turn help to shape future sessions.

Auxiliary Means

For many exercises, working with technical aids (e.g., data projector, overhead projector, blackboard, flip chart, paper, different colored pens) is suggested. The verbal level of communication can be supported by visual aids for catching and increasing attention. These auxiliary means also help to structure the groups.

Therapy Materials

The original therapy materials have been modified, extended, and differentiated, based on experiences in various therapy groups. The degree of standardization differs according to the demands of the subprograms. When working with the materials described in the Appendix, take this into account as well as fact that the materials are designed in a very practical manner; also note that the various institutions carrying out the program differ considerably from one another. For these reasons, it is usually necessary to modify and complement the materials according to the needs of a specific institution and group. The materials presented in the Appendix are intended to be a pool from which adequate exercises can be specifically and carefully selected.

The conception of the materials is based on the contents of the therapy, whereby the relevant areas of therapy as well as the different categories of emotions played a decisive role.
- *Different areas of therapy:* Leisure, clinic, living, work, family, friends, and acquaintances.
- *Categories of emotions:* Happiness, contentment, hope, curiosity, insecurity, anger, aggression, sadness, fear, and horror.

In order to make the following section less complicated, we do not mention this additional division again. As emphasized in Chapter 4.1, the therapeutic relevance lies mainly on the division into "task-oriented" or "emotionally neutral" versus "emotionally loaded" material.

B5: Implementation

All therapy exercises should begin with materials considered to be emotionally neutral. Only after group members have achieved some mastery of the exercises with emotionally neutral materials, should the therapist increase the degree of task difficulty by introducing more emotionally loaded task stimuli. If the group members find the emotionally loaded task stimuli too stressful, the therapist should revert to more emotionally neutral task stimuli in the next session. The same procedure is used for the presentation of therapy materials (see Appendix).

The division is a result of expert judgment as well as practical experience. It is the therapists' task to judge the extent to which even emotionally "neutral" material has affective connotations for the members of the group. The division mentioned here should, therefore, not be seen as generally mandatory. As mentioned previously, the implementation of the "right" therapy materials depends largely on the group.

5.2 Cognitive Differentiation

The description of this subprogram is divided into two sections. The first section presents considerations on how to introduce the subprogram to the therapy group; the second part describes the individual exercises of this subprogram.

We now give examples for therapy implementation. It is important to keep in mind that it is impossible to illustrate all possible situations that may arise in the course of therapy. The examples were chosen so as to provide a look at all essential instructions for conducting the exercises. The Appendix contains a detailed description of the exercise materials used in the Cognitive Differentiation subprogram.

5.2.1 Introducing the Subprogram

The purpose of this subprogram is to improve basic cognitive processes, which are prerequisites for learning. They also serve as the cognitive substrates for social interaction and problem solving.

Motivating Patients to Participate

The group members are normally introduced to the Cognitive Differentiation subprogram the first time they meet as a group. Each participant should be well prepared for participating in the therapy. This is best insured through individual contact with the therapist before the group begins. Assessment of a group member's motivation should take into account the type and intensity of an existing disorder as well as the degree of chronicity. As mentioned earlier (see Chapter 5.1), the FCQ or ESI can be used for motivational purposes; these questionnaires measure cognitive abilities, among other things, which allows a direct link to the first subprogram designed for the amelioration of cognitive deficits. An exhaustive discussion of each patient's subjectively experienced distress usually leads to a sufficient level of motivation to participate in the therapy program.

Frequency and Duration of Therapy Sessions

Most therapists prefer to begin with two or three sessions weekly of 30 to 45 minutes, and to then increase the duration of the sessions to 60 minutes after a few sessions (e.g., when beginning with the subprogram of Social Perception). When introducing the Cognitive Differentiation subprogram it is important always to begin with Step 1 (card-sorting exercises). Once the group members are familiar with the card-sorting exercises, Step 2 (verbal concept exercises) may then be introduced. The sequence for conducting Step 2 exercises should be retained as described in the manual, although the order of their presentation can be modified based on considerations concerning the degree and types of difficulties group members are experiencing. Step 3 exercises (search strategies) may be introduced immediately after having introduced Step 2. Previously mastered exercises, however, should be repeated continually, in order to maintain the therapeutic effect.

5.2.2 Description of the Subprogram's Different Steps

In the following sections we present excerpts in order to describe specific exercises taken from a group including six members (Andy, Sally, Kevin, Walter, Bob, and Lucy) and two therapists (Mr. S. and Ms. B.).

Step 1: Card-Sorting Exercises*

The therapy materials consist of 2.8-inch × 2.8-inch cards, printed with designs that differ on the dimensions shape, color, number, and days of the week (see Worksheet 1). The group members sit in a circle, and each group member, except for the primary therapist, receives 10 to 15 cards. Group members might find it difficult to keep this many cards in their hands, and it may be helpful to perform this exercise on a table where the cards can be laid out.

In the first session, the cards are laid out on the table, and group members identify the characteristics of the cards (red, 2-digit number, blue, rectangle, etc.). When all the characteristics have been identified, the therapist explains the meaning of a common characteristic or property; for example, "The number 4 is a common characteristic if it appears on at least two cards." Subsequently the therapist asks the group members to pick up their cards and sort the cards according to a single characteristic. For example, the therapist says, "Find all the cards with a yellow background and put them on the table in front of you." Once everyone has sorted their cards and laid them out, each

---

* The cards can be ordered from the first author.

group member checks his/her neighbor's cards to see if the task has been carried out correctly. The number of sorting criteria is gradually increased, as group members get more familiar with the task. For groups with average intelligence, the maximum number of sorting criteria is usually four or five. As the number of sorting criteria increases, the probability of finding a card meeting the criteria decreases. It may be necessary to increase the number of cards given to each group member for exercises involving four or five sorting criteria.

A number of variations of the card-sorting procedure are possible for advanced groups. For example, instead of the therapist, the group members can generate the sorting criteria, or the therapist can set one criterion and have each group member add one or two other criteria. Subsequently, group members can define their own criteria and share them with the group. Another type of exercise involves increasing the number of criteria by removing or adding a card. For example, the therapist says, "Which card do we need to remove from Walter's cards so that the remaining cards have five characteristics in common?" (Originally Walter had four cards with four common characteristics.)

When working with a group of low-functioning members, it is useful to lay all the cards on the table and ask the group members to take out all the cards containing certain characteristics, for instance, all cards that are blue with a rectangle on them.

The following example further illustrates card-sorting exercises; all group members were present. Ms. B. was the primary therapist. It was the group's seventh session:

Example

Course of Action in a Card-Sorting Exercise

Therapist: Good morning everyone. Thank you for being on time. Today we will do the card-sorting exercises again. Let me hand out some cards to each of you (she distributes the cards). Sally, would you please name two characteristics for the group to sort their cards by? Once Sally has named two characteristics, each of you decides on a third characteristic for sorting the cards. OK? Sally, have you decided on the two characteristics?

Sally: Yes, red and a two-digit number.

Therapist: Thank you, Sally. That was quick. Lucy, could you repeat the task instructions?

Lucy: We should lay down all our cards with red and a two-digit number.

Therapist: Yes that is correct, Lucy. What is the second part of the task Bob?

Bob: Everyone is to pick out a third sorting characteristic.

Therapist: That is correct Bob. Andy, how many characteristics do we have to sort for?

Andy: Uh, red . . .

Therapist: Yes, red and what else?

Andy: (Silent)

Therapist: Kevin and Walter, can you help Andy?

Kevin: And a two-digit number. The third characteristic everyone chooses himself or herself.

Therapist: Is that correct Walter?

Therapist: OK, that is correct. So we are to sort according to three characteristics. Andy, can you repeat the three characteristics? (Andy correctly repeats the three characteristics.) OK, now everyone lay down your cards please.

It is very important for the therapist to always make sure all group members understand the task before attempting to complete it.

(All group members now have their cards laid out on the table in front of them.)

Therapist: Bob, would you please check if your neighbor has completed the task correctly and tell us what his third characteristic is?

Bob: Yes, the task is done correctly.

Therapist: Correct. Now please tell us once more the first and second characteristics.

Bob: Red and a two-digit number.

Therapist: That is correct. And what, in your opinion, is your neighbor's third characteristic?

Bob: A rectangle.

Therapist: OK, Bob. There is a rectangle on all three cards. Was that your third characteristic, Walter?

Walter: No, it was . . .

Therapist: Just a minute Walter, don't tell us what your third characteristic was. First we'll ask the group. Who sees another characteristic?

Sally: All three cards contain the word "Saturday."

Walter: Yes, that was it.

Therapist: OK, now we have found four common characteristics in Walter's cards: red, two-digit numbers, "Saturday," and rectangle. Walter, will you please check your neighbor's cards? (etc.)

The therapist reinforces all relevant responses given by group members in an informative manner and offers feedback throughout the task so all group members clearly understand the task as it proceeds. If a group member does not have any cards with common characteristics, that member should be given additional cards or be excused when correcting the task. If all group members perform poorly on the card-sorting task (e.g., because of attention/concentration deficits), the selected characteristics can be written on the blackboard before beginning with the task, in order to simplify the memory component of the task.

Step 2: Verbal Concept Exercises

The materials consist of different exercises including conceptual hierarchies, synonyms, antonyms, word definitions, and word clue exercises based on the use of word cards (Worksheets 2 and 3) as well as words with different meanings depending on the context.

A. Conceptual Hierarchies Exercise

The therapy materials consist of different words or fragments of sentences, considered to be emotionally neutral or emotionally loaded. The therapist should start the exercise with emotionally neutral words or phrases.

The therapist writes down a word or sentence on the blackboard, for example, "packing for a camping trip." The group members sit in a semicircle and are asked to name related words (nouns) as they come to mind. The cotherapist or a group member writes the words on the blackboard. At the beginning of this exercise, the number of words should be limited to 25 or 30 so as not to exceed information processing capacity. Later, the related word list might include up to 50 or 60 words. All words are written on the blackboard without evaluating whether they match the context or not. As soon as about 30 words are listed (the group members are requested to count them), the therapist asks a group member to read all the words aloud. He then asks which words form a category and how they decided which words go together. Subsequently, they are asked to find a hypernym for the words that go together. Along with the words belonging to the group, the hypernym is written on a second blackboard, or on a large piece of paper in a specific color. For example, "toiletries" might be the hypernym and words belonging to that category would include toothbrush, toothpaste, and nailfile. This process is repeated until all the related words are organized in hypernyms. New words may be added to previously identified categories. For example, aftershave and soap might be added to toiletries. Conceptual hierarchies can also be used as homework. For example, one or two group members could write a packing list for a camping trip, with the assistance of a cotherapist, and copy and distribute it to the other group members. Whenever the patients are given homework, it should be discussed at the beginning of the next session.

B. Synonyms Exercise

The therapy material consists of words considered to be either emotionally neutral or emotionally loaded. The procedures for conducting the synonym exercise are illustrated in the following therapy excerpt; Mr. S. is the primary therapist and Ms. B. the cotherapist. Two group members (Bob and Lucy) are absent:

Example

Therapists' Approach for the Synonym Exercise

Therapist: Today we will do an exercise using synonyms as we did in our last session. Walter, do you remember what we did in our last session?

Walter: Yes, we looked for words with a similar meaning as "decision."

Therapist: Correct, everyone wrote down words similar in meaning to "decision." What did we do next, Sally?

Sally: We made sentences with the words and decided whether they really had the same meaning.

Therapist: Well done! You remembered the task correctly. Today I am going to write the word "work" on the blackboard. Everyone should write a synonym for "work" on his or her paper. Andy and Kevin, what are we going to do now?

Andy: We are going to write down words similar to "work."

Kevin: How many should we write down?

Therapist: That's a good question, Kevin. Perhaps everyone should begin by writing down one word. Now that Andy has correctly repeated the task, we can begin. (Therapist waits while group members write.) So, would you please begin by reading your word aloud, Sally?

Sally: Job.

Therapist: Yes. Now I will ask everyone in turn: Andy?

Andy: Labor.

Therapist: Good. And Kevin?

Andy: Occupation.

Co-therapist: I also wrote "job," like Sally.

Therapist: OK, now it's your turn, Walter.

Walter: Employment.

Therapist: Good. Ms. B., would you please write all the words mentioned on the blackboard? And now everyone please write a sentence using his or her synonym for "work."

As the example illustrates, all group members are asked to find synonyms for a specific word and to write them on their paper. Then each group member shares their synonym with the group; all synonyms are written on the blackboard, and group members make up a sentence using their synonym. Each group member's sentence should also be written on the blackboard. The synonym in the sentence should be replaced by the original word, and the group members then decide which of the synonyms is closest to the original, and justify this decision.

C. Antonyms Exercise

Again, the therapy material consists of words considered to be either emotionally neutral or emotionally loaded. The exercise starts with emotionally neutral ones.

Initially, the procedures are similar to the synonym exercise: A word is given and everyone writes down a word with the opposite meaning. Group members read their antonyms aloud and the words are written on the blackboard. The group members then judge whether the words given as antonyms actually have an opposite meaning. At this point, working with examples is recommended in order to clarify the meanings of words. It is often necessary for the therapist to provide additional structure and explanations in this exercise. For example, group members may suggest "boy," "baby," and "woman" as antonyms for "man." The therapist's task is to help the group members to understand that there are various dimensions to the word "man," and that it is possible to find a number of words with an opposite meaning:

– Man–boy: dimension(s): age, developmental stage, size
– Man–woman: dimension(s): sex
– Man–baby: dimension(s): age, developmental stage, size

It is important that the tasks not be too difficult. Therapists should decide in advance which level of task difficulty meets the abilities of the group members.

B5: Implementation

D. Word Definitions Exercise

As with the previous exercises, the therapy material for this exercise also involves words that vary on the dimensions of emotional loading and level of abstractness. The therapist should begin the exercise with emotionally neutral, concrete objects, in order to start with easy tasks.

This exercise involves some role-playing by the cotherapist, as the following example using the word "door" illustrates.

The group members and primary therapist form a semicircle around the cotherapist, who is introduced to the group as someone from another civilization who does not know what a door is. The primary therapist asks the group members to explain to the "foreigner" what a door is, in a precise and understandable manner. The primary therapist supports the group members by describing the important aspects of concrete objects and writing relevant conceptual aids, such as material, location, size, color, function, and shape, on the blackboard. The object is then described based on these aids. For example:

– "A door is a panel made of wood, plastic, glass, or metal." (material)
– "To enter or leave a room, there is a large hole in one of the walls of every room. With this panel this hole can be opened or closed." (purpose/function)

After some initial description, the "foreigner" can ask group members questions if she or he does not really understand what kind of an object is being described. After every round in which each group member gives an explanation, the cotherapist tells the group what she/he has learned so far about doors, given their descriptions. In an advanced group, a group member can take over the role of the "foreigner" in this activity.

With the use of concrete, emotionally neutral objects, the group members usually experience this exercise as relatively easy. Significant difficulties can occur when abstract, more emotionally loaded concepts are introduced.

E. Word Clue Exercise

The therapy materials consist of cards with two words printed on them, one of which is underlined (example: pen – pencil). Words are still considered either emotionally neutral or emotionally loaded. As before, emotionally neutral words are used to introduce this exercise, and as they progress in the therapy, the group members should be able to deal with emotionally loaded words.

The therapist hands a card to patient A and asks him to read both words aloud without revealing which of the words is underlined. His task is then to think of a one-word clue to help the other group members to identify the underlined word. The clue has to be a noun and cannot contain the underlined word. In the above example, using pen – pencil, the clue word could not be, for instance, ballpoint pen. Once the clue has been given, the group members write down the word they think is underlined. As soon as everyone has finished writing, all group members read their guesses aloud and justify their choice.

For example: Group member A gave the clue, "ink." Group member B wrote down "pen," reasoning that pens write with ink but pencils do not. If the majority of the group members choose the same word, group member A is asked to reveal the underlined word. If the group members' choices are about equally split between the two words, group member A is asked to give a second clue and again everyone is asked to write down their guess, read it aloud, and justify their choice. This procedure can be repeated three or four times if necessary. Once the underlined word has been identified, the group is asked to think of other clue words that could have been used. If group members show severe attentional problems, the two words on the card may be written on the blackboard (omitting the underlining).

F. Context-Dependent Words Exercise

The therapy material consists of concrete objects or specific words with more than one meaning. The exercise can be illustrated with the word "bulb." The purpose of this exercise is to determine the different meanings a word can have depending on the context it is used in. A "bulb," for instance, can be used in the sense of a "flower bulb" or a "light bulb." Again, during the first sessions introducing this exercise, the therapists work with concrete objects, minimizing the degree of abstractness. For this exercise it is useful to bring the objects or at least pictures of the objects that depict the different meanings of a word.

The group sits in a semicircle, and the objects or pictures are placed in the center. Each group member is instructed to come up with a sentence containing the word "bulb," but without using any of the words that define the various meanings. For example, with "bulb," the words "light" and "flower" should not be used in the sentence. However, the sentence should clearly bring out which type of bulb was meant. For example:

– "A bulb can be planted." (flower bulb).
– "The bulb burned out." (light bulb).

Each group member reads his or her sentence aloud and the other group members decide whether or not the meaning of the word "bulb" is clear, given the context of the sentence. Finally, the group members discuss the similarities and differences concerning the two types of bulbs and write them down on the blackboard. In order to do this, previous exercises – like hypernyms – can be used.

Context-Dependent Words Exercise

Differences:

	Flower Bulb	**Light Bulb**
Origin:	natural plant	industrial product
W8:	heavy	light
Use:	for esthetic reasons	to produce light
Material:	plant cells	glass and metal

Similarities:

Shape:	pear-shaped	pear-shaped
Color:	sometimes white	almost always white

With an advanced group, it is not necessary to use concrete objects or pictures. The therapist merely writes a word on the blackboard (e.g., "bulb") and asks the group members to come up with sentences including the word. The participants are then asked to find out themselves the different meanings, depending on the context, using the context as a cue. In this variation of the exercise, the support of the cotherapist may be necessary. The subsequent procedure is analogous to the previous example.

Step 3: Search Strategies Exercises

No therapy materials are needed for this exercise. Group member A and the cotherapist constitute a team, which chooses an object. Initially the object must be in the room; however, as the group members master the task, the area from which the object may be chosen can be expanded (hospital ward, hospital grounds, city, etc.). The name of the object is written down on a piece of paper for control purposes, but this information is not shared with the other group members. The group's task is to identify which object has been chosen, through a series of yes/no questions. The cotherapist assists group member A as necessary. Each group member is allowed to ask a· maximum of two questions consecutively (because of the attentional demands of the task). If the answer to the first question of a group member is "yes," he or she can ask a second question. If, however, the answer to the first question is "no," it is the next person's turn to ask a question. The group member who guesses the name of the object correctly gets to pick a new object and is then questioned by the group.

Usually the group members start with asking very concrete questions (e.g., "Is it the yellow shoe?" or "Is it the red curtain?"). Conceptual questions, such as "Is the object on the floor?" or "Is the object on the left side of the room?" occur quite rarely. If group members do ask conceptual questions, the therapist should recognize and reinforce them. The therapist can also make the group aware that conceptual questions lower the probability of getting a no answer, and the object can be identified more quickly. At a later point in the exercise the therapist encourages the use of conceptual questions by devoting an entire session to generating and listing conceptual questions. This is particularly useful before extending the object search area beyond the therapy room. The use of conceptual questions can also be encouraged by occasionally conducting a competitive game in which group members get to ask an unlimited number of questions as long as they are answered with a "yes." The group member who asks the highest number of questions in a row is the winner.

As indicated above, the difficulty of the task is increased over time by extending the object search area. In some groups the definition of the word "object" may need to be discussed. It is important for the group members to understand that the objects they choose have to be visible. Objects such as "ghost" and "air" are, thus, not permitted.

5.3 Social Perception

The description of this subprogram is divided into two parts. First, there is an introduction to the subprogram as well as to the requirements in terms of form and content, and subsequently we describe the three steps of the therapeutic procedure using examples of therapy excerpts. It is important that the three steps of the subprogram be conducted in the sequence given. The therapy materials are presented in the Appendix.

5.3.1 Introducing the Subprogram

Knowledge About the Patients and Their Disorders

At the beginning of the subprogram, it is important for the therapist to be familiar with the group members and their problems as well as histories. The purpose of the therapy can be made more tangible to the patient if one refers to his/her own experience and complaints concerning, for instance, distorted perception. In our studies, endorsed items of the Frankfurt Complaint Questionnaire (FCQ, see 5.1; Süllwold, 1977) are used to determine the characteristic complaints of group members (e.g., "Sometimes I have to fix my eyes on one point, otherwise everything disappears" or "Sometimes I see something and am not sure whether I am dreaming."). In order to motivate the patients to participate in therapy, it can be helpful to present them with one of the slides used in therapy as an example. This is especially true if they are then able to spot details on the slide they otherwise might have overlooked.

Knowledge About the Content of Slides

It is mandatory for the therapist(s) to be familiar with the content of the slides before beginning the therapy. Preparatory role-plays between therapists before beginning the therapy have proven to be useful for identifying potentially important details of the slides.

Although it is not absolutely necessary in this subprogram, the presence of a co-therapist is recommended to provide technical assistance with the projector, while the primary therapist focuses on observing the different therapy steps, for instance.

Slides Used*

A new set of slides has recently been published (Roder et al., 2008). A more intense inclusion of (burdening) emotions differentiates this new set of slides from the previous ones (from 1988 and 1997). Each slide contains an identifiable expression of an emotion. For pedagogic reasons, the emotions depicted on the slides refer only to basic

---

* The slides can be ordered from the first author.

B5: Implementation

Table 5.1 Characteristics of the 80 randomly selected raters

Age (years)		Sex	
Average	32.2	Male	51.2%
SD	12.2	Female	48.8%

Distribution of the raters' age

Age (years)	Absolute frequency	Relative frequency (%
15	1	1.3
18	1	1.3
20	3	3.8
21	4	5.0
22	2	2.5
23	4	5.0
24	7	8.8
25	6	7.5
26	8	10.0
27	4	5.0
28	4	5.0
29	5	6.3
30	2	2.5
31	4	5.0
32	1	1.3
33	1	1.3
35	2	2.5
38	1	1.3
39	2	2.5
42	1	1.3
43	1	1.3
44	2	2.5
46	2	2.5
47	2	2.5
48	1	1.3
49	2	2.5
52	1	1.3
54	1	1.3
58	1	1.3
60	1	1.3
62	1	1.3
70	1	1.3
72	1	1.3
Total	80	100.0

emotions: happiness, surprise, anger, sadness, and fear. These basic emotions were adopted from Ekman and colleagues (Ekman, Friesen, & Ellsworth, 1972; Argyle, 1988). The new set of slides (see Worksheet 4) was evaluated according to the previous sets; however, additionally the kind of emotions depicted in each slide were assessed. "Naive," (psychiatrically) normal judges rated the slides on the dimensions "cognitive complexity" (see Worksheet 5), "emotional load" (see Worksheet 6a), and "expressed emotion" (see Worksheet 6b). The dimension "cognitive complexity" measures the degree of difficulty for an observer to perceive what is on the slide (e.g., how many details are in the picture). "Emotional loading" describes the extent to which a slide can trigger a specific emotion in an observer, and the dimension "expressed emotion" discriminates which of the five mentioned emotions is depicted in a slide.

Initially, experts chose 40 out of almost 800 pictures for the new set of slides. By means of a standardized questionnaire, 80 evaluators then rated these 40 slides (Table 5.1) according to the three dimensions. Moreover, a concise title was proposed for each picture.

The values for each slide (low cognitive complexity, moderate cognitive complexity, high cognitive complexity) are indicated in the table on Worksheet 5, "Ratings of the Slides' Cognitive Complexity." The values for the dimension emotional load (not/barely emotionally loaded, somewhat emotionally loaded, highly emotionally loaded) are indicated on the respective Worksheet 6a. For each slide the percentage frequencies of emotions named by the observers can be gathered from Worksheet 6b. On average, the observers detected 81.8% of the emotions shown in the slides correctly (Table 5.2). This very high rate of recognizing emotions (compared to those found by Ekman, for instance: 60% [Argyle, 1988; Ekman et al. 1972]) underlines the therapeutic usability of the slides. Moreover, a title is included in the respective table of the appendix for each slide (see Worksheet 7). The titles chosen were those which the highest number of observers had given to each respective slide.

The succession of slides in the tables is random and does not represent the order in which they are to be used in therapy groups. In fact, the therapist needs to carefully determine the order of presenting the slides, depending on the problems (i.e., needs and competency) of group members as well as according to the parameters given in the tables. At the beginning of the subprogram "Social Perception," the therapists should choose "easy" slides, which have been rated as "cognitively simple" (high percentage of this category for the respective slide) as well as "not/barely emotionally loaded" (high percentage of this category for the respective slide) by most of the observers. As therapy progresses, the degree of complexity as well as the emotional load can be increased successively. Additionally, at the beginning of therapy, it is important to choose slides depicting easily detectable emotions, i.e., the emotions shown in slides with a high percentage of observers (80% and more [see Work-

Table 5.2 Frequency of correctly recognized emotions presented in the pictures

	Average	SD
Correct recognition of emotions	81.8%	16.2
Wrong recognition of emotions	17.9%	16.3

sheet 6b]) who correctly identified the category of emotions. The emotion of a slide is unambiguous if the parameter of one identified emotion is significantly higher than the values of other emotions detected. If, however, the difference between these parameters is small, the slide is considered to be emotionally ambiguous. For these slides, even "naive" observers find it difficult to correctly distinguish the depicted emotions, so that they should be used only in later therapy sessions once the patients have mastered the task. Moreover, it is best to choose slides depicting positive emotions (e.g., happiness) at the beginning of therapy (see Table 5.2).

Preparations Before Beginning the Therapy

The materials needed in addition to the slides are a projector and a computer as well as a screen for projecting the slides. The therapist needs to be familiar with the use of these materials before starting the therapy, and their functionability should be verified prior to each session. Furthermore, the lighting conditions need to be adequate for the use of a projector (darkened room): The room needs to be dark enough for the slides to be clearly visible but light enough for the therapist(s) and group members to see each other well. The seating plan is also important: During the therapy session the group members and therapist(s) should sit in a semicircle facing the screen where the slide is being projected. Ideally the primary therapist sits in the middle, and the chairs are arranged so that each group member and the therapist(s) are able to make eye contact with each other.

Therapy sessions last approximately 60 minutes. At the beginning of this subprogram, gathering information (Step 1) about one single slide may take one to two sessions. Later on, after six or seven slides, it is possible to complete all three steps for one or two slides in a single session. If a session is planned to include both the social perception exercise as well as an exercise from the cognitive differentiation subprogram, the social perception exercise should be conducted first since the time to complete the three steps for any slide can vary considerably (between 20 and 40 minutes).

Although group members may initially find it difficult to distinguish Step 1 (gathering information) and Step 2 (interpretation), they usually quickly become familiar with the steps of the subprogram as well as their sequence, and are easily able to stick to it. Once the group members are familiar with the steps of the subprogram, it is up to the primary therapist to judge whether or not there is further need for him to refer explicitly to the sequence of steps.

5.3.2 Description of the Subprogram's Different Steps

The Social Perception subprogram is characterized by a high degree of structure, requiring the therapists' approach to be directive but not authoritarian. It is important to complete each step and adhere to the sequence of the steps because fragmented or incomplete information gathering may hinder a subsequent interpretation of the slides because of a lack of arguments. Furthermore, an incomplete or fragmented gathering of information may maintain or even reinforce dysfunctional patterns of perception. For example, if the interpretation commences prematurely, before all the information needed has been gathered, some group members may be fixated on only certain details of the picture; their thoughts may become dominated by those details and they lose the ability to focus their attention on other aspects of the picture. Such fixations can be avoided by closely adhering to the steps of the subprogram. Dysfunctional perceptual habits should be corrected in order to construct new possibilities of interpretation. The main aim of each slide is the adequate perception of social interactions and expressed emotions.

Step 1: Gathering Information

The therapist presents the group with a slide and encourages each of the group members to help in identifying the relevant details of the picture. The primary therapist points out relevant details that have not yet been mentioned by the group members, emphasizes particularly important details, and summarizes the relevant details mentioned. He reinforces the details noticed by group members by repeating them and gives explanations as needed. With complex slides it can be helpful to divide the picture into different parts, assisting group members to gather visual information in a systematic way. For example, group members could be directed to focus first on the left upper quadrant of the picture. Other possibilities for such division are background versus foreground, people, clothing, etc. These points of focus help the members' perception and make the number of stimuli manageable for them. The therapist always begin by focusing on things that are less important (e.g., houses and streets), building up to more important details and finally to the most important ones (expressed emotions of persons/interactions).

The following therapy excerpt illustrates a typical first session of the Social Perception subprogram. The group consists of six group members (Sam, Phil, Helen, Paul, Will, and Steven) and a therapist. The picture displays a young woman with a frightened expression on her face standing by a window looking outside. The following statements illustrate some therapeutic techniques:

– *Focusing:* "Now let us look at the center of the slide and describe it."
– *Pointing out ignored details:* "Can anyone describe the face in more detail?"
– *Guiding attention to relevant details:* "Can anyone describe how the girl is opening her mouth?"
– *Reinforcing:* "You did a good job examining the girl's mouth, Paul. This is a very important detail you have just described."
– *Summarizing:* "Helen, you have pointed out a lot of details. A woman with long brown hair and hazel eyes is wearing a necklace that could be made of silver or something similar. She is wearing a purple dress."

B5: Implementation

Example

Therapist: Now let us focus on the center of the slide and only describe this part.

Will: You mean we should just look at her face?

Therapist: Yes, Will, exactly, just the face for now (therapist pauses, giving the group members time to examine the face). Can anyone describe the face? Steven?

Steven: Well yes. I mean, no I can't.

Therapist: Sam, can you help Steven?

Sam: She has brown hair and a dark complexion. Actually the hair is dark brown, indeed, very dark brown hair.

Therapist: Well done, Sam

Sam: Yeah, I know, I was always good at school. She is wearing a skirt. That's all I have to say.

Therapist: Yes, Sam, you've pointed out something very important to us.

Sam: Yeah, there are no other important things to say.

Paul: Well, she's got long hair.

Will: Yes, long brown hair.

Helen: Like I used to have.

Therapist: Fine, so up to now . . . (Steven interrupts him).

Steven: Her hair could be brown, but then again it might actually be black. I don't think so though, more like brown since there are small freckles or something on her cheeks. She's got a necklace or a small chain around her neck.

Therapist: Good, Steven, you took a very good look. Quite right.

Will: Yes, it's made of wood or something like that, something brown in any case. And there's a second one too, but that one is made of silver.

Helen: And her skirt is purple.

Therapist: Good, Helen you've pointed out something else, but for now let's concentrate on the face. Steven, Sam, Paul, and Will have discovered many things in this picture: a woman with long brown hair, dark brown eyes, and a dark complexion. She has freckles or something like that on her cheeks and is wearing two necklaces, one of which is longer than the other. One is probably wooden, and one is made of silver.

Helen: Oh dear, she doesn't have any teeth.

Paul: That's true, you can't see her teeth at all.

Therapist: Good, Helen and Paul, you've pointed out something important that hasn't been mentioned yet.

Sam: Yes, but probably you just can't see her teeth, and it's not as if she didn't have any.

Will: When your mouth is open, I can't see your teeth either, because your lips cover them.

Therapist: Very good, Will, you've pointed out that if the mouth is open one doesn't necessarily see the teeth. (Pause)

Therapist: Can anyone describe the woman's open mouth in more detail?

> **Sam:** Well, I'd say it's half open.
> **Phil:** You can see the lips covering the mouth, and you can see the dark inside of her mouth.
> **Helen:** Yes, the mouth is open, otherwise you couldn't see inside her mouth.
> **Therapist:** That was a good observation Helen and Phil.
> **Phil:** Helen is right. If the mouth were closed, you wouldn't see a dark spot. The girl's or woman's mouth is half open just like mine (he demonstrates), but there is not much else to say about her really.
> **Therapist:** Good, Phil, you've shown what her mouth looks like in the picture (pause) – and Paul, what do you think?
> **Paul:** Well yeah, there is nothing special about her than the fact that her mouth is open.
> **Helen:** The girl has her mouth open because you can see the lips around the mouth and the darkness inside her mouth.

Especially for patients with a perceptional deficit, the introduction into this exercise should be quite clearly structured (e.g., focusing the attention on a certain point). If the exercise is not structured enough, it can become confusing. Furthermore, the therapist needs to provide feedback to every statement coming from a group member.

Example

Ineffective Approach for Information Gathering that Should Be Avoided: Imprecise Introduction

> **Therapist:** Ok, let us start. What can we see here? (Silence) Adam, what do you see?
> **Adam:** A red piece of cloth.
> **Therapist:** And Barbara?
> **Barbara:** Yes, a red piece of cloth.
> **Therapist:** Clive?
> **Clive:** Yes, that is what I see too.

The method of questioning in the example above is confusing especially for persons with perception disorders. The therapist neither provided a structure by asking group members to focus on various parts of the picture nor did he give any feedback concerning their verbal contributions. Because of their inability to distinguish relevant from irrelevant stimuli as well as their distractibility, the group members can easily become overburdened and confused by an unstructured approach. The patients typically react either with silence, because they are incapable of finding the correct stimulus within the multitude of stimuli, or they respond with disinterest and might even become oppositional to further instructions from the therapist. Another reaction of group members to such a therapeutic approach may be the repetition of previous statements serving as internal anchors, which helps in organizing stimuli and resolving uncertainty. Rather

B5: Implementation

than improving visual perceptional skills, the method of questioning mentioned may actually reinforce disturbed visual perception.

Example

Ineffective Approach for Information Gathering That Should Be Avoided: Rejection

Therapist: What details do you notice about the woman's face?
Adam: The woman is unhappy.
Therapist: Now, Adam, you've given us an interpretation. However, as you know, right now we are just gathering visual information.

When interpretations are expressed in the first step, the group member should not be corrected, as this may be perceived as hurtful and might discourage further contributions.

Example

Appropriate Approach for Information Gathering

Therapist: That is a very important point, Adam. However, it is an interpretation, and we will come back to that later in Step 2. For now we are just gathering visual information: details we can see in the picture. Is that OK, Adam, to come back to your interpretation later?

Step 2: Interpretation and Discussion

In practice, it is difficult to separate the interpretation of a picture's content and the discussion of these interpretations. It has proven useful, however, to discuss interpretations of pictures continuously right after concluding the first step of gathering information. In general, the group finds one or two interpretations of a slide (in rare cases of very complex and ambiguous pictures even three) and is capable of coming to an agreement concerning these interpretations. The therapist should remain noncommittal throughout the interpretation phase, so that the group members cannot easily identify a "correct" interpretation, but rather engage in thoughtful reflection and consideration. This is possible only if the details from Step 1 can be used consistently as arguments to defend the different opinions. By means of such discussions, cognitive dissonances in group members can be resolved instead of their just adopting group consensus. As the discussion progresses, the therapist relates the different interpretations and arguments to one another, summarizes what has been said so far, asks if there is now consensus, and invites the members to enumerate the details of the picture again.

Step 2 should be continued until all group members accept and understand one or two (maximum three) comprehensible interpretations based on the visual information gathered in Step 1. Important therapeutic techniques are illustrated using the picture used previously as an example for the information gathering, and a rather long therapy excerpt is used to demonstrate the structured course of action implicated in the interpretation and discussion.

– *Facilitating interpretation:* "Yes, Paul, can you tell us, which expression you see in her eyes?"
– *Testing the interpretation:* "Very well, Paul, how do you account for that?"
– *Encouraging group discussion:* "What do the rest of you think?"

The following therapy excerpt illustrates the procedural techniques mentioned above. The slide used for the example is the one used in the previous example of information gathering.

Example

Therapist: What expression is in her eyes?

Steven: Maybe she's about to call out to someone.

Therapist: Yes, that's a possibility. And how did you decide that?

Steven: Well, she might be calling out to someone because she's got her mouth open, because she's turned away from us, and because you can see the darkness in her mouth.

Paul: No, I don't think so.

Therapist: Why is that, Paul?

Paul: Because of her eyes.

Steven: Yeah, but the way she's looking through the window, maybe she's calling her child.

Will: Yes, she's turning toward her child and is shouting something.

Therapist: Those are interesting thoughts, Steven and Will, but do we see any children in the picture?

Will: Hmmm . . .

Therapist: We see only a woman at a window. Let's look at her face again. What is the expression of her face, Sam?

Sam: She seems frightened.

Steven: I agree, she's scared. Just look at the eyes, you can see the whites of her eyes.

Therapist: And what do you think, Paul?

Paul: I agree, she's shouting something out the window. She is standing right at the window and her mouth is open.

Therapist: Paul suggested studying the eyes more closely. That's a good suggestion, Paul. One can indeed see the whites of her eyes. Does that tell us something about the expression on her face?

Will: Yes. If you can see the white, that's a sign of fright.

Therapist: What do you think, Sam and Phil? What is your opinion about her eyes and the interpretation offered by Steven and Paul?

Sam: No, that doesn't fit. I don't think so. I think that she's looking at something in the street that frightens her.

Therapist: What's the most important clue to your impression that she's frightened?

Sam: Well, first of all her eyes. They're so wide open you see the whites.

Paul: Yes, that is the way I see it too. If you're just calling out to someone, you don't open your eyes so wide you can see that much white.

Therapist: Fine, Paul, your reasoning is quite clear. What do you others think about it?

Phil: I don't believe that the woman is calling out to someone either. I think she's frightened. When I shout, I don't open my eyes this wide. Also her cheeks are very tense. People don't have such tense cheeks when they are calling out to someone, unless they are shouting really loud.

Therapist: That's a very good and detailed explanation. Helen, what do you think?

Helen: Phil is right. If the woman were calling out to someone, she would have put her hands around her mouth and use them like a megaphone. To me, her eyes are open too wide and her eyebrows are raised too high. When you're frightened, you automatically push up your eyebrows. When calling out you don't.

Therapist: Helen, that was a clear explanation. What do you think Steven?

Steven: Well, hmm, the others are right. When shouting, the eyes close, the pupils don't open, and the cheeks aren't all that tense.

Therapist: It seems that you all agree that her face has an expression of fear because of her wide-open eyes with dilated pupils and the whites showing, her wide-open mouth, and her tense cheeks. (Therapist looks around the group, and all nod.)

Therapists should never give interpretations of slides nor should they take sides with one of the patients. It is the patients' task to come up with interpretations – not the therapist's. Whenever this is not the case, the patients no longer need to actively deal with cognitive dissonances between details, interpretations, and reasoning, so that the goal of an active reconstruction of interpretational schemata would be missed.

The following examples serve to illustrate frequently observed errors in therapeutic techniques:

Example

Ineffective Approach for Interpretation and Discussion that Should Be Avoided: Therapist's Interpretation

Therapist: Until now, we've only gathered information. Now that we've described the situation thoroughly, let's go on to the interpretation step. For me, the picture shows an astonished or frightened woman, because her mouth and eyes are open very wide. Her eyes are so wide open you can even see the whites all round her pupils. Do you agree, Adam?

Example

Ineffective Approach for Interpretation and Discussion that Should Be Avoided: Therapist Taking Sides with Someone

Barbara: She's calling out to someone. Her mouth is open.
Clive: No, that's wrong. With shouting the eyes aren't open so wide.
Therapist: Yes, Barbara, I agree with Clive. You should take a closer look at the eyes.

Discussions about facts that cannot be resolved, given the information on the slide, are seldom productive. In all stages of the exercise, it is important for the group members to deal with visible elements of the picture. When the discussion degenerates into speculation, the therapist needs to intervene. The following example clarifies procedures for dealing with this problem.

Example

Therapist's Intervention when Patients Speculate During Interpretation and Discussion

Barbara: The woman is frightened because she sees an unexpected guest.
Clive: No, she's frightened because she sees a canary fly by.
Barbara: No, that's wrong. She sees an unexpected guest.
Therapist: Clive and Barbara are discussing the causes of the woman's fright. Now, we only have the picture. Can we determine what is causing the fright by looking at the picture? What do you think Dave?
Dave: No, we can't.
Emily: That's right, it's only a single picture, not a whole movie.
Clive: Of course we can't tell for sure, but it's possible that a canary flew by.
Barbara: Sure, but it's just as possible that she has a visitor.
Therapist: As I've noted, we all understand that we cannot know the reason for her fright. It is, after all, only one single picture. Possibly the cause is as Clive or Barbara says, but we can't decide from the information in the picture.

Step 3: Assigning a Title

Once Step 1 and Step 2 have been completed, the therapist asks the group members to find a title for the picture. The title should reflect the most important aspects of the picture (especially the interpersonal aspects, if the picture contains more than one person). Each group member should think of a title, and the titles are then written on the blackboard. If there are cotherapist(s), they give their title(s) last in order not to influence the group members. Then the group discusses which is the most appropriate title.

If a title is given that appears to have little to do with the visual information in the picture, the therapist should inquire as to how the group member came up with that title. This inquiry may generate new group discussion.

Example

Therapist's Approach to Assigning a Title

Therapist: Very good, now let us all think about a title for this picture.
Phil: A Frightened Woman.
Sam: Maybe *The* Frightened Woman would be better.
Helen and Phil (simultaneously): Yes, The Frightened Woman.
Will: I like that too.
Paul: Well, it doesn't matter to me whether it's "a" or "the." They're both OK.
Therapist: I feel the same way. OK then, we will end our session for today.

Concluding this section, we give some therapeutic methods and guidelines that are applicable to all the subprograms, but are especially important in conducting the Social Perception subprogram:

- *Addressing by name:* Group members should always be addressed by name. The impersonal "you" can cause confusion.
- *Acknowledging contributions:* Acknowledge all contributions of group members through a brief repetition of the information/opinion, to affirm the importance of their contributions and reinforce their participation.
- *Reinforcing long-term patients:* Especially at the beginning, long-term patients need a lot of social reinforcement from the therapist in order to make verbal contributions. The mere courage to make verbal contributions should be reinforced.
- *Preventing dominance and caginess:* Both therapists and cotherapists need to make sure that none of the group members become too dominant or withdraw themselves too much. Higher functioning group members who tend to dominate should be given special duties like summarizing the statements made in the group, so they do not get bored.
- *Relaxed posture:* The therapist(s) should assume an easy-going, relaxed style in the group. A stiff, authoritative manner may convey insecurity and fear, which makes it difficult to lead the group.
- *Introduce short role-plays:* Difficulties in understanding interpretations (especially regarding facial expressions) are often resolved by a brief role-play by one of the therapists containing the problematic facial expression.
- *Let details be pointed out:* In order to clarify visual details as well as to establish group activities and interactions, it is useful to ask group members to go directly to the screen and point out details. For example, "John, would you please show us where you see that?"
- *No devaluating comments:* Therapists should never respond to "wrong" or inadequate interpretations in a pejorative way. This is especially important in regard to

the discussion of interpretations that are not based on the visual information in the picture.

– *Intervention:* The therapist(s) should intervene if group members make hostile or demeaning comments about another group member's interpretation. For example, "Every interpretation is useful in learning to understand social situations. For this reason we will listen to all interpretations."

– *No rush:* The structured and directive procedures for dialog should provide ample time for group members to reflect and formulate responses. Some group members need extra time to organize their thoughts. Continually asking group members to voice their thoughts may be counterproductive.

– *Summarizing:* Consolidating summaries have an important role in all of the subprograms. Repetition of important information is especially helpful for group members with attentional deficits or deficits of sensory-motor information processing, and can improve their attentional focus and memory for significant details

– *Not getting gridlocked:* Inexperienced therapists may easily get stuck with vague or ambiguous details in Step 1. If the detail in question is not highly relevant to the interpretation, allow some vagueness to persist and direct the group members' attention to another part of the picture.

– *Goal:* The main therapeutic objective of the Social Perception subprogram is to learn how to adequately perceive people and interpret social situations (emotions and affects, social interaction). Therapeutic procedures should be directed toward attaining this objective. For example, it is not important to describe the picture's background in detail if these details are irrelevant to understanding the social content of the picture.

– *"Irrelevant" details are often the precondition:* For the description of a slide (Step 1) it is possible to start with "irrelevant" contents, since they are often the prerequisite for an adequate perception of people.

5.4 Verbal Communication

The description of this subprogram is divided into two sections. The first section provides information and examples on how to prepare group members for the Verbal Communication subprogram in order to motivate them to accomplish it. The second section describes the five steps of the subprogram in detail. The complete therapy materials can be found in the Appendix.

5.4.1 Introducing the Subprogram

The Verbal Communication subprogram acts as a transitional link between the practice of basic cognitive functions and the more complex skills involved in social competence. Thus, the completion of the first two subprograms is often a prerequisite for beginning the first part of the Verbal Communication subprogram (Step 1 an 2). During this subprogram the highly structured exercises, which are particularly helpful for schizophrenia patients to support the group setting, decrease and group interaction increases. This means that the group members need a higher level of mental resilience than in the previous subprograms.

As in the previous subprograms, two or more exercises may be conducted during a single session (e.g., Social Perception for 30 minutes, Verbal Communication for 30 minutes).

Visual Aids

The therapists should make as much use as possible of visual aids, such as overhead projector, blackboard, and individual notepads, in order to provide additional structure and assistance in focusing attention.

Motivating the Patients

Before conducting the first Verbal Communication exercise in the group, patients should be motivated with the following procedure: The therapist explains to the patients that the cotherapist will whisper a sentence into his neighbor's ear that will then need to be passed on around the circle. The last patient to receive the message then writes it on the blackboard.

Example

Therapist's Approach to Introducing Verbal Communication

Therapist: Did everyone understand the task? (No reaction.) Roger and Zoe (low-functioning group members with attentional disorders), did you understand the task? (They nod.) Zoe, can you please repeat the task so that it is clear to everyone what we will be doing?

Zoe: Whisper a sentence to one another around the circle.

Therapist: Correct. You are to pass on a sentence. What is Wanda (the last person in the circle) to do, Roger?

Roger: Write the sentence on the blackboard.

Therapist: This is correct. Mr. A. (the cotherapist), would you please whisper the message to Ms. O.?

(The co-therapist whispers a sentence, for example, "The fish in the village lake will be fed tonight at six p.m." to Ms. O., who passes it on to Jake, etc., until it eventually reaches Wanda, who then writes it on the blackboard.)

Therapist: Thank you Wanda. Mr. A., would you write the original sentence on the blackboard? (Usually there is a large discrepancy between the two sentences.)

The therapist explains, "Often the information in a message changes and is passed on incorrectly, since it has been passed on a number of times. Incorrect messages create misunderstandings between people. In the following sessions we will be practicing how to listen, understand, and pass on information."

The explanation of Step 1 of the Verbal Communication subprogram can be given directly after this exercise. As shown in the example, the therapist does not accept "yes/no" answers. He insists on getting a concrete answer, in order to ensure that the patients really understood the task. In groups it is often noticed that some "clever" members answer the question with "yes" whether or not they have understood the task. This is why it is important to ask open questions that cannot be answered with a single word. For instance, after a statement given by Jim, the therapist asks John: "John, what do you think about Jim's statement?" (open question), rather than: "John, do you agree with Jim?" (question requiring a "yes/no" answer). The therapist might also discuss examples of communication difficulties experienced in previous groups as a means of motivating group members to participate in the exercises.

The extent to which the group needs to be motivated at all to participate in this new subprogram depends greatly on the group's experiences with the first two subprograms. Group cohesion, the value of the group as a form of social reinforcement, and feeling toward other group members and the therapist(s) play important roles in determining the level of motivation to participate. Even if the group members are motivated to participate in the program, the introductory exercise should be carried out, since group members usually enjoy the exercise.

5.4.2 Description of the Subprogram's Different Steps

The subsequent examples illustrate the different steps of the Verbal Communication subprogram. They are excerpts from an actual therapy group with five group members (Jake, Victor, Wanda, Roger, and Zoe) and three therapists (Mr. K., Ms. O., Mr. R.).

Step 1: Literal Repetition Exercise

The therapy material for this exercise consists of cards with one or more sentences written on them. The sentences vary on two dimensions: number of words (5–10, 11–15, and 16–20) and emotional content (emotionally neutral and emotionally loaded, see Worksheet 8). At the beginning of the exercise emotionally neutral sentences with 5–10 words should be used. As group members start mastering the exercise with short, emotionally neutral sentences, one can increase the length of the sentences. Once the patients master longer, emotionally neutral sentences, short sentences with emotional content are introduced into the exercise.

The following example is an excerpt of a therapy session in which all group members were present. Mr. K. was the primary therapist, Ms. O. the cotherapist; Mr. R. was not present. In the previous session, the therapists introduced the Verbal Communication subprogram to the group with the "whispering exercise."

B5: Implementation

Example

Therapist's Approach to Literal Repetition of Given Sentences

Therapist: I would like to welcome all of you to this session. Last time we met, we did an introductory exercise in which we passed on a message from one group member to the next. Do you all remember? (General agreement.) Today, just like the last time, we will practice transmitting information correctly. Jake, may I give you this card? There is a sentence written on it. (Jake nods.) It is your job to read the sentence slowly to the whole group. Ms. O. (the cotherapist) will then try to repeat the sentence literally. Jake, I would like you and the other members of the group to listen carefully to see if Ms. O. is able to repeat the sentence, word by word. Okay? (Mr. K. turns to Zoe, who seems somewhat distracted).

Therapist: Zoe, today we are starting a new exercise. Could you please repeat the task for today?

Zoe: (Hesitates and appears anxious.) Jake is to read a sentence aloud. (Hesitates, is unsure of herself.)

Therapist: That is correct. Jake is going to read the sentence on his card aloud. What will you do then, Jake?

Jake: I listen to see if Ms. O. repeats my sentence correctly.

Therapist: This is correct. Ms. O. is to repeat the sentence, literally. And what should the group do, Wanda?

Wanda: We are to listen and find out whether she repeats the sentence correctly word by word.

Therapist: Is that correct, Roger and Victor? (They both nod.) Right, that is correct. Is the exercise clear to you now Zoe? (She nods in agreement.)

As in all the exercises of the therapy program, it is very important for the therapist to give informative feedback. All verbal comments (with the exception of obvious attempts to disrupt the group, which are ignored) should be reinforced immediately.

This is of particular importance for low-functioning, withdrawn group members. Higher-functioning group members should be requested to perform the exercise first, in order to provide role models for low-functioning, insecure, or fearful group members. If low-functioning group members are reluctant to participate, the therapist should not push them, though the therapist does need to make sure all group members have understood the task before starting with the exercise (as in the example with Zoe). As mentioned before, once the patients have adequately reproduced short, emotionally neutral sentences, the group continues with longer sentences – and only once the group has also mastered longer neutral sentences can the emotionally loaded sentences be introduced.

Step 2: Paraphrasing Exercise

Similarly to the previous step, the therapy materials used in the phrasing exercise consists of small cards containing stimuli that vary in emotional load. However, this time only one or two words are written on the cards. One of the group members is asked to formulate one or two sentences including the word(s) written on the card. Another group member then reproduces the sentence(s) analogously. The task of the other group members is to control whether or not the analogously reproduced sentence is correct. As in the previous exercise, it is important to start with emotionally neutral, single-word cards (Worksheet 9).

The following example, illustrating the paraphrasing exercise, is drawn from the same group as in the previous example (Ms. O. is the primary therapist and Mr. K. is the cotherapist). The example begins in the middle of a session. The group has already carried out a social perception exercise as well as a literal repetition exercise and is in the midst of the paraphrasing exercise.

Example

Therapist's Approach to Paraphrasing Sentences

Therapist: Wanda, I will hand you this card. Could you, please, read out the word written on it to the group?

Wanda: "Summer"

Therapist: Yes, "Summer." Would you formulate one or two sentences containing the word "summer," please? Your neighbor, Jake, is then to reproduce these sentences analogously.

Wanda: Summer is too hot for me. I always stay in the ward then, because I don't like to go out.

Therapist: Now, Jake, would you please give us a sentence or two that has approximately the same meaning as Wanda's sentences?

Jake: Summer is too hot for me. I always stay in the ward then, because I don't like to go out.

Therapist: Thank you, Jake. Wanda, was that correct?

Wanda: Yes it was exactly correct.

Therapist: Do the rest of you agree? (They nod.) Jake, you paid very close attention. You repeated the sentences word by word, even though the idea was for you to come up with a sentence with similar meaning.

The above example illustrates several therapeutic steps: First of all, the word on the card is read to the group aloud; subsequently, the patient forms a sentence with that exact word (verb stays verb, etc.); a different group member then paraphrases this sentence. Either the therapist or a patient assigned to do so decides whether or not the sentence was in fact correct. As illustrated in the example, a group member may repeat the sentence literally instead of paraphrasing it. Rather than saying the answer was "wrong," the therapist tells the patient that he did more than he needed to do. To prevent the patients from literal reproductions, the therapist can ask the group members to form longer sentences.

If the tasks of Steps 1 or 2 are not fulfilled completely, the therapist can either ask the other group members for corrections or the group can start the exercise over. If, however, the exercises of Steps 1 and 2 overburden the group, the therapist should first provide visual aids (overhead projector/blackboard). During Step 2 it is helpful in any case if the cotherapist writes down the sentences formed (better means of control).

Furthermore, the example illustrates that the group is engaged in two subprograms (Social Perception and Verbal Communication) as well as in two steps (1 and 2) in parallel. This is useful, on the one hand, in order to maintain prior learning effects over time; on the other hand, it encourages generalization to other areas. In addition, the practical application of the program shows that repetition of familiar exercises involves a great deal of reinforcement. This is the case because patients successfully perform exercises they already know well. For this reason, it is also recommended to repeat familiar exercises if new elements provoke fear and insecurity.

Finally, a structured order of answering during Steps 1 and 2 can also reduce fear in the patients. A useful way of structuring the exercise is to go around the circle and always have the person next to the speaker repeat or paraphrase the formed sentence. This structure also makes it easier for the therapist to keep track of who has already contributed in the exercise and who has not. A different way of making the exercise more predictable would be to tell the group who will be asked to give an answer before explaining the task. The opposite strategy (name after explaining the task) requires the greatest amount of attention.

Once the group has started mastering the tasks to the point that they no longer provoke fear, it makes sense to drop the high degree of structure and apply the latter strategy: If the degree of structure is too high, the patients might get bored with the exercise and lose their motivation. If, however, the group starts getting chaotic and several members speak at the same time, returning to more structure by reintroducing an order of speaking (e.g., in a clockwise circle) is recommended. This makes it easier to focus on the tasks again. Step 3 should be introduced only after all group members have mastered the two previous steps. The following steps are all based on one another, so that the therapist can return to a previous step if an exercise still seems difficult.

Step 3: W-Questions

The therapy material for this exercise consists of question words beginning with "w" (see Worksheet 10) as well as cards on which the group members can write down words. The therapist and the group members generate emotionally neutral and emotionally loaded themes, and the group is then asked to think of words associated with that theme. Again, it is important to start the exercise with emotionally neutral themes.

In the beginning, the primary therapist introduces a topic and writes it on the blackboard. To facilitate participation and motivation, it is very important to choose a topic all group members are interested in. The related words generated by the group members (approximately 30) are also listed on the blackboard. The therapist should make sure each group member generates at least one word associated with the theme. For each word listed, the group needs to decide whether the word is really associated with the topic. Question words beginning with "w" (why, when, who, what, etc.) are listed on a second blackboard or on an overhead.

Each group member is asked to pick a word from the related-words list and a question word from the other list and then combine them into a sentence, asking a question about the chosen topic. Group members take turns asking and answering the questions.

The evaluation of adequate communication is an important aspect of this exercise. The cotherapists monitor whether the question was related to the topic and whether the answer fits the question. Later, high-functioning group members can assume the functions of the cotherapists.

In the following example, the group was already acquainted with the exercise from previous sessions. All group members and three therapists were present. The primary therapist was Mr. R.

Example

Therapist's Approach to Formulated "W"-Questions and Answers

Therapist: Good morning everyone. Two days ago, at the end of the session, we agreed to talk today about environmental pollution. What do you think of when you hear the word pollution? Let's all take turns in stating a word or two that comes to mind. Ms. O., would you please write the words on the blackboard. Let's try and come up with about 30 words related to pollution. Wanda, why don't you start? (The group members rapidly call out words occurring to them: water, air, oil slick, radioactivity, dead fish, etc., until the cotherapist signals that 30 words have been gathered.) So, now each of you will receive four pieces of paper. Please write down one or two of the words written on the blackboard on each piece of paper, and form a question with a related word and a question word beginning with "w," as we have done previously. Has everyone understood the task? Victor, could you please repeat what you are asked to do now?

Victor: I have received four pieces of paper, and I am to write one of the words written on the blackboard on each paper.

Therapist: Correct, and what then, Roger?

Roger: Then we are to make up questions with the words on the paper.

Therapist: Exactly. Let's begin. (All participants write their words related to the topic on their papers.) Ms. O., would you please check whether the questions are related to the topic? And Mr. K., would you make sure the answers fit the questions? Zoe, please read out your first word related to the topic and the question you have written using a question word beginning with "w." (Question words beginning with "W" are written on the blackboard or overhead projector.)

Zoe: Water (long pause) – how does water get to the earth?

Cotherapist: Stop, the question does not fit the topic.

Therapist: Zoe, could you please explain how your question relates to the topic? (No answer.) What is the theme, Zoe?

Zoe: Oh, I forgot.

Therapist: Victor, do you know what the theme is?

Victor: Environmental pollution.

Therapist: That's correct. Zoe, you are supposed to use the word "water" and one of the "w" words on the blackboard to formulate a question fitting the context of environmental pollution. (Zoe nods.)

Zoe: What is water polluted by?

Therapist: Yes, that's correct. And who would you like to answer your question, Zoe?

Zoe: Wanda

Wanda: For example, in the ocean by the oil leaking from ships.

Therapist: Good. The question is related to the topic, and the answer fits the question. Roger, would you please ask the next question?

The therapist(s) should use expressions the group members are familiar with, and their instructions need to be short and precise. Moreover, they need to give feedback.

In some groups the transition from the paraphrasing exercise to the w-question exercise may be difficult. If group members find it difficult to form a question using a related word and a w-word, the therapist needs to jump in and assist. It is also possible to have two group members work together. Once the group masters the task of asking questions, Step 4 can be introduced:

Step 4: Asking Questions About a Topic

No standard therapy materials are used in this step. This exercise is not only closely related to everyday life, but also very demanding for the group members. It is best to direct the questions to a team consisting of a single group member and a cotherapist. Rather than in the usual circle, the group now sits in a semicircle around the cotherapist and the group member who have to answer the questions. Initially, the exercise consists of group members asking questions of the cotherapist and the designated group member about a topic the group has agreed on at the beginning of the exercise. As the group members become more comfortable with this exercise, they may answer questions without the assistance of the cotherapist. The therapist should divide the topics the group has chosen into an emotionally neutral and an emotionally loaded category, and initially use only emotionally neutral themes. Topics might include newspaper headlines the group is interested in, with the group members asking questions in order to find out more about the article. Other possible topics might be weekend activities recently experienced by the group members, short trips planned, etc. The idea is to pick topics that are relevant and of interest to the group members. The group should be challenged by the topic but not overburdened. If the group or certain members do not want to deal with a particular topic, they should not feel forced into it. Question and answer evaluations, such as "Is the question relevant to the topic?" or "Does the answer respond to the question?" are initially performed by the cotherapist. Later higher functioning group members can take on this task.

The following example, which commenced 15 minutes after the beginning of the session, is an excerpt from an exercise in which the group questioned the cotherapist (Ms. O.) and the group member Roger on a newspaper article with the headline "Multiple Car Crash on the Highway." The cotherapist and Roger have already read and briefly discussed the article in order to prepare themselves. All group members and three therapists were present. Mr. K. was the primary therapist.

Example

Therapist's Approach to Questioning Group Members About a Specific Theme

Therapist: Wanda, we have now heard a lot about the accident. Could you please summarize what we know?

Wanda: The accident happened at 7 p.m. last Friday in vacation traffic. During a heavy rain 31 cars ran into one another. (Pause.)

Therapist: Thank you, Wanda. That was a lot of information already. Victor and Jake, is there anything more to say?

Victor: The drivers didn't keep enough distance from each other. The accident caused material damage of US$20.000.

Jake: And 9 persons were slightly injured.

Therapist: Very well, you remembered that very precisely. That's probably all, or have we forgotten anything? (Looks around the group.)

Zoe: The accident caused a traffic-jam of about 30 miles.

Therapist: Well done for remembering all that. You listened very carefully. Zoe, would you like to ask the next question?

Zoe: Was the highway closed?

Therapist: Roger, this question is for you.

Roger: Well, I think so, but I'm not sure.

Co-therapist: (helping him) The highway had to be closed completely on the side the accident happened.

Therapist: Jake, now it's your turn to ask a question.

Jake: How long was the highway closed for?

Roger: I don't remember.

Co-therapist: Four and one-half hours.

Therapist: Good, Victor, why don't you ask the next question?

As the example shows, the interrogated group member should always be the first to respond. The cotherapist helps out only if the group member is unable to answer the question. If two group members are interrogated, they should take turns answering the questions. It can be helpful to periodically summarize the information presented. If group members are experiencing difficulty formulating questions or remembering information presented, use visual aids, such as the blackboard, for listing the w-question words or to sum up all the information. It is best to start the final step of the subprogram only after the group has mastered Step 4 quite well, without the use of visual aids.

Step 5: Focused Communication Exercise

This step is the conclusion of the subprogram Verbal Communication. The aim is to learn how to communicate adequately about a given topic. It is important for the group members to learn how to focus questions and comments on only one aspect of a topic. The evaluation of the communication process is central to this exercise. With particularly high functioning groups, the goals of this exercise can be broadened to include the evaluation of nonverbal aspects of communication (i.e., eye contact, tone and volume of voice, etc.) in addition to verbal aspects. This is, however, completely dependent on the group's level of functioning.

The primary therapist is highly challenged in this exercise, must firmly guide the discussion, and decide on the focus of the discussion. At the same time, however, it is important not to determine the direction of the discussion too strictly, since this may affect the group members' motivation and involvement. Initially, the cotherapist(s) evaluate whether the question asked is focused on the particular aspect of the topic being discussed, and whether the answer, in fact, fits the question. Later in the exercise these roles can be assigned to higher functioning group members.

In the following examples, all group members and three therapists were present. Ms. O. had the role of the primary therapist, and Mr. K. did the evaluation. The topic was "radioactive fallout from the explosion of the nuclear plant in Chernobyl." A number of newspaper articles on this topic had already been discussed in earlier sessions.

Example

Therapist's Structured Approach to Focused Communication

Therapist: We have now discussed this theme for about 10 minutes. At the beginning, I asked the question, "What would each of you do if an accident similar to Chernobyl were to occur within 40 or 50 km of your home?" Everyone gave an answer. There were several suggestions, and I think it would be good if we discussed Wanda's suggestion in more detail. After that we can talk about other suggestions. Wanda, could you please repeat your suggestion?

Wanda: I would be particularly cautious with food.

Therapist: Yes, that was your suggestion. What do the rest of you think about this suggestion? Mr. K., could you please listen to see if we only discuss being cautious with food? Zoe, what do you think?

Zoe: Nuclear plants are very dangerous.

Cotherapist: Stop. That comment is not related to food.

Therapist: Zoe, your comment is related to our general theme of the nuclear accident in Chernobyl, but now we are only discussing Wanda's comment about being cautious with food. (Zoe has a blank look on her face.) Wanda, could you please explain your suggestion again?

As the example shows, in most groups the therapist needs to provide structure and to animate the group to narrow the topic down to certain aspects.

The following example is the sequel to the previous one, occurring after 15 minutes of discussion about being careful with food.

Example

Setting a Focus During Communication

Therapist: I think we have thoroughly discussed this aspect now. What other aspects of the nuclear accident in Chernobyl would you like to discuss? Mr. A. has written the other suggestions on the blackboard. (Silence.) Roger, could you read aloud all the suggestions that are written on the blackboard? (Roger reads them aloud.) Thank you, Roger. So, what shall we discuss now? (More silence.) What does your silence mean? Are you interested in discussing further suggestions? Perhaps each of you could tell me your opinion on this.

Roger: As far as I'm concerned, I've had enough for today. I'd rather know what we do about radioactivity nowadays and discuss what could be done about it in the future.

Therapist: Are you talking about the radioactivity from Chernobyl that traveled to us in the cloud?

Roger: Yes.

Therapist: I think that is a good suggestion of how we can continue our discussion about this theme. Are there other suggestions? Does anyone want to join Roger in this discussion? (General agreement from the group.) Roger, could you and Victor listen to see if we only talk about the aspect of our topic you suggested? If we talk about other things, please raise your hand. (Roger and Victor nod in agreement.) Is the theme clear to everyone? (Agreement from the group.) So, who would like to say something about this matter?

The group has to generally accept the discussion focus the therapist has chosen, though if the group remains task-oriented and demonstrates great interest in some unplanned direction, the therapist should follow the interests of the group whenever possible. The therapist's task is then to provide structure and to give feedback about the communication process. Even though it is important to thoroughly plan each session, the direction a discussion finally takes depends on the group's interests and motivation. As in the previous step, it can be helpful to use articles from newspapers, short stories, figures of speech, or proverbs in order to find topics. Furthermore, it is possible to view finding a topic as the first theme of this step; this way the therapists usually receive a multitude of topics the group can talk about subsequently.

5.5 Social Skills

The description of the Social Skills subprogram is divided into two sections. The first section introduces the subprogram and outlines general considerations. The second section describes specific social skills training techniques via therapy excerpts. Therapy materials are listed in the Appendix (Worksheet 11–13).

5.5.1 Introducing the Subprogram

Group Size

The Social Skills subprogram is best carried out in small groups of four to five participants. Larger groups generally do not provide enough opportunities for practicing skills in the group setting. Smaller groups, however, are largely unproblematic. In a modified form, the social skills subprogram (and all other subprograms of IPT) can be used for individual therapy as well.

Team of Therapists

Ideally, three therapists carry out the Social Skills subprogram – one primary therapist and two cotherapists. However, the presence of two cotherapists is often not possible. If only one cotherapist is present, the primary therapist assumes the duties of the second cotherapist. In more advanced groups, a group member can often assume the actor role in place of a cotherapist.

Frequency and Duration of Therapy Sessions

Generally, the Social Skills training sessions are held twice a week, and they are best spaced in a way that there is enough time between sessions for group members to carry out in vivo exercises. The nature of the therapeutic work in this subprogram, which involves role-plays, often requires longer sessions, which can take 90 minutes; group members will need at least one break during such sessions. For this reason group members should be informed in advance about the need for longer sessions and planned breaks.

Decreasing the Degree of Standardization

To the extent that the significance of group processes increases over the course of the subprograms, the therapy material as well as the degree of standardization become less important. The therapy sessions are no longer characterized by given materials, but rather by a given course of action. The Appendix provides a choice of important exercise situations for Social Skills. All situations are grouped into categories depending on their content, and they have all proven useful in practice. However, it is important to see them merely as *suggestions* rather than as a standardized program. In practice, the situations should be adapted to the group's desires and can be expanded or decreased accordingly.

Gradual Increase of Emotional Level

As for the other subprograms, a steady increase of emotional load of the therapy's contents is important for the success of the Social Skills subprogram. Therefore, the therapeutic approach of this subprogram also consists of a low level of emotional load at the beginning and a steady increase thereafter. The emotionally neutral standard situations are characterized by a low degree of strain, the outcomes not being that risky.

Low-Risk Situations
Situations with a low risk factor are situations in which social interactions are highly predictable. The outcome of such situations is largely independent of the receiver's reaction. In other words, there is a high probability that the receiver will act according to the interactional goal. Within this category, it is possible to vary the degree of difficulty of exercise situations as follows:
– *Facilitation:* Rather than merely using the given descriptions of a situation, a concrete dialog can be formulated.
– *Obstruction:* The interactional goal, explicitly formulated in the defined situation, can instead be denoted implicitly.

Examples for low-risk situations are given in the Appendix (Worksheet 11). They are sorted according to their content of social interactions.

Higher Risk Situations
Once the group has truly mastered the role-plays, the situations can be drawn from the patients' actual lives (e.g., adequate interaction with other patients) in order to deal with them in a therapeutic setting. The outcomes of social interactions in higher risk situations do not necessarily lead to the desired interactional goal, since they are largely dependent on the receiver's reaction. The interactions are, therefore, much less predictable and a successful outcome much less probable than in low-risk situations. Of course, as before, it is possible to vary the degree of difficulty in such situations. In addition to the strategies already mentioned, the receiver can act contrary to the interactional goal. This severe manipulation of the exercise situation obviously also changes the goal of the therapy: It is now important to learn how to cope with frustrated interactional outcomes.

This method of complicating the task brings with it many risks. The therapy as a whole could be perceived as aversive, and the patients might feel guilty for not having reached the interactional goals, which in turn can foster negatively attributing failures to themselves. However, this seems to be a very important experience with respect to better generalizing therapy effects to daily life: The patients learn how to face and cope

B5: Implementation

with frustrating real-life social interactions. Nevertheless, it is important that only experienced behavioral therapists introduce such obstructions: The therapist needs to know how to assess and to minimize the risks such a situation can bring about. Furthermore, even in such exercises, the focus needs to be put on the successful outcome of the standard situation.

Examples of higher risk situations are given in the Appendix (Worksheet 12). Again they are sorted according to their content of social interactions.

Complex Situations

In complex situations, the demands made upon the social skills of the conversational partners are particularly high. This is because it is difficult to anticipate the essential parameters (e.g., number of interactions) that take place in normal conversations and, therefore, also in exercises that reflect daily life. Accordingly, it is difficult to estimate, or vary, the generally high degree of complexity in such situations. Moreover, it is hard to account for complex situations cognitively. Usually, only the central and vital contents of interactions can be written down in an abstract manner. Role-plays, which are based on such exercise-situations, can therefore often only be used therapeutically as an additional technique in the course of Interpersonal Problem Solving. Guidelines for the category "complex situations" are given in the Appendix (Worksheet 13). It can be helpful to explain the general idea of this subprogram in the introductory session, in order to minimize the fear of expectations and to increase motivation.

Video Equipment

Video equipment is a valuable tool for social skills training. It permits recording and playing back role-plays during therapy sessions. Video feedback effectively fosters the therapist's intentions of shaping the patients' behavior. It is easier for group members to understand verbal feedback about their performance if it is supported visually and they can see how they actually behave. In order to minimize the group members' concern caused by video recording, it is not recommended introducing it as a part of therapy before the group members have mastered the subprogram (from the fifth session on). It is important not to problematize the use of video recording beforehand. The more naturally the therapists handle the medium, the smaller the risk for patients to become frightened. It is generally possible to lead confused patients back to task-oriented contents by asking directive questions. The sequence in the following paragraph deals with the therapist's approach to such matters.

5.5.2 Description of the Subprogram's Different Steps

The following example, which illustrates the introduction of video equipment, is drawn from a relatively early social skills training session. The group consisted of three therapists, Mr. W. (primary therapist), Ms. B. (first cotherapist) and Ms. M. (second cotherapist), and five group members (Alice, Julie, Brian, Warren, and Mark). The session should always begin with a short review of the most important aspects from the previous session. The following sequence illustrates how the primary therapist can initiate such a review. Moreover, it shows the casual use of the video equipment.

Example

Introductory Review of Social Skills

Therapist: First, I would like to welcome all of you to this session. Today, we are in the video room because we will be taping this session. But you are all acquainted with video recording, aren't you? Some of you have already noticed that the camera is running. Warren . . .

Warren: Yes, the red light on the camera went on.

Therapist: Exactly. You're a good observer. So the camera is running now. Let's begin. Alice, could you please tell us what we did in our last session?

Alice: Role-playing. First you showed us something and then we practiced it.

Therapist: That is correct. And does anyone remember what the role-play situation was?

In this example the entire session was videotaped, though usually only short role-play sequences are recorded. During the Social Skills subprogram, videotaping makes sense in order to provide feedback for role-plays. In order to structure the patients' expectation of the therapy session, it is important to review (mainly) the central aspects of the last therapy session (technique, contents, goals, and objectives). In later parts of the Social Skills subprogram, reviewing consists of recalling and discussing homework exercises assigned in the previous session. Homework exercises may be perceived as stressful and should be introduced only after group members seem to master the role-play situations in the group quite well.

Step 1: Setting Up the Role-Play

After a review of the previous session and/or homework exercises, the therapist introduces a new role-play situation. One group member is asked to read out a role-play situation printed on a card. An example for such a situation would be the following:

"A patient from the ward who loves painting is in the common room, hanging up a picture he has just finished painting. You like the picture a lot." This situation deals with the topic of praise and appreciation: paying someone a compliment. This is a low-risk situation drawn from the Appendix. The difficulty of this example is that the interactional goal is not mentioned. In the standard model, however, the interactional goal is mentioned explicitly. In addition to the situation described, the goal is described as follows:

"You would like to tell the painter that you like his picture a lot, and for this purpose you approach him." If several situations dealing with the same topic have been discussed in previous sessions, one could leave out the description of the interactional goal, in which case the patients need to define goal of the situation themselves.

If some group members have a low level of functioning, the role-play situation should be written on the blackboard. This makes it easier to discuss the situations and their goals. The situation should be described in as much detail as possible by the patients.

Example

Therapist's Approach to Specifying Situations to Exercise

Therapist: Alice, could you please describe the situation as you might see it?
Alice: Well, a resident is hanging up a picture, a beautiful picture.
Therapist: Correct. What kind of picture is it?
Alice: One he has painted himself.
Warren: But we don't know what he has painted.
Therapist: That's true. We only know that he has painted a pretty picture. But we could imagine that it is a pretty landscape picture. So, the resident is hanging up the picture. Where does he hang it, Brian?
Brian: In the common room.
Therapist: Right. So he is hanging up his picture in the common room. Can you see the situation in your mind, Warren?
Warren: Yes.
Therapist: Would you please try to describe the situation once again in your own words?

When asking the group members to describe the role-play situation, it is important not to get caught up in time-consuming discussions of unnecessary details. In the previous excerpt, the therapist's suggestion to imagine the content of the picture demonstrates this danger. The reason for the therapist's suggesting imagining the content of the picture was that the therapist had brought a landscape picture to the session in order to carry out the role-play as realistically as possible. Later on, in the description of the role-play situation, the group members talked about the possible identity of the painter, presuming they were dealing with another resident they all knew well – who, in fact, did paint quite well. The therapists chose to leave the identity of the painter unclear since the resident they all knew was considered to be rather rude and gruff and may have affected the group members' motivation to complete the role-play. Instead they instructed the group members not to imagine anyone in particular.

If the interactional goal is not explicitly stated in the role-play situation, it is important for the group members to discuss possible objectives, decide on a specific goal, and determine the behavior needed to reach that goal, before starting the role-play.

While setting up the role-play, the therapist should explicitly state the association between the specific goal of a role-play and the respective abstract concept. For example, the therapist might say, "The specific goal for this role-play, 'Tell him I like the picture,' is one example of giving a compliment." Linking specific examples to abstract concepts is very important since abstraction plays a major role in generalization processes.

The following excerpt is a continuation of the example used to illustrate introduction of the role-play; once the group has decided on the goal, the next step is to have the group prepare a possible dialog to accomplish the goal.

Example

Therapist's Approach to Helping Define a Common Interaction Goal

Therapist: Who are the people who take part in the situation in the recreation room?
Alice: The painter.
Julie: And one of us. We are to imagine that we are there. That we see him put up the picture.
Therapist: You are both right. The painter is in the common room hanging up his picture and – this is very important – one of you is there too! So imagine you are watching him put up his picture. What would you do in that situation, Mark?
Mark: I would look at the picture.
Therapist: Uh-huh. As we said, you are looking at the picture and you like it. And what would you do then?
Brian: One could help him hang up the picture.
Therapist: OK, but let's imagine he's almost done hanging up the picture and doesn't need any help from us.
Julie: I would tell him that I like his picture.
Therapist: That's a good idea. So you would tell him you like his picture. What did we call that type of statement last time, Warren?
Warren: Giving a compliment.
Therapist: Right, exactly. Last time, we called this "Giving a compliment" or "showing recognition." Do you think you would also give a compliment, Mark?

Example

Therapist's Approach to Working Out a Dialogue Leading to the Defined Goal with the Group

Therapist: How would you begin the conversation with the painter?
Julie: First of all, I would ask him whether it really is his picture. Whether he really painted it himself.
Therapist: Fine. Now go ahead and ask. Imagine that Ms. M. is the painter.
Julie: Did you paint that yourself?
Second cotherapist: Yes, I did it myself.
Therapist: Thank you. Can all of you imagine starting out the conversation this way? Yes? Good, let's write Julie's suggestion on the blackboard.

The group members can develop dialogs for all the persons in the role-play or, as is often the case, just their own contributions. The following example demonstrates how each group member comes up with his or her own answer. The passive cotherapist takes the role of the painter. This is usually the way this subprogram is introduced.

Example

First cotherapist: I'll write "A" to indicate the sentences group members will say and "B" to indicate the sentences the painter will say. Could you please repeat the group member's sentence Mark?
Mark: Yes. Is that your picture?
First cotherapist: Was that correct Julie?
Julie: No. I said, "Did you paint that yourself?"
First cotherapist: Good. But the meaning is more or less the same, don't you think, Brian?
Brian: Yes, It's the same.
First cotherapist: Let's write both possibilities on the blackboard.
(He writes:
A: Did you paint that yourself?
A: Is that your picture?
B: Yes, I painted it.)

If group members have very different ideas about how the interaction should begin or proceed, preparation of possible dialogs may be difficult. The therapists should work with no more than two suggestions at a time – and that only if the suggestions are oriented toward achieving the same interactional goal. However, often several very similar suggestions are made concerning how to conduct the discussion, which makes the decision on how to continue the dialog relatively easy. Final decisions concerning the dialog are left up to the group members.

Continuing with the above example, group members decided on the following dialog:

A: I really like that!
B: Oh really?
A: Yes, I think you paint very well.
B: I am pleased to hear you like it.

Once the dialog has been written on the blackboard for everyone to read, the group members should give the role-play situation a title that describes its most important aspects. Group members are already familiar with this procedure from the Social Perception subprogram. The subject of the title should be the person initiating the interaction. In the example given above, group members assigned the title, "I give a compliment to a painter and his picture." Assigning a title to the role-play situation provides a last chance for the therapist to check whether all group members have indeed understood and retained the basic points of the role-play, before beginning the actual role-play. If a group member seems to have a very different view of what the title should be or simply agrees with others, without giving a reason, the therapist might need to inquire further as to their reason for assigning a particular title.

The next step involves a discussion of anticipated difficulties. It serves to decrease group members' fears and related anxieties. Persons with chronic schizophrenia frequently voice fears related to cognitive difficulties they experience, for example:
– "I'm afraid I will suddenly lose track, that I'll have a blackout concerning my text."
– "I'm scared that I might start getting twitches all of a sudden."
– "There's one long sentence, I'm sure I'll mess up."

In our example, group members who judged the role-play situation to be "fairly difficult" feared they would suddenly blush or start laughing. Such fears are often present at the beginning of the Social Skills subprogram. However, they appear to be associated with the relative novelty of performing role-plays and "revealing themselves" rather than with the actual difficulty of the role-play. The therapist should respect the fears voiced by group members and translate them into observable behavior, as accurately as possible. In our example, group members were assigned to observe different aspects of the speaker's behavior, such as the volume of the voice, how fast a person spoke, and whether or not the tone of voice was friendly. ("Please observe whether the person giving the compliment speaks in a friendly way or whether he or she sounds grumpy or even angry.") Usually a group member is assigned to observe whether the actors can keep up their roles or whether they start laughing. However, blushing and other kinds of uncontrollable behavior should not be observation criteria.

The last step before starting the role-play is to have the group members judge the difficulty of the role-play situation on a scale from 1 (*very easy*) to 6 (*very difficult*). To decrease anxiety and provide role models, it is recommended that higher functioning group members – who judge the role-play situation to be less difficult – commence the role-plays. In the previous example only one group member (Julie) considered the role-play to be "very easy," whereas all other members chose level 3 for the role-play situation. Because of the nearly equal ratings, the results of the self-judged level of difficulty could not be used to determine the order in which the group members should begin the role-play. In such cases, group members, together with the therapists, should work out the order in which the role-plays are carried out.

Another reason to ask group members to rate the perceived level of difficulty before engaging in the role-play is that it provides a comparison if the role-plays are rated again afterward. Group members usually tend to perceive the role-plays as less difficult after having played a situation, and this change in perception can sometimes be useful for reducing extreme, unwarranted anxiety. If, however, a group member judges the degree of difficulty to be greater after completing the role-play, this is a serious indicator that the group member is highly stressed and measures need to be considered to decrease the level of stress for this group member.

B5: Implementation

Step 2: Enacting the Role-play

A small "stage area" is prepared for performing the role-plays. The normal circle is opened up into a semicircle to make enough room to carry out the role-plays and to record them with the video camera.

First, the two cotherapists serve as role models: They perform the role-play before asking group members to participate. The following order has proven useful for giving feedback: first the group member (or the cotherapist) performing the role-play, followed by the group members observing specific aspects of the role-play performance, and then the other actor(s) (usually a cotherapist and/or higher functioning group members). Finally, the primary therapist summarizes all the feedback comments. The therapists should make sure all their feedback is of positive nature. In a demonstration role-play, the cotherapist, playing the person giving the compliment, purposely spoke very quietly. In the subsequent feedback, the group member responsible for observing the volume of voice promptly criticized him for his soft voice. The primary therapist reframed the negative comment of the observer into a positive request for increasing the volume of voice and the cotherapist re-enacted the role-play with a louder voice.

After the role-play has been performed by the cotherapists and the subsequent feedback session is held, group members participate in the role-plays themselves.

In the following excerpt, a continuation of the example above, a group member stands in the "common room" near the wall where the painter is hanging the picture.

Example

Therapeutic Approach to Enacting a Role-Play

Therapist: So, now it is your turn. Julie, would you like to carry out the first role-play?

Julie: Yes.

Therapist: Very good. And what have you been assigned to observe?

Julie: How fast people talk.

Therapist: If Julie is taking part in the role-play, she can't really attend to how fast people talk. Who would like to take over this role for her?

Brian: I can do that.

Therapist: You haven't been assigned anything else to observe?

Brian: No.

Therapist: OK, then you will be responsible for observing how fast people talk. Who are the other observers?

Mark: I am responsible for observing how loud people talk.

Alice: I am also an observer. I'll check if she sounds friendly or not.

Therapist: Fine. A final request to our observers. Pay close attention to what happens during the role-play, but please wait until the end of the role-play to discuss what you have observed.

Alice: After the role-play?

Therapist: Exactly. OK, Julie, could you perhaps stand over here? From here you can also see the blackboard.

Alice: I don't need to see the blackboard. I can remember what to say.

Therapist: Even better. Remember, you don't need to repeat what is written on the blackboard. The sentences written there are intended to help you in case you can't decide what to say. Try to speak freely and to use your own words as much as possible. Is everything clear or are there any questions? No? Well, then you can start, Julie.

After these instructions, the role-play starts. Ms. M., one of the cotherapists, is putting up a landscape poster on the wall, using adhesive tape.

Julie (observing her from some distance, her hands on her hips): Hello! Did you paint that picture yourself?

Cotherapist (Painter): Yes, I did.

Julie (looks at the picture with her head cocked to one side): I think it's a very good picture.

Cotherapist (Painter): You do?

Julie (with a rather serious look on her face): Yes, I do. I really like it.

Cotherapist (Painter): I'm really glad you like it.

Once the role-play is over, the actors remain where they are and the feedback discussion starts.

Example

Feedback for Patients' Role-Plays

Therapist: Thank you, Julie. Now let us begin our feedback discussion. How did it go for you, Julie?

Julie: Pretty well I think.

Therapist: Was it difficult for you?

Julie: Well . . . I found it quite easy.

Therapist: Good, as you expected, the role-play wasn't so hard for you. Let's see what the others observed. What did you observe, Brian?

Brian: I think she talked normally. I could understand her well. I think it was good what she did.

Therapist: Uh-huh. And you, Mark, what did you observe?

Mark: The volume of their voices.

Therapist: And how was the volume?

Mark: It was loud enough.

Therapist: Good. What did you observe Alice?

Alice: I would have spoken a little bit more kindly. You could understand it, but it could have been a little bit friendlier.

Therapist: How is that?
Alice: You mean, how could it be more friendly?
Therapist: Yes.
Alice: Oh, I don't know. Maybe she could have smiled more when speaking.
Therapist: I think that's a good idea. So you would make a suggestion that Julie smiled when speaking the next time.
Alice: Yes.
Therapist: Fine. Did you make any other observations, Warren?

The therapists' feedback has two main goals: to provide positive reinforcement and to make constructive suggestions for behavior modification. Problems like long-lasting self-doubt and strongly held negative self-statements can often be reduced or eliminated by the use of positive feedback. Following the observations of the group members, the therapists give their own feedback, making sure their statements are positive and clear. It is important to give specific and concrete suggestions for changes in behavior and to reformulate any negative statements of group members.

After the feedback, the therapist should propose playing the videotape of the role-play so the role-play participant(s) can examine their performance with reference to the feedback given. The videotape should be played only if the role-play participant(s) agrees to watch it. In our example, Julie agreed to have her role-play scene played back to her and the other group members. By means of the video, Julie was able to understand and accept the therapist's suggestions for behavioral modification, and she agreed to integrate them into a second role-play that followed immediately. In order to save time as well as for therapeutic reasons, the primary therapist should be the only one offering feedback if a group member participates in more than one re-enactment of the same role-play.

Group members now take turns carrying out the role-play and receiving feedback. Once all group members have completed a particular role-play, the therapist again asks the group members to judge the difficulty of the role-play. In the role-play illustrated above, Julie was the only group member who stuck with her original estimate of difficulty. All other group members judged the role-play as being easier than they had originally expected.

In order to help group members generalize the social skills they are learning, each therapy session ends with the assignment of a homework exercise to be completed for the next session. It is best to keep the homework task on an abstract level, such as "giving a compliment" or "making a request," to allow more freedom and flexibility in completing the task. Group members' experiences with completing homework should be discussed in the following session. The therapists should positively reinforce all efforts to complete homework assignments, in order to promote generalization of behaviors practiced in the role-plays. Group members who did not complete the exercise or who report having "failed" should receive encouragement. For group members who consistently refuse to do their homework, individual operant reinforcement programs can be motivating. In this subprogram, the role of the passive cotherapist can be progressively taken over by a group member.

In this subprogram, the social reinforcement should stick closer to everyday life than the previous subprograms. Intermittent and motivational reinforcement are used increasingly.

5.6 Interpersonal Problem Solving

The Interpersonal Problem Solving subprogram is the least standardized and structured one of all the subprograms. Our description of the subprogram is divided into two sections: The first section provides general information for conducting the subprogram, and the second section provides a description of the problem-solving steps through a series of therapy excerpts, drawn from a timespan of several sessions. The examples offered are meant to encourage and guide the reader in developing similar problem-solving strategies to address the particular problems of their group members. Unlike the descriptions of the previous subprograms, we want here to provide the reader with input on how to solve problems, rather than with a standardized procedure. An example of the therapeutic guideline is given in the Appendix. This guideline consists of a "problem list" that can be used to identify potential problems that can occur when living in a community.

The Interpersonal Problem Solving subprogram is behaviorally oriented and addresses personal problems identified by group members. This subprogram does not contain standardized therapy materials, however; rather, the procedure is defined in six steps leading to the solution of a problem which need to be conducted in sequence:

- Problem identification and anylysis
- Problem description
- Generating alternative solutions
- Evaluating alternative solutions
- Deciding on a solution
- Implementing the chosen solution(s)
- Subsequent feedback

5.6.1 Introducing the Subprogram

Setting

For the Problem Solving subprogram – as for the other subprograms discussed – a small group size has proven useful. It is easier in small groups to create an open and anxiety-free atmosphere, so essential for developing the confidence base needed to analyze personal behavior and work on problem solving. In order to find solutions, it can be useful to work with role-plays, which can subsequently be transferred into everyday life. The use of role-plays with the Social Skills subprogram implies that every group member is offered the same opportunity to practice their skills.

Team of Therapists

Because of the relatively unstructured and complex nature of this subprogram, it is important for the therapists to be well trained and experienced. Furthermore, it is recommended that two therapists lead the group and carefully coordinate their way of working together.

Duration of Therapy Sessions

Therapy sessions are normally held twice a week and are usually limited to 90 minutes (including breaks). As with the Social Skills subprogram, homework tasks are frequently assigned and require sufficient practice opportunities between sessions.

Increasing the Level of Emotional Strain

The Interpersonal Problem Solving subprogram focuses on identifying specific behavior patterns that are problematic for certain group members. This is why it is so important to adapt the approach to the patients' needs rather than applying highly structured methods. In order to slowly increase the level of emotional strain, it is recommended to start this subprogram with emotionally neutral contents that are not very stressful. If group members find it difficult to identify this type of problem, the therapist might choose a problem that is not necessarily directly related to the patients' situations. Starting with problems that are easy to solve enables the group members to familiarize themselves with the different steps of problem solving. As a general rule, highly emotionally loaded problems should be reserved for more "advanced" or stable patients. It is possible, for instance, to use important phases of rehabilitation as problem situations and approach them in a therapeutic, behavioral manner.

Standardized "Problem Lists"

In order to provide a basic repertoire of problems, the therapists can work with so-called "problem lists"; several North American researchers have developed such standardized lists with which most patients are familiar (e.g., Kopelowicz et al., 2006; Liberman et al., 1993). In practice, these problem lists can be implemented in very different ways. On the one hand, they can be used as memory aids for problems that certain aspects of rehabilitation might implicate. On the other hand, they can help therapists decide which problems might be worth addressing in the group. The Appendix contains various examples of such problem lists for the rehabilitation phase regarding preparation for life outside of the hospital (Worksheets 14–18). These lists can be used as inspiration for creating other such lists. In this example, the process of preparation is divided into different parts: "Activities outside the hospital and skills in everyday life," "Looking for an apartment," "Furnishing the apartment," "Living and working in a community," and "Moving."

B5: Implementation

5.6.2 Description of the Subprogram's Different Steps

The following therapy excerpts, drawn from several subsequent sessions, illustrate the six steps of problem solving and their proper sequence. The group consisted of two therapists (Mr. W. and Ms. M.) and three group members (Emma, Peter, and Daniel). Group members were being prepared for living in a community outside the clinic. During this preparation, all group members had begun voicing increased feelings of feebleness and fatigue. Behaviorally, these feelings manifested themselves in increased tardiness and decreased participation in the therapy.

Problem Identification and Analysis

A further analysis of the problem revealed that the feelings of feebleness and fatigue were generalized and affected a number of areas of functioning. Family members and other attachment figures noted a change in attitude and a general drop of motivation regarding the planned move into the living community. In individual sessions, the three group members expressed feelings of stress and fear of failure. By expressing these feelings, the group members even seemed to reinforce one another in a very subtle way. Moreover, the occupational therapist noticed a decline in productivity, and the exercise therapist observed an increased clumsiness in two of the three group members.

We responded to this situation with a number of interventions: We broached the issue of fears in supportive individual sessions, individually reinforced punctuality, and suspended the preparations for the move to living communities in favor of working with the problem of feebleness. In order to prepare the therapeutic work, we developed a questionnaire for self-observation and self-assessment, resembling a timetable. The patients were asked to evaluate their subjective level of energy once an hour (from 7 a.m. to 7 p.m.) over the course of a week. The answers were given on the following 3-point scale:

0 = "During the past hour, I was far too tired and too slow."
1 = "During the past hour, I was a bit tired and a little slow."
2 = "During the past hour, I was not tired. I felt full of energy."

The self-evaluation form, which provided a quantitative expression of subjective energy levels, allowed group members to calculate both daily and weekly totals. The daily and weekly totals were used to monitor energy level changes in the course of therapy. Each group member's range of subjective fitness was used as a guide to the potential range of modification.

There were several goals associated with the use of the evaluation form. The first goal was to determine the extent of energy loss and its relationship to specific situations, for instance, to stimulus control. The second goal was to increase the patients' awareness of fluctuations in their energy level, which could be helpful in assessing the problem more realistically. Finally, based on research results concerning "self-handling," we hoped that the mere act of monitoring their own energy level would increase

B5: Implementation

their sense of self-control and associated feelings of well-being. Furthermore, this instrument was used to assess the progression of therapy.

Problem Description

One week before we started the therapeutic work on fatigue, the group members received a "fitness form" for self-evaluation, with clear, brief instructions. This detailed weekly overview of the group members' subjective energy levels marked the beginning of the problem description. The therapists decided to choose the concept of sports for future discussions of "fatigue" in relationship with well-being. For example, words like "fitness," "power," "efficiency," "lack of energy," and "exhaustion" were to be used to discuss their problem of fatigue and possible problem-solving strategies. The patients should first become acquainted with the possibilities and the significance of the "fitness form":

Example

Therapist's Approach to Cognitive Problem Description (I)

Therapist: So now we've added up your daily totals, what do you think about them?
Emma: I am amazed how fit I was that one day!
Peter: And how bad things were on another.
Therapist: Correct. Both of you have noticed something very important. Emma, you said that your daily total showed you how fit you were on a particular day. And you, Peter, noticed that your daily totals were very different. So you see which days you were the least fit and the least efficient.
Daniel: And you can see when we had the most energy.
Therapist: Exactly, Daniel. Now, I would like you all to do something for me. Would each of you please choose the day on which you felt the least fit?

As illustrated in this excerpt, a discussion about the ratings on the self-evaluation form allowed group members to gain a clearer understanding of the problem. After comparing the daily totals, we had a look at the fluctuation of fitness throughout a day. The insight that the fluctuations were sometimes remarkable motivated the patients to search for the reasons for such fluctuations. Even though it was not possible to determine clear situational reasons for subjective fitness to rise and fall, the patients worked out that a high level of fitness was related to general well-being and enjoyable experiences. Therapeutically, the most important consideration the patients came up with was the fact that the fluctuations could be due not only to medication: The fluctuations were not compatible with the effects of the medication, which is supposed to be continuous. Consequently, we interpreted the difference in subjective levels of fitness the patients experienced as evidence that personal potential is manipulable and, therefore, treatable.

> **Example**
>
> **Therapist's Approach to Cognitive Problem Description (II)**
>
> **Therapist:** Have you thought about the fact that you have various levels of fitness? As I recall Daniel, you had daily totals ranging from 11 to 19.
> **Daniel:** Yes, that is a big difference.
> **Co-therapist:** Was that what you expected?
> **Daniel:** Well no. I didn't expect it to be so different.
> **Therapist:** Uh-huh. And what do the rest of you think about this?
> **Emma:** My span was not as big. I have a large total over the entire week.
> **Therapist:** It must have been a good week for you then.
> **Emma:** Yes, it was a good week for me.
> **Peter:** My values vary widely, too. I only had one good day. I had 18 points on that day.
> **Therapist:** On Thursday.
> **Peter:** Yes.
> **Therapist:** Earlier you had said that you hadn't noticed till then that Thursday had been such a good day for you.
> **Peter:** That's true.
> **Therapist:** You seem surprised that you had such a high daily total.
> **Peter:** Well, I guess I didn't expect it.
> **Co-therapist:** Do you think that means something good?
> **Peter:** Having 18 points?
> **Co-therapist:** Yes.
> **Peter:** Yes, I think it's good.
> **Co-therapist:** I think your ratings show that feebleness and fatigue are not something constant, but that there are apparently great variations. Do you think you can help yourself to feel strong and fit, Emma?

Through the discussion of daily totals and daily variations in energy levels group members were able to work out a number of ways to positively influence feelings of feebleness and fatigue. The group came up with several ideas on how to raise the energy level, such as getting a sufficient amount of sleep, drinking coffee, partaking in common activities (e.g., talking to each other), taking a shower, doing enjoyable things (e.g., listening to music), engaging in sports, and eating a healthy diet (e.g., salad and lots of vegetables).

Generating Alternative Solutions

The patients seemed to have obtained the knowledge about strategies to help them deal with low energy states. However, they did not seem disposed to the respective behavior. These relatively unsystematic and general ideas of dealing with problems were used to prepare the starting point for the next therapeutic step of generating possible solutions. We ended this session by discussing the objectives of the therapy with the patients, as the following excerpt illustrates.

Example

Therapist's Approach to Generating Alternative Solutions (Preparation I)

Therapist: Now, at end of today's session, let's talk about your expectations for the therapy. We would like to know what you expect from the next few weeks. What are your goals?

Daniel: I would hope to have more energy again.

Peter: And I would hope I'm not so tired anymore.

Therapist: Could one say that you want to become fitter? To better your overall condition?

Daniel: Yes, exactly.

Emma: I think if I lost some weight I would also feel fitter.

Therapist: So it is also your goal to have more energy in the future?

Daniel: Yes, to simply feel stronger – or less weak.

Therapist: Could you describe this more precisely? What could you do more or better if you were stronger?

Peter: For example, I could go to occupational therapy.

Therapist: Aren't you doing that now?

Peter: Yeah, but recently I've been coming in late and I can't make it through to the end.

Therapist: Uh-huh. So you would see yourself being more punctual and having the ability to stay till the end of occupational therapy.

Peter: Yes, you could put it that way.

Daniel: If I were more energetic, I could also do better in exercise class.

Therapist: Do you mean you would be more agile?

Daniel: Yes.

Therapist: So your major goal for the therapy would be to help you feel better physically?

Daniel: Yes, just not always feel so weak.

Therapist: Fine. Emma, you haven't said anything.

Emma: Well, to be honest I would be happy if I would just weigh less. I've gained so much weight in the past few years.

Therapist: Being fitter for you means losing weight?

Emma: It would certainly be the most important thing for me.

Therapist: Uh-huh. Let's continue. Can someone tell me what exactly would change for the better in daily life if she or he were fitter?

In the course of the discussion, we tried to reformulate the group members' goal statements into concrete, behavioral goals. We ended the first therapy session by handing out new self-evaluation fitness forms; each group member was asked to think about what he or she could do in order to reach the defined goal.

It is crucial to prepare the following steps of therapy carefully. Doing so can reduce the risk of being taken by surprise with suggestions that are counterproductive (e.g., reducing medication) or impracticable (e.g., vegetarian diet). The responsibility for the course of therapy lies completely in the hands of the therapists. This is a very important point, especially considering the fact that the concepts of personal responsibility and nondirective methods can be misleading in this context. As a consequence, it would be conceivable that no practicable solutions to the problems can be found. This risk is especially high with chronic schizophrenia patients that are easily overburdened. Such a failure could challenge the whole approach of creatively solving problems. However, if the session is well-planned, it is easier to encourage possible solutions and to discuss how to put concrete, realistic alternatives into action. Nevertheless, the therapist should be careful not to set too narrow boundaries to the course of therapy: If the planning is too rigid, it may have the effect of restricting group members' decisions and potential actions. Interpersonal Problem Solving could then be seen as an instrument for communicating decisions that have been already made and could then reduce the patients' feeling of being directly involved in the process of choosing possible solutions, which may further reduce their motivation for putting them into action.

While preparing the subsequent therapeutic steps, the therapists discussed the group members' ideas of potential solutions and possible ways of continuing group sessions with the direct care staff. We decided to continue using the self-evaluation fitness forms since the group members had accepted them very well.

The discussion led to the decision to clearly encourage any solution associated with sports or exercise. We decided to guide suggestions concerning the abstract concept of sport toward concrete behavior. Moreover, we felt the need for the group members to realize that only real and consistent efforts over a longer period of time (at least 6 months) could lead to their reaching the goal (perceivable and lasting amelioration of the subjective level of energy). We, therefore, decided to introduce an exercise called "trainer game." The following excerpt illustrates the session in which possible solutions were generated.

B5: Implementation

Example

Therapist's Approach to Generating Alternative Solutions (Preparation II)

Therapist: Good morning everyone and thanks for being on time today.
Cotherapist: Emma, would you like to start today by summarizing the last session for us?
Emma: We looked at the fitness forms and added up our daily and weekly totals.
Cotherapist: Very well. You remembered that precisely. Peter, is there anything you would like to add to that?
Peter: Yes, we also looked at when each of us felt especially good or particularly bad. And on which day this occurred.

> **Cotherapist:** Correct. We picked out the days on which you felt fit and the days you felt less fit.
> **Daniel:** I am especially tired in the morning before I get up and after lunch.
> **Cotherapist:** Uh-huh. You remember that we also looked at the differences in fitness throughout the day.
> **Daniel:** Yes.
> **Cotherapist:** Fine. At the end of the last session we handed out new fitness forms, which we will look at in a week's time. Now I would like to know if anyone had any trouble filling out the forms this time?
> **All:** No.
> **Therapist:** Fine. We also discussed what each of you expects from the therapy and what your goals are. Do you remember, Peter?

At the beginning of the session we discussed all of the major points of the previous session in order is to reinforce prior learning and to provide continuity in the problem-solving process, which extends over a number of sessions. A review is particularly important for schizophrenia patients, who tend to forget about previous steps because of their cognitive disabilities. This is the only way to help them to remember the logical context of a therapy extending over several sessions. However, this review should not take up more than one-sixth of the total time of any one session.

Following this review of the previous session, we discussed the homework assignment, which in this case was to generate solutions.

Example

Therapist's Approach to Generating Alternative Solutions

> **Therapist:** Let's discuss which solutions crossed your minds. As you will remember, the assignment was to write down all the ways you can think of to solve the problem of feeling low on energy.
> **Peter:** I thought of getting enough sleep regularly, that is, going to bed earlier.
> **Co-therapist:** I'll write that on the blackboard, "Going to bed earlier." All right?
> **Peter:** Yes. And perhaps taking a nap in the afternoon.
> **Co-therapist:** Afternoon nap (she writes it on the blackboard).
> **Therapist:** Fine. Any other ideas . . .?
> **Emma:** If we move into a house in the community, we could cook for ourselves. We could eat more salad and vegetables.
> **Therapist:** Uh-huh. Let's write down, "Eat a lot of salad and vegetables."
> **Daniel:** But not only that!
> **Therapist:** Daniel has an objection. Daniel, let's discuss each suggestion later in more detail. Right now, you remember, we are just gathering ideas that have crossed every one's mind.

B5: Implementation

Daniel: Sports! Maybe we're so tired because we didn't exercise all winter. We hardly ever went outdoors.

Cotherapist: And when there were opportunities to go out, you were too tired or didn't want to go most of the time.

Daniel: That's true. But if we don't do anything, we'll get even weaker and lazier.

Therapist: I think you've mentioned something very important. I totally agree with you. OK, let's write "Exercise" on the blackboard.

Peter: I thought of drinking lots of fruit juices. It's healthier than coffee.

Therapist: Very good. I think it's remarkable that this thought occurred to you since you almost exclusively drink coffee.

Emma: I feel that it helps to take a shower immediately after getting up in the morning. That's when I really wake up. Also, I always get up as soon as the alarm clock goes off, rather than staying in bed forever.

Therapist: Uh-huh. If I understand you correctly, you've made two suggestions: "Getting up immediately after the alarm clock goes off" and "Taking a shower right after getting up."

Emma: Yes.

The cotherapist should write the suggestions on the blackboard so that everyone can see them. In some cases, it may be necessary for the therapists to complete the list with other possible solutions in addition to those suggested by the group members. In our example, it was not necessary, as our favored solution, "exercising," had already been suggested.

Evaluating Alternative Solutions

The next step is to evaluate the different solutions suggested by the group members. The group discusses the advantages and disadvantages of each solution in turn. With our group, we decided to discuss the solution "exercise" last, because we thought of it as the best and most practical solution. Moreover, the suggestion to exercise more can thereafter be used to introduce the "trainer game," which we had planned for the end of the session. We, therefore, discussed the other suggestions first:

All group members agreed that "go to bed earlier" was a good means of increasing their energy level. Everyone understood the connection between getting enough sleep and feeling rested. As it turned out, patients usually went to bed quite late because they watched TV until late at night. We, therefore, made a written agreement beforehand concerning the TV shows the patients could watch and at what time. As a general rule we agreed that the patients should be in bed by 11 pm, with the exception of one night a week. The direct care staff was encouraged to control whether the patients observed these rules.

The group, however, rejected the idea of taking an afternoon nap. All group members said that they were even more tired after such a nap. Another argument was the danger of oversleeping and, therefore, being late for occupational therapy in the afternoon.

Emma's suggestion to eat lots of salads and vegetables was rejected vehemently by the male group members. They did not want to do without their meat, rice, or noodles. We decided not to encourage the whole group to implement this idea, since it did not seem practical while the patients were still hospitalized. However, we decided to bring this point up again at a later point of time in connection with living and cooking in a living community. Moreover, we encouraged Emma to implement this solution for herself.

The suggestion to "drink lots of fruit juice" was broadly accepted. It was agreed that in the future everyone should drink a glass of juice after the morning meeting.

As expected, the group members were skeptical about the suggestion of "getting up quickly" and "showering" in the morning. However, all group members eventually agreed on a slightly softened rule on getting up and showering, which they were all willing to try out "in vivo" (and thereafter proved to be quite effective and well accepted).

Deciding on a Solution

These examples demonstrate that the discussion of possible solutions may lead directly to decisions about which solutions to implement. In some cases, however, it may be necessary to first evaluate the advantages and disadvantages of all solutions in order to decide whether or not to put a solution into practice. A particular decision may be valid for all or for only one of the group members, depending on the advantages of a particular solution for each individual as well as his or her motivation to implement it.

Only after having discussed all other possible solutions did we talk about "exercising." In order to help group members cognitively process the required effort needed to improve fitness, we introduced the "trainer game." In this exercise, group members are asked to imagine they had to prepare their favorite athlete for an important event in 6 months. The trainer game demonstrates that exercising is a meaningful solution only if effective exercises are carried out over a long period of time and on a regular basis. The group members came to understand that their own fatigue and feebleness could not be improved through sporadic, ineffectual exercises. With this information in mind, group members were given a homework assignment of putting together their own 6-month fitness-training program.

We started the next therapy session by discussing the self-evaluation fitness forms in detail. Both male group members, Daniel and Peter, reported an obvious improvement in their ratings over the past week, and their improved sense of well-being had a positive influence on their cooperation. Emma had maintained her relatively high fitness ratings. All group members agreed to keep filling out the self-evaluation forms after we decided to have them rate themselves only twice a day.

Subsequent to discussing the self-evaluation forms, we talked about the group members' ideas of their individual training programs. All group members had worked out a 6-month program, which was clearly a result of the trainer exercise completed in the previous session. Suggestions included regular morning gymnastics (all group members), jogging and joining sports groups (Emma), swimming (Daniel), regular walks

(Daniel and Peter), and regular cycling (Peter). Emma's suggestion was to gradually increase the demands of her workout, which consisted of a long-term commitment to jogging individually and joining a sports group thereafter. The other two group members developed similar suggestions in the course of the discussion.

The remainder of this session was dedicated to planning these programs as precisely as possible and to working out the organizational structure needed to implement the plans. Training schedules were arranged in accordance with their daily treatment schedules and were entered into their daily timetables. In order to reduce "start-up difficulties," we arranged for the direct care staff to take part in the initial phases of the group members' exercise training programs. Finally, we invited each group member individually to develop written therapy contracts that outlined the requirements of their training program.

Implementing the Chosen Solution(s)

The transfer of the chosen solutions into real life was done as realistically as possible, and help was provided as needed. After concluding the topic of fatigue and feebleness in the Interpersonal Problem Solving subprogram, we turned the focus of therapy back on preparing for life in the community. However, the group continued to meet weekly to provide reinforcement for continuing their exercise training programs and to discuss the self-evaluation fitness forms.

Subsequent Feedback

Once a month booster sessions were held to discuss group members' experiences with their chosen solutions for dealing with fatigue and to make any necessary adjustments.

5.6.3 Revised Therapeutic Procedures for Interpersonal Problem Solving

Reasons for Modification

A number of problems arose from the practical implementation of the Interpersonal Problem Solving subprogram:

- The subprogram puts a strong emphasis on cognitive aspects. As a result, high demands are made on therapy participants concerning abstract and logical thinking, attentiveness, and concentration. Because schizophrenia patients often show an impairment of information processing, Interpersonal Problem Solving often seemed to overburden them.
- The participants usually did not implement the solutions to problems discussed in therapy in real-life situations. We, therefore, have to assume that not enough consideration is given within the subprogram to transferring cognitively developed problem solutions to concrete behavior put into action.
- Many patients often did not show the empathy needed to understand the problems

of other patients. Consequently, they also could not give any suggestions for solving other patients' problems.

– Therapy participants recurrently showed resistance to even sharing their problems with the group and to participating in role-plays at all (e.g., because of anxiety). It is, therefore, important to put greater emphasis on emotional processes and patients' reactions as well as on carefully dealing with them in therapy (group processes).

In a modified version of the Interpersonal Problem Solving subprogram, we gave greater consideration to the above-mentioned aspects. We now put a greater emphasis on a problem-centered and more behaviorally oriented therapeutic approach, with a particular focus on emotional processes. Very complex themes, such as preparing therapy participants for community living (see above), are not the subject of this subprogram any longer. Instead, they are dealt with in the Social Skills subprogram. The modified version of the Interpersonal Problem Solving subprogram deals exclusively with patients' individual problems.

Carrying out the Modified Procedure

Warm-up exercises are conducted during the first therapy sessions of the Interpersonal Problem Solving subprogram to establish and to strengthen trust, openness, and cohesiveness among the group members (e.g., Antons, 2000). To reduce anxiety, the therapist should also establish the basic rules and standards to be adhered to by all group members (e.g., confidentiality, mutual respect, and acceptance).

Beginning of a Therapy Session

– Group members report on their homework assignments or name new problems that have come up.
– The therapist focuses on one particular problem brought up by a patient. The discussion of a chosen problem situation – and with it of the patient who brought it up – needs to be guided by hypotheses (e.g., individual processes of that patient, urgency of discussing the matter for the patient, respect for the momentary group processes).

Treating a Chosen Problem

– The designated group member discusses the problem with the therapist in detail.
– Group members share similar problem situations and experiences, increasing the cohesiveness of the group. For example, "Who has had a similar problem?"
– The designated group member and the therapist discuss strategies to solve the problem. Other group members are also encouraged to generate possible solutions.
– Following a discussion of the various advantages and disadvantages of each possible solution, the designated group member selects a solution.

- The designated group member enacts a cognitively prestructured role-play with a clearly defined content. Cotherapists or other group members assist the patient.
- The therapist gives feedback and makes concrete suggestions on how to improve the performance.
- A second re-enactment of the role-play can be performed (same procedure as in the first role-play).
- At the end of the session, homework is assigned to provide the opportunity to practice the skills and knowledge acquired in therapy in the natural environment.

Subsequently a different problem situation of a different group member is treated analogously, and if time permits a third situation can be treated as well. Again, the choice of the situation is made by the therapist and needs to be guided by hypotheses. It is important to pay attention to only treating the problem situation in the here and now (e.g., if a patient is talking about problems on the job, childhood is not taken into consideration). In doing so, the therapist prevents patients from disclosing methods and interpretations that are counterindicated.

Generally, group members do not present all aspects of a problem the first time they bring it up. Resolving a problem is a lengthy process that can take weeks or even months. The therapist should carefully encourage group members to explore their feelings and thoughts leading to their own solutions. This procedure enables the patients to gradually develop a greater connection to reality and to improve their quality of life.

5.7 Group Processes Considerations

Two problems are inherent in conducting group therapy with schizophrenia patients (mainly in the subprograms Social Skills and Interpersonal Problem Solving):
1) Opposition to self-disclosure and to active participation (e.g., enacting a role-play, bringing up a problem situation).
2) Maintaining an optimal balance between motivation, anxiety, and participation.

The following therapeutic techniques are useful in dealing with these difficulties:

Joining

To establish an emotional bond, giving individual attention to each group member at the beginning of the sessions is recommended. The contact should not be associated with the task or problem. For example, "Did you enjoy the noon concert at the park yesterday, Phil?"

Sharing

If the level of anxiety in the group is still rather elevated (posture, eye-contact, spontaneity, etc.) and a group member is asked to present a problem situation, the therapist

B5: Implementation

should ask whether other group members have experienced similar problems. This technique is effective in reducing social isolation and in increasing the group's sense of cohesiveness.

Auxiliary Ego

In difficult role-play situations, the cotherapist may be used as an auxiliary ego for the person performing the role-play. The cotherapist stands beside the designated person and assumes their posture while assisting him/her in a difficult conversation. This supportive technique is particularly effective when the designated person is anxious about the problem situation.

Modeling

If a patient is openly resistant to acting out the problem in the group setting (fearful), even with the cotherapist acting as an auxiliary ego, the cotherapist should take over the role of the designated person. The patient, however, now instructs the cotherapist on how to act out his/her role. Subsequently, the designated person role-plays the situation (if needed, with an auxiliary ego).

Role Reversal

In groups consisting of persons with psychotic disorders, role reversal is feasible only to a limited extent because they are often incapable of taking another person's perspective in a situation. An example of a role reversal might involve a group member who is ambivalent about how to solve a problem situation. The therapist asks the group member to swap roles with the cotherapist. The cotherapist and the group member switch place and sit in each other's chair. The therapist then briefly describes the role of the "new" cotherapist (patient), e.g., "Now we will have you and the cotherapist swap roles. You will play the part of the cotherapist. We have been working together since this group started. Phil, the cotherapist, will play your part and is wondering how to solve this problem."). The "new cotherapist" is then asked to suggest a course of action considered to be practical and effective in solving the problem situation. Because the "new cotherapist" is no longer so directly involved in the problem – both cognitively as well as emotionally – it often seems easier to arrive at an effective solution to a given problem. Such a role reversal is possible only in groups with cognitively flexible and intelligent patients. Generally speaking, role reversal becomes more difficult the more aversive and, therefore, emotionally loaded the role is each person needs to adopt.

Mirroring Ambivalence

Group members often have mixed feelings about decisions to be made. In high-functioning groups (i.e., groups demonstrating cohesiveness, a mild degree of peer anxiety, and a theme-oriented approach to solving problems), two cotherapists can mirror ambivalence. They put forward arguments for and against the decision alternately. The group member attempting to take the decision briefly states his or her opinion about each argument voiced. It is important not to overtax the group member taking the decision.

Reframing and Positive Appraisal

Group members tend to magnify failures and appraise events from a negative and self-critical point of view. The therapist should help them to explore negative self-statements, assist the group members in reframing problems more realistically, and offer positive approaches to dealing with problems.

For example, a group member says, "Nobody in my unit likes me anymore." Inquiring about the situation more closely, the therapist finds out that the patient had lately had several arguments with her roommate: The patient had been trying to sleep at night, but could not because the roommate listened to music so loudly. The therapist, who has known the group member for a long time, says: "You are trying to stick to the objectives we established and want to get a good night's sleep so that you feel fit the next day. Your roommate cannot understand that since you used to like staying up late. We should spend some time in therapy talking about the problems you are having with your roommate so that you can learn how to resolve such difficulties."

Structured Organization

Organizational structure decreases the ambiguity of the group process and clarifies expectations. Group members' anxiety, their motivation for therapy, and their ability to participate in therapy determine the degree of structure needed (see Figure 5.1): Clinical experience shows that when schizophrenia patients show a high level of fear (overload), their level of physiological arousal (not task-related) runs equally high. Furthermore, these patients usually show resistance to taking part in group activities (low level of motivation). Increasing the amount of organizational structure may significantly decrease anxiety in these patients; however, if the structure is too rigid, it is difficult to instill sufficient motivation for behavioral change (mentally underchallenged). The therapist's management of structure should, therefore, be based on a close observation of the group process and group members' level of anxiety (ideally low) and arousal (ideally moderate) as well as their motivation for therapy (ideally high) (see Figure 5.1).

B5: Implementation

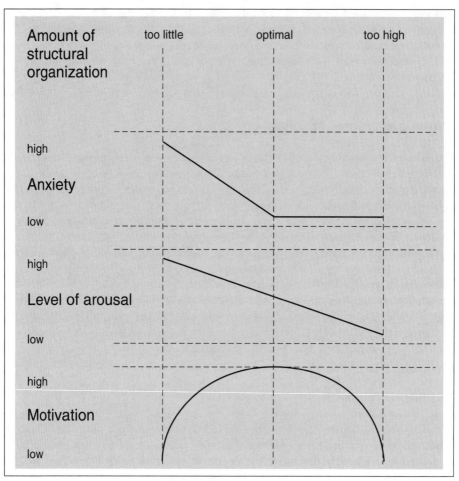

Figure 5.1 Anxiety, arousal, and motivation as related to structural organization in groups with schizophrenia patients

The therapist needs to regulate the level of motivation, fear, activation, and structure in order to meet the needs of the group. Techniques to strengthen the group's structural organization include:
– Directive and leader-oriented communication
– Addressing group members by name before making a request
– Providing sequential procedures for tasks (i.e., asking group members to respond in sequence clockwise or counterclockwise rather than randomly asking group members to respond)
– Avoiding long periods of silence
– Employing a task- or theme-oriented approach
– Establishing clear rules and standards to be adhered to by all group members
– Providing constant feedback

– Summarizing and repeating information
– Keeping the contents of therapy fact-oriented
– Speaking in short, clear sentences
– Avoiding ambiguous statements and interpretations

Three Phases of a Group Session

In addition to the therapy techniques listed above, dividing each session into three phases of group activity facilitates the group process:
1) Warming-up
2) Working out the theme
3) Positive ending

At the beginning of each session, it is important to establish a relaxed, supportive atmosphere. This allows the patients to work in a task- and theme-oriented manner (see "joining"). In the second stage, the task or problem providing the topic of the session is addressed. In the final phase, the therapist should clarify possible ambiguities, address problems, offer reassurance and support, and end the session on a positive note.

B5: Implementation

6 Assessment and Therapy Planning

All people with severe mental illness have certain things in common; yet each is also a unique individual with a unique combination of problems and treatment needs. Historically, this was not a major clinical issue before the advent of broad arrays of highly defined treatment procedures because everyone got the same treatment anyway. Even after the appearance of a diversity of chemically distinct antipsychotic medications, controversy persisted as to whether any medication was functionally distinct from any other. Gradually, as assessment and treatment technology became more advanced, the importance of tailoring treatment to individual characteristics ("personalization" in current mental-health policy discussions) also became more widely accepted.

This chapter provides an overall approach and discusses specific tools for assessing the problems and behaviors found in seriously mentally ill persons, pertinent to planning and providing Integrated Psychological Therapy. The process of translating assessment data into an individualized treatment approach is termed *treatment planning* in conventional mental-health services, and *case formulation* in more behaviorally and/or psychologically oriented services.

With the growth of the recovery movement (discussed in Chapter 1), treatment planning and case formulation took on an important new dimension. Historically, conventional assessment systems focused on problems and deficits. For example, psychiatric diagnosis focused on the symptoms of illness, and behavioral assessment focused on problem behaviors. Advocates in the recovery movement point out that this neglects the positive aspects of a person's functioning as well as, most importantly, personal desires and goals relevant to treatment. In the recovery perspective, these should be the first steps in assessment and should guide the treatment process throughout.

This is a compelling point of view, but the reality in mental-health treatment settings is that often the patient (or consumer or survivor or participant or however identified) is unable to identify or articulate such goals or desires. Historically, this was the main reason to disregard the patient's perspective. In the wake of the recovery movement, however, it has become a reason to target those abilities in treatment. The cognitive processes that support a person's ability to identify goals, to envision and hope for a better future, and to realize the promise of recovery, are processes that can be restored and strengthened in modern treatment and rehabilitation, especially in Integrated Psychological Therapy.

The assessment, formulation, and planning approach described in this chapter incorporates methods of proven usefulness, informed to varying degrees by the recovery perspective. Many of the most useful methods predate the recovery movement, yet are not incompatible with it. It is important that the reader keep in mind that an overriding purpose of modern assessment, treatment, and rehabilitation is to help the person to identify and pursue personally relevant recovery goals, building on the strengths and assets their illness has not taken away. Over the next few years we may expect that our assessment and treatment methods will reflect increasing sophistication in our ability to do just that.

6.1 Problem Analysis

In the light of the importance of identifying a person's strengths and assets, the approach described in this chapter reflects the general principles of behavior-analytical assessment (e.g., Kanfer, Reinecker, & Schmelzer, 2000), familiar to many mental health professionals. However, the distinguishing features of schizophrenia-spectrum disorders demand a certain degree of specialization, mostly to accommodate the multiple problems and causal factors usually encountered across biological, psychological, and social levels of functioning. Comparable specializations of behavior-analytical assessment are described elsewhere (e.g., Hunter, Wilkniss, Gardner, & Silverstein, 2008; Roder, Brenner et al, 2008; Spaulding et al., 2003). Readers interested in developing a full understanding of this approach should consult these sources as well as the broader literature on behavioral-analytic assessment. The concepts and methods presented here represent a synopsis, well suited to people with schizophrenia-spectrum disorders. Table 6.1 gives an overview of the whole process of assessment and treatment planning.

6.1.1 Behavior and Problem Analysis

Problem Description

The first step in behavioral-analytic assessment is the "identification and description of a problem." A "problem" here means a behavior or other component of biosystemic functioning (thoughts, emotions, psychophysiological responses) that poses a barrier to personal effectiveness and/or independence. Typically, such problems are the reasons people seek out mental-health professionals. For that reason, problems are also termed "behaviors of interest."

In behavioral-analytic assessment, a problem must be operationally defined and measurable. If it is not, there is no way to determine whether it has changed, i.e., whether treatment is, in fact, effective. Therefore, problems cannot be abstract concepts such as "schizophrenia" or inferential constructs that can be defined or measured in various different ways, such as "thought disorder." Problems must be able to be defined in terms of observable social behaviors, for example, instances of aggression; or as quantitative performance measures, for example, instances of derailment in a speech sample; or as subjectively reported specific internal experiences, for example, feelings of hopelessness or cognitions – as long as they can be quantitatively measured in some way. Later in this chapter we describe various instruments for quantifying observations and subjective reports.

Table 6.1 Behavior and problem analysis as well as treatment planning

a) **Behavior/problem analysis**

    1. Description of problem areas

        1.1. Behavioral indicators

        1.2. Cognitions

        1.3. Emotions

        1.4. Special aspects of problem description

    2. Analysis of conditions maintaining the problems and setting up hypotheses (functional analysis)

        2.1. Antecedents

        2.2. Consequences

        2.3. Hypotheses

    3. Analysis of motivation

        3.1. Related to the problem areas

            3.1.1. Discrepancy between self- and expert-rating

            3.1.2. Motivation of the patient for change

        3.2. In general

            3.2.1. Personal (rehabilitation) goals of the patient

            3.2.2. Possible reinforcers

    4. Unproblematic behavior (Behavioral resources)

    5. Current social relationships

        5.1. Inside the hospital

        5.2. Outside the hospital

b) **Sociocultural background**

    6. Analysis of past personal history (particularities during childhood or adolescence that might be related to the present problems)

    7. Recent life events (e.g., loss of spouse, job)+

c) **Classificatory diagnostics**

    8. Psychological assessment+

    9. Psychopathological assessment (DSM-IV-TR diagnosis etc.)+

    10. Somatic assessment (physical conditions that might be related to the problems)+

d) **History of past problems and treatments**

    11. Psychotherapy and sociotherapy+

    12. Pharmacological treatment+

e) **Treatment plan**

    13. Selection of treatment methods+

    14. Setting time lines and prioritizing therapy goals+

B6: Assessment/Planning

A person may have any number of distinct problems worthy of attention in the course of treatment and rehabilitation. Almost by definition, people with severe mental illness have a multiplicity of problems. An initial challenge to the practitioner is to determine whether a particular combination of behaviors represents a single problem or multiple problems. Pragmatically speaking, it is a (single) problem if its causes are distinct and responsive to a distinct treatment approach, whereas multiple problems respond independently to different treatments. Often, this can only be determined by administering the treatment and assessing what responds and what does not respond. In this sense, identification of problems is a hypothetico-deductive process. In fact, the entire treatment process can usefully be understood as a partially controlled experiment. Initial problem definitions represent an initial hypothesis, which is tested by treatment.

Functional Analysis

A core principle in behavioral-analytic assessment is that any behavior of interest is controlled by some combination of antecedents and consequences. Antecedents are events that precede the behavior of interest; consequences are events that follow it. Originally, in the operant learning theory that gave rise to behavioral-analytic assessment, antecedents, behaviors of interest, and consequences were all assumed to be observable environmental events. The sequential relationships of antecedents, behaviors, and consequences came to be known heuristically as "the ABC's of functional behavioral analysis." With the advent of social learning theory, inferred cognitive events could be introduced at any point in the sequence. As the biosystemic paradigm became accepted in psychology, this was extended to biochemical and neurophysiological events as well.

Today, functional analysis can potentially incorporate biological, cognitive, emotional, behavioral, or environmental events at any point in the ABC sequence. For example, neurophysiological dysregulation can be hypothesized to be the antecedent of psychotic symptom behavior. The hypothesis is tested by manipulating the antecedent (i.e., pharmacologically) and measuring the behavioral effect (i.e., with a quantitative measure of the symptom). Alternatively, the same behavior can be hypothesized to be the result of social reinforcement (an environmental consequence), which in turn can be tested by manipulating social responses to symptom behavior. Thus, functional analysis is a powerful and versatile method for determining the causes of identified problems and thereby identifying the effective treatment. The scope of functional analysis is limited only by the practitioner's repertoire of behavioral measures and potential treatments.

Motivational Analysis

Low therapy motivation and compliance represent a basic problem concerning patients with schizophrenia. Therapists often reach the ethical limits of their decision-making ability with regard to the determination of therapy goals by the patient or by others. Discrepancies result from the hypothesis and cognitive functioning referring to two different levels: the level of recognizing and describing the problem as well as the level of attributing causes to a problem. If there is a consensus on both levels through the description of the patient and others, one can expect the patient to be(come) motivated for change. Without any consensus, the therapy motivation is probably low.

When functional behavioral analysis reveals a particular behavior of interest to be under the control of a specifiable consequence, we understand that behavior to be motivated by the consequence. Antecedents may also be motivating factors if they signal the availability of a valued consequence. For example, the availability of a job may be a motivating antecedent if a person believes that a consequence of working the job is a paycheck.

Motivation can be common and concrete, such as the motivation to work at a job for the consequence of receiving a paycheck; or it can be idiosyncratic and subjective, such as the motivation to behave consistently with privately held convictions and beliefs. We all have a tendency to assume that other people are motivated by the same antecedents and consequences as we are, both concrete and abstract. However, a moment's reflection would compel us to question the validity of such an assumption. Motivation is often complex and counterintuitive, especially for people in extraordinary circumstances. As the saying goes, "one man's meat is another man's poison."

Recovery models strongly demand that patients' goals be self-determinated. To take the patients' point of view and expectancies into account for therapy planning supports therapy motivation. If patients with a low activation-level are not motivated, we suggest a systematic assessment of activities that may function as incentives and that also allows for realizing the treatment goals by the use of incentives.

People with severe mental illness are often in extraordinary circumstances, and they often have convictions and beliefs most other people are not familiar with. Their behavior can, thus, appear counterintuitive or even irrational to an observer who assumes motivation is the same for everybody. Failure to appreciate the idiosyncratic nature of motivation often leads to an erroneous understanding of behavior, especially the behavior of people with mental illness. If the behavior appears irrational, it is simply attributed to the mental illness, as if that were a satisfactory explanation. Ironically, sophisticated perspectives on the neurophysiology and psychopathology of schizophrenia can make us even more prone to this error: Without careful functional analysis to identify idiosyncratic or circumstantial motivation, it is easy to misattribute behavior to dopamine dysregulation or thought disorder or schizophrenia.

Motivational problems are abundant in severe mental illness, and they are very different from both neurophysiological and neurocognitive problems and skill deficits. They do not respond to medication or cognitive remediation or skills training; they respond to changes in the circumstances that motivate the behavior of interest. The safety and social support of the institution or hospital, the attention of hospital staff (even negative attention can be motivating to someone who is used to being completely disregarded), and disability benefits are motivational factors that, if not sufficiently considered, are especially prone to producing incorrect interpretations of behavior. Taken together, such motivational factors support the generalized social role of a "hopeless and helpless mentally ill patient" – and produce the well-known behavioral syndrome of institutionalization.

At the same time, neurophysiological and neurocognitive problems can certainly contribute to the circumstances that motivate a person to perform the social role of

B6: Assessment/Planning

"mental patient." When people repeatedly experience defeat and frustration as a result of psychotic relapses or cognitive impairment, they can understandably develop a belief system in which the role of a "mental patient" is safer and more beneficial than the role of a more independent and competent adult. People make very complex calculations about the advantages and disadvantages of specific social roles, including people with SMI (serious mental illnesses), even though they may not be able to easily articulate the details. Self-perceived liabilities such as risk for psychotic relapse or cognitive deficits can influence these calculations. Therefore, changes in liabilities can also influence one's motivational calculations. If a person believes that liabilities can be overcome, the social role of "mental patient" is less compelling. *Overcoming liabilities is a key goal in rehabilitation and recovery.* To this end, every aspect of treatment and rehabilitation is potentially relevant to motivation. Assessment and reassessment of motivation is a crucial aspect of the recovery process, as treatment and rehabilitation progress.

Behavioral Resources

Dysfunctional behavior and experiences are of importance for both the entire rehabilitation process and for resources. When describing problems and negative life events, it is essential that they are viewed in contrast to the positive aspects – the successful events and coping skills – of patients' current lives. Therefore, a description of unproblematic behavior, experiences, and the patient's resources has to be included in problem analysis as well. These behavior resources should be reported to patients as feedback concerning their competencies, in order to stabilize desirable and functional behavior, and to strengthen their self-confidence.

Current Social Relationships

Another element of problem and behavior analysis lies in the patient's social network. All important social relationships within and outside of the hospital are assessed. It may be necessary to include special persons in the therapy process in order to enhance the therapy success.

6.1.2 Sociocultural Background

The patient's social history is an extremely important source of information for behavioral and motivational analysis, especially early in the course of treatment and rehabilitation. A thorough social history often reveals many of the antecedent-behavior-consequence relationships that drive problem behaviors. Patterns in the patient's social history are helpful in inferring the kinds of social role choices the patient has made in the past – and whether and how those role choices were influenced by internal factors (e.g., symptoms, deficits) and environmental factors (e.g., family support, access to institutional resources, disability benefits). Patients' sociocultural background is often an important factor in their social history. Different sociocultural backgrounds lead people in different directions when they choose and develop their social roles.

6.1.3 Classificatory Diagnostics

The information necessary for a complete problem analysis usually comes from multiple sources. The most familiar is the psychiatric diagnosis, which in a sense is a summary of the person's liabilities (symptoms, course of illness, social deficits) and assets (premorbid functioning, social achievements, current personal and social functioning). Diagnosis is a starting point for categorical clinical decisions, such as ruling out somatic factors (e.g., specific neuropathology) and initial medication choices.

6.1.4 History of Past Problems and Treatments

Treatment history, including past response to pharmacological and psychosocial interventions, often provides key information for problem analysis and other aspects of treatment and rehabilitation planning. However, care must be taken to correctly interpret records of treatment response. Too often, treatment trials are insufficient to support a conclusion of nonresponsiveness. Pharmacological interventions are especially vulnerable to this pitfall (e.g., inadequate dosage or trial length), though it happens with psychosocial interventions as well, especially when the person's motivational factors have not been thoroughly assessed.

6.1.5 Treatment Plan

The initial formulation is essentially a list of various problems identified by the treatment team. The treatment plan consists of the specific interventions assigned to the respective problems. Together the problems and their associated interventions suggest assessment measures or key indicators that can quantitatively reflect responses to the interventions. Some of these key indicators may be the measures used to identify and operationally define the problem in the initial assessment; others may be new measures especially well suited to particular interventions.

When the initial formulation and the treatment plan have been completed, the treatment team must ensure that every one of its members understands and supports both. In psychiatric rehabilitation, numerous practitioners are usually involved in providing treatment, and a common understanding is necessary for optimal coordination and cooperation. Also, it is especially important that the patient be involved as a key member of the treatment team. The treatment team must effectively communicate a "plausible model" that helps the patient to understand the treatment plan as a logical strategy for meeting recovery goals (Reinecker, 1987). As with articulating recovery goals in the first place, progress in treatment may be necessary before such communication can be accomplished. When that is the case, the treatment team must weigh the imperative of

B6: Assessment/Planning

proceeding with treatment against the desirability of optimal engagement of the patient in the treatment process. Continual motivational analysis plays a key role in the treatment team's progress toward optimal engagement.

In keeping with the concept of treatment as a systematic test of initial hypotheses, the treatment team analyzes the data generated by the key indicators to determine whether treatment is having the expected effects. Failure to fulfill expectations, i.e., failure to support the initial hypotheses, gives occasion for reformulation. Often, only a subset of the behaviors of interest or deficits responds to a specific treatment, which suggests there is more than one problem requiring differential interventions. For example, some psychotic symptoms may respond to antipsychotic medication, while others do not. This stimulates the hypothesis that the nonresponsive symptoms are driven by other factors, such as positive environmental consequences associated with performance of a "mental patient's" social role. A reformulated treatment plan is then constructed to test the new hypotheses with a revised treatment regimen.

6.2 Assessment Instruments

This section describes a variety of instruments and measures commonly used to assess severe mental illness at the neurophysiological, cognitive, emotional, behavioral, and social levels of functioning. The various instruments can be usefully categorized as self-report questionnaires, observational questionnaires and ratings, structured interviews, and performance-based instruments. Observational measures are usually intended for ratings by mental-health professionals or specifically trained staff, whereas some others are designed for family members or other lay observers. Structured interviews rely on specifically trained professionals or staff, who rate responses to predetermined sets of questions. Performance-based instruments are psychological and neuropsychological tests administered by specifically trained professionals or staff in laboratories or comparable settings.

6.2.1 Psychiatric Symptoms and Mental Status

Although all of the instruments in this category measure observable behavior and/or patients' responses to questions, by inference they are *indirect* measures of the neurophysiological processes associated with psychiatric illnesses.

Structured Interviews

– **SCAN** – Schedules for Clinical Assessment in Neuropsychiatry (WHO, 1999)
– **SCID** – Structured Clinical Interview (First, Spitzer, Gibbon, & Williams, 2002)
– **IRAOS** – Instrument for the Retrospective Assessment of the Onset and Course of Schizophrenia and other Psychoses (Häfner, Löffler, Maurer, Riecher-Rössler, & Stein, 2003)

These instruments are designed primarily to render reliable psychiatric diagnoses. The SCAN is based on the diagnostic criteria in the World Health Organization's International Classification of Disease (ICD-10). The SCID is based on the American Psychiatric Association's Diagnostic and Statistical Manual (DSM-IV). The IRAOS elicits more detailed information concerning the onset and early course of psychotic disorders. Use of these instruments requires interviewers specifically trained to administer them.

Observational Ratings

- **BPRS** – Brief Psychiatric Rating Scale (Overall & Gorham, 1976)
- **SANS** – Scale for the Assessment of Negative Symptoms (Andreasen, 1983; Andreasen et al., 1981)
- **SAPS** – Scale for the Assessment of Positive Symptoms (Andreasen, 1984, 1987)
- **PANSS** – The Positive and Negative Syndrome Scale (Kay, 1991; Kay, Opler, & Lindenmayer, 1989)
- **NOSIE-30** – Nurses Observational Scale for Inpatient Evaluation (Honigfeld, Gillis, & Klett, 1966)

These instruments are designed to provide quantitative ratings of symptom severity and related aspects of social behavior. The BPRS, SANS, SAPS, and PANSS are all based on observations gleaned from dyadic interviews. However, the questions are not as specifically determined as in structured interviews, and information from collateral sources (e.g., records, clinical staff informants) may also be used to determine the ratings. For these reasons these instruments are also termed *semistructured interview measures*. As the names imply, the SANS and SAPS focus on schizophreniform symptoms, while the BPRS includes dimensions of mood and anxiety. PANSS is a broader-based assessment instrument measuring 30 symptoms categorized into positive, negative, and general symptoms. Considerable training is required to maintain reliable ratings. The NOSIE-30 is based on ratings of clinical staff who have observed the patient in an inpatient unit or comparable setting for a specified period (usually three work shifts over 72 hours). It comprises 6 subscales and a total scale, reflecting various aspects of social behavior. A modest degree of staff training and quality monitoring are required to maintain reliability.

Self-Report Instruments

- **FCQ** – Frankfurt Complaint Questionnaire (Süllwold, 1991)
- **ESI** – Eppendorf Schizophrenia Inventory (Mass, 2001)
- **SCL-90-R** – Symptom Checklist (Derogatis, 1977, 1994)
- **DWMS** – Dysfunctional Working Models Scale (Perris, Fowler, Skagerlind, Chambon et al., 1998; Perris, Fowler, Skagerlind, Olsson, & Thorson, 1998)

The FCQ and the ESI measure schizophrenia patients' subjectively experienced symptoms; the ESI includes a validity subscale. The SCL-90-R and its short form, the Brief Symptom Inventory (BSI) (Derogatis, 1993) cover nine symptom domains, at least two of which (paranoia, psychoticism) reflect positive symptoms of psychosis. The DWMS assesses cognitive schemata of the self and others, often targets for treatment in cognitive therapy for schizophrenia.

6.2.2 Cognitive Functioning

The recent proliferation of cognitive and neuropsychological instruments for use with severe mental illness makes it difficult to provide an updated inventory. Also, changing boundaries between neurocognitive and social cognitive functioning make classification difficult (discussed in Chapter 1). The information provided here is from a reasonable survey of the area, however, as for the assessment of social functioning, ongoing consultation with experts in this domain of assessment, specifically applied to severe mental illness, is necessary for both research and clinical applications.

As discussed in Chapter 1, the MATRICS initiative has had an important influence on overall assessment and especially on neurocognitive assessment for severe mental illness. It is important to note, however, that the priority for developing the MATRICS battery was for research and development of psychiatric pharmaceuticals. The considerations in choosing assessments for case formulation, treatment planning, and progress evaluation in psychiatric rehabilitation can be very different.

For most clinical programs that serve people with severe mental illness, the ideal situation is to have access to a fully functional clinical neuropsychological assessment laboratory. The laboratory should have instruments and professional staff capable of providing evaluations comparable to those needed for progressive neuropathy and traumatic head injury, comparable neurocognitive impairments being common in the schizophrenia-spectrum population. In addition, the laboratory should be able to provide assessments of executive functioning and social cognition beyond those typically used in clinical neuropsychology. This is because patients with schizophrenia-spectrum disorders often have deficits in those domains more subtle than the deficits caused by neuropathy or head injury, yet still very relevant to recovery and treatment planning.

Performance-Based Measures of Cognitive Functioning

– **MCCB** – The MATRICS Consensus Cognitive Battery (Kern et al., 2008; Nuechterlein et al. 2008)
– **NAB** – The Neuropsychological Assessment Battery (Stern & White, 2003)
– Measures of Social Cognition (see Table 6.2)

The NIMH-MATRICS committee has made an effort to reach a consensus in selecting a test battery to assess cognition. The goal of the test selection was to establish a well-accepted standard to assess each of the initially defined seven cognitive domains relevant for schizophrenia patients (Nuechterlein et al., 2004). The test battery had to be brief – 1 hour of assessment time. From a pool containing over 90 tests, the MATRICS committee selected a beta-version of 36 tests for validity and reliability testing (Nuechterlein et al., 2008). In the meantime, the final MATRICS Consensus Cognitive Battery

(MCCB) includes 9 tests that have undergone a conorming and standardization procedure (Kern et al., 2008) (see Chapter 1). Recently, the committee began establishing the final test battery as a worldwide standard. The tests were translated into several foreign languages, and have been already or will be standardized in local populations in other countries. Further information on the MATRICS Consensus is available online at http://www.matrics.ucla.edu.

The commercially distributed Neuropsychological Assessment Battery (NAB) (Stern & White, 2003) represents an example of a comprehensive assessment package measuring neurocognition. NAB includes a modular battery of 33 neuropsychological tests grouped into five main modules: attention, language, memory, spatial, and executive functions. A comprehensive test battery increases the clinicians' flexibility to focus on specific areas of concern. A subpart of the memory module was included in the beta-version of the MCCB as a candidate test to assess verbal learning and memory. A major goal of the NAB development was in minimizing the amount of manipulation necessary for testing. Demographically corrected norms and U.S.-census-matched norms of neurologically healthy controls are available. A software portfolio automates the use of these norms.

Measures of Social Cognition

The MCCB includes only one assessment of social cognition addressing emotion management. This is surprising, on the one hand, since the MATRICS committee defined five separate social cognitive domains (Green et al., 2005); and on the other hand, since there is now generally accepted empirical evidence claiming that social cognition represents a strong mediating factor between neurocognition and functional outcome (see

Table 6.2 Selection of tests to assess social cognition

Domain	Test	Stimuli
Emotion Perception	Pictures of Facial Affect PFA (Ekman & Friesen, 1976)	Pictured faces
	Face Emotion Identification Task FEIT (Kerr & Neale, 1993)	Pictured faces
	Bell-Lysaker Emotion Recognition Task BLERT (Bell, Bryson, & Lysaker, 1997)	Video
Social Perception	Half-Profile of Nonverbal Sensitivity PONS (Rosenthal, Hall, DiMatteo, Rogers, & Archer, 1979)	Video
	Social Cue Recognition Test SCRT (Corrigan & Green, 1993)	Video
	Social Perception Scale SPS (Garcia, Fuentes, Gallach, Ruiz, & Roder, 2003)	Pictured social scenes
Theory of Mind	Hinting Task (Corcoran, Mercer, & Frith, 1995)	Written vignettes
	The Awareness of Social Inference Test TASIT (McDonald, Flanagan, Rollino, & Kinch, 2003)	Video-taped vignettes
Social Attribution	Ambiguous Intentions Hostility Questionnaires AIHQ (Combs, Penn, Wicher, & Waldheter, 2007)	Written vignettes
Social Schema	Schema Component Sequencing Task SCST-R (Corrigan & Addis, 1995)	PC-based test

Chapter 1). Consequently, it is important for clinicians as well as for psychotherapy researchers to have standardized, objective instruments for assessing the domains of social cognition. However, there are fewer standardized tests available to assess social cognition than to assess neurocognition. Some of them that have been used in research projects and clinical settings were initially developed to assess social cognitive functioning of patients suffering from disorders other than schizophrenia (e.g., brain injury, autism, etc.). In some of these tests, norms for schizophrenia patients are still missing. Table 6.1 includes a selection of tests to assess social cognition.

The test selection in Table 6.2 shows a wide range of stimuli used to assess the five social cognitive domains defined by the MATRICS initiative (Green et al., 2005). The PFA is the most commonly used test to assess emotion perception. It is based on pictures from the well-known Ekman pictures set, distributed by Paul Ekman (www.paulekman.com). The standardized pictures comprise culturally independent basic emotions in facial affects. In the PFA as well as in the FEIT, patients have to correctly recognize the emotion on a pictured facial affect. The BLERT, on the other hand, consists of video scenes in which an actor shows emotionally salient facial expressions and vocal prosody while speaking and acting.

In the Half-Profile of Nonverbal Sensitivity (PONS), gestures, facial expressions, and voice intonations are presented in videotapes to measure social perception. A similar procedure is used in the SCRT: The perception of concrete and abstract cues is measured by analyzing videotaped vignettes of interacting people. Another procedure characterizes the SPS: The social situations depicted are analyzed to measure social perception. Most of the pictures used in this test are taken from the therapy material of the social perception subprogram of IPT.

The Hinting Task test comprises short stories presenting an interaction between two characters. Each short story ends with one of the characters dropping a very obvious hint. Theory of Mind (ToM) functioning is measured through patients' ability to identify the real intentions behind indirect speech statements. Another ToM-related test is the TASIT. It consists of videotaped vignettes and standardized response probes. The TASIT is divided into three parts with alternative forms for retesting: emotion evaluation, minimal, and enriched social inference. Patients have to recognize basic emotions in an ambiguous context and be sensitive to conversational inferences (a person may say one thing and mean another) in order to make specific judgments about the speaker's intentions, feelings, beliefs, and the meaning of their statement.

The AIHQ includes a series of written vignettes describing ambiguous and non-ambiguous social situations. Social attribution is measured in a questionnaire addressing patients' estimation of the actor's intentions and their own response to the situations. The SCST-R is also available as a PC-based version, consisting of a series of social scripts, each of which is drawn from daily life situations and includes a sequence of actions and behaviors. The sequence is divided into different parts. The social schema is measured through the patients' ability to reproduce these parts of the sequence in the correct order.

Interview-Based Assessment and Self-Rating of Cognitive Abilities

- **SCoRS** – Schizophrenia Cognition Rating Scale (Keefe, Poe, Walker, Kang, & Harvey, 2006)
- **CGI-CogS** – Clinical Global Impression of Cognition in Schizophrenia (Bilder, Ventura, & Cienfuegos, 2003; Ventura, Cienfuegos, Boxer, & Bilder, 2008)
- **CAI** – Cognitive Assessment Interview (Ventura, Bilder, Seise, & Keefe, 2008)
- **MIC-CR, MIC-SR** – Measure of Insight into Cognition (Clinician Rated or Self-Report) (Medalia & Thysen, 2008; Medalia et al., 2008)

Interviews and questionnaires are the source of further information about patients' cognitive resources and deficits. However, these assessment formats present a challenge because it is generally difficult for schizophrenia patients to estimate their own cognitive performance. In other words, the insight of schizophrenia patients into their own cognitive functions is low, and self-reports of the level of own cognitive functions have generally low correlations with objective test performance. Interview-based expert ratings, on the other hand, have mostly higher correlations to test performance than do self-ratings (Green, Nuechterlein et al., 2008; Keefe et al., 2006; Medalia & Thysen, 2008; Medalia et al., 2008; Moritz et al., 2004). Nevertheless, self-reports and interview-based assessment of cognitive abilities can be strong indicators of a cognitive disorder – not because these measurements represent unrealistic estimations, but because self-rating and interview-based expert ratings provide information about patients' awareness of cognitive functioning in daily living, which is linked to everyday social functioning. Consequently, such measures do give valuable information concerning cognitive capacity referring to important intervention topics.

The SCoRS is an interview-based assessment of cognitive deficits and the degree to which they affect day-to-day functioning. The administration of the SCoRS includes three sources: an interview with the patient, an interview with an informant (e.g., caregiver, family members), and a rating by the interviewer. SCoRS measures the neurocognitive domains of attention, memory, reasoning and problem solving, working memory, language production, and motor skills. The CGI-CogS represents a similar assessment instrument with the same sources of information. However. the assessments specify all six neurocognitive domains and one (global) social cognitive domain defined by the MATRICS initiative. Both SCoRS and CGI-CogS were recently evaluated in the MATRICS Psychometric and Standardization Study (PASS) (Green, Nuechterlein et al., 2008). The CAI is based on the conceptual work of CGI-CogS and SCoRS and represents a new semistructured interview that is still under evaluation. The assessment comprises patient and informant input. The CAI specifies all six neurocognitive domains defined by the MATRICS initiative.

The MIC-CR and MIC-SR measure patients' awareness of problems with attention, memory, and executive functioning. The MIC-CR is a clinician-rated interview and the MIC-SR a patient self-report measurement instrument. While the MIC-CR examines insight into cognitive symptoms and the attribution of cognitive deficits to mental illness, the MIC-SR assesses only the awareness of cognitive deficits by the reported occurrence of cognitive difficulty.

6.2.3 Social Functioning

Social functioning is a very broad domain for assessment and generally difficult to measure (Bustillo et al., 2001; McKibben et al., 2004). Self-report measures are limited by patients' ability to give accurate appraisals of their performance (Green, Nuechterlein et al., 2008). Observational measures of social functioning are difficult to administer, and as with other types of observational instruments, staff training and continuous quality monitoring are often required to maintain reliability. Performance-based assessments in contrived settings are generally easier to administer and are more reliable, but they may not accurately reflect performance in the natural environment. These factors should be carefully considered when selecting an assessment battery for a particular clinical or research application. Recent reviews by Yager and Ehamann (2006) and Kurtz and Mueser (2008) provide helpful detailed information for this purpose.

Structured Interviews

– **DAS** – Disability Assessment Schedule (WHO, 1988)

The Disability Assessment Schedule (DAS) uses information from collateral sources, such as family and mental health professionals familiar with the patient's social functioning. The DAS measures various aspects of social functioning including specific abilities associated with work, leisure time, and housing.

Observational Measures

– **ILSI** – Independent Living Skills Inventory (Menditto et al., 1999)
– **ILSS** – Independent Living Skill Survey (Wallace, Liberman, Tauber, & Wallace, 2000)

These two very similar instruments are based on staff observations of patient functioning in a variety of functional domains, ranging from personal finances to cooking to housekeeping and occupational functioning. The ILSS provides more quantitative ratings and has well-established psychometric properties. The ILSI is more categorical, but distinguishes between "competence" and "performance" – as (theoretically) knowing how to perform the skill and actually performing it at the appropriate time in a natural environment. Therefore, the ILSS may be more suitable for measuring change, while the ILSI may be more useful for clinical assessment and treatment planning.

Performance-Based Assessments

– **AIPSS** – Assessment of Interpersonal Problem Solving Skills (Donahoe et al., 1990)
– **MASC** – Maryland Assessment of Social Competence (Bellack, Sayers, Mueser, & Bennett, 1994)
– **UPSA** – University of California at San Diego UCSD Performance-Based Skills Assessment (Patterson, Goldman, McKibbin, Hughes, & Jeste, 2001)

The AIPSS and MASC are similar instruments, specifically designed to measure the cognitive and behavioral aspects of interpersonal skills. Both involve having the patient view recorded videos of role-played interpersonal problems or conflicts. The patient's understanding of the social situation is then assessed with a structured interview, and the patient is instructed to role-play a solution to the problem or conflict with the interviewer. The patient's performances in the interviews and the role-plays are then rated to yield separate cognitive and behavioral dimensions of interpersonal skills.

The UPSA measures independent living skills across multiple domains, like the ILSS and the ILSI. Instead of using ratings based on unsystematic observation or collateral informants, the UPSA is based on performance in contrived situations that emulate natural situations, e.g., a home kitchen, albeit in a laboratory-like setting.

MASC and UPSA were both selected by the NIMH-MATRICS initiative as co-primary measures (besides cognitive measures) for clinical trials in schizophrenia. Both were evaluated in the MATRICS Psychometric and Standardization Study (PASS) (Green, Nuechterlein et al., 2008). More relevant information are available on the MATRICS homepage at http://www.matrics.ucla.edu.

6.3 Self- and Expert-Rating System

We developed a self- and expert-rating system for a precise therapy follow-up (Roder, Brenner et al., 2008). This offers the therapist the possibility of continuously judging the patient's cognitive and social skills as well as reality reference. Besides providing a therapy follow-up, it functions well for the whole therapy planning with regard to long- and short-term goals within a multimodal treatment approach. The construction of the rating system was oriented to typical social and cognitive deficits in schizophrenia and the necessary skills for integration outside the hospital.

The following sheets can be used for ratings:
- BT (Behavior in the Therapy Group)
- HM (Household and Maintenance)
- MT (Movement Therapy)
- WT (Work Therapy)
- GA (Planned Group Activities)
- CG (Cookery Group)
- HG (Hygiene and Grooming)
- Self-assessment sheet in two parallel forms

The following sheets can be used for evaluation:
- Evaluation of Self-Assessment Questionnaires P1 and P2
- Rehab Evaluation 1
- Rehab Evaluation 2
- Summary of Rehab Evaluation 1
- Summary of Rehab Evaluation 2

B6: Assessment/Planning

A description and operationalization of the scales and the evaluation procedure togeth-
er with all assessment and evaluation sheets are in the Appendix (see Worksheet
19–33). For every patient eight process curves can be illustrated on the basis of the
ratings. They refer to:
– Attendance
– Punctuality
– Proactivity
– Therapy contents
– Work
– Self-Care

These single curves result in one average curve. The self-assessment sheet covers all
six fields as well and can be used to generate a self-assessment curve. A comparison
of the average with the self-assessment curve allows for conclusions about the patient's
correspondence with reality (under- or overestimation).

7 Description and Discussion of Empirical Results

The IPT manual has been published in 13 languages, and IPT studies have been conducted in 12 countries in North and South America, Europe, and Asia. To date, 35 independent studies with a total sample size of 1,529 schizophrenia patients (diagnosed according to ICD or DSM) have evaluated IPT or a combination of IPT subprograms. IPT was compared mainly to standard care (pharmacotherapy and social therapy), a placebo-attention condition (nonspecific group activity), or both of these control conditions. Furthermore, three studies were conducted in which IPT was compared to a different therapy approach. The 35 IPT studies are summarized in Table 7.1.

Table 7.1 35 Evaluation studies of IPT (1529 patients)

	Author	Country	N	Setting	Centers
1)	Brenner, Stramke, Mewes, Liese, & Seger,1980; Brenner, Hoder, Kube, & Roder, 1987	Germany	43	inpatients	academic
2)	Brenner, Stramke, Hodel, & Rui, 1982	Germany	28	inpatients	academic
3)	Stramke & Brenner 1983; Stramke, Hodel, & Brauchli, 1983	Switzerland	18	inpatients	academic
4)	Bender et al., 1987	Germany	28	inpatients	nonacademic
5)	Brenner, 1987	Germany	18	outpatients	nonacademic
6)	Hermanutz & Gestrich, 1987	Germany	64	inpatients	nonacademic
7)	Kraemer, Sulz, Schmid, & Lässle,1987	Germany	30	inpatients	mix
8)	Roder, Studer, & Brenner, 1987	Switzerland	17	inpatients	nonacademic
9)	Funke, Reinecker, & Commichau, 1989	Germany	24	inpatients	nonacademic
10)	Heim, Wolf, Göthe, & Kretschmar, 1989	Germany	65	inpatients	nonacademic
11)	Peter, Glaser, & Kühne, 1989; Peter, Kühne, Schlichter, Haschke, & Tennigkeit, 1992	Germany	83	inpatients	academic
12)	Kraemer, Zinner, Riehl, Gehringer, & Möller, 1990	Germany	43	inpatients	academic
13)	Olbrich & Mussgay, 1990	Germany	30	inpatients	academic
14)	Roder, 1990	Schweiz	18	inpatients	nonacademic
15)	Schüttler et al., 1990, Blumenthal et al., 1993	Germany	95	inpatients	nonacademic
16)	Hubmann, John, Mohr, Kreuzer, & Bender, 1991	Germany	21	inpatients	nonacademic

Author	Country	N	Setting	Centers
17) Van der Gaag, 1992	Netherlands	42	inpatients	nonacademic
18) Takai, Uematsu, Kadama, Ueki, & Sones, 1993	Japan	34	inpatients	mix
19) Theilemann, 1993	Germany	45	inpatients	nonacademic
20) Hodel, 1994	Switzerland	21	inpatients	academic
21) Hodel & Brenner, 1996	Switzerland	15	inpatients	academic
22) Spaulding, Reed, Sullivan, Richardson, & Weiler, 1999	USA	91	inpatients	academic
23) Roder, Zorn, & Brenner, 2000	Switzerland, Germany, Austria	143	mix	mix
24) Vallina-Fernandez et al., 2001	Spain	35	outpatients	nonacademic
25) Vauth et al., 2001	Switzerland	57	inpatients	academic
26) Vita et al., 2002	Italy	86	outpatients	nonacademic
27) Penadés et al., 2003	Spain	37	outpatients	academic
28) García et al., 2003; Fuentes, Carcia, Ruiz, Soler, & Roder, 2007	Spain	23	outpatients	nonacademic
29) Lewis, Unkefer, O'Neal, Crith, & Fultz, 2003	USA	38	outpatients	nonacademic
30) Ueland & Rund, 2004	Norway	26	inpatients	academic
31) Briand et al., 2005, 2006	Canada	90	outpatients	mix
32) Alguero, 2006	Panama	12	inpatients	nonacademic
33) Zimmer, Dunsan, Laitano, Ferreira, & Belmonte-de-Abreu, 2007	Brazil	56	outpatients	academic
34) Tomas, 2009	Spain	39	outpatients	academic
35) Gil Sanz et al., 2009	Spain	14	outpatients	nonacademic

The different studies included inpatient as well as outpatient settings in academic and nonacademic contexts, using various sample sizes and methodological rigor. Patient characteristics are presented in Table 7.2. Two-thirds of the patients were male, the mean age being 35 years and the mean IQ over 90 standard points. The duration of illness and hospitalization as well as the daily dose of antipsychotic medication were largely heterogeneous. As presented in Table 7.3, the mean duration of therapy was more than 40 hours, i.e., three sessions per week over almost 17 weeks. The therapy setting also differed considerably in the 35 studies: In the 1980s and 1990s a higher number of weekly therapy sessions was preferred, whereas nowadays two weekly IPT sessions are the norm. This is supported by empirical results showing that two weekly sessions have higher treatment effects compared to only a single session per week; three or more sessions, on the other hand, have no decisive additional effect (see Figure 7.1).

Table 7.2 Patient characteristics

	M	95% CI
Gender: % male	68.2	62.4 < δ < 74.0
Age	35.4	33.5 < δ < 37.3
IQ	92.5	88.3 < δ < 96.7
Duration of hospitalization (months)	74.9	39.2 < δ < 110.6
Duration of illness (years)	10.6	8.6 < δ < 12.6
Chlorpromazine equivalents	826.8	386.3 < δ < 1267.3

CI = confidence interval.

Table 7.3 Therapy setting (IPT)

	M	95% CI
Duration of therapy (weeks)	16.6	11.8 < δ < 21.4
Duration of therapy (hours)	42.4	33.1 < δ < 51.7
Weekly number of therapy sessions	3.0	2.5 < δ < 3.5

CI = confidence interval.

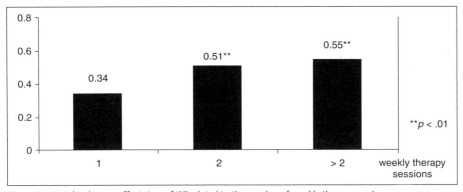

Figure 7.1 Weighted mean effect sizes of IPT related to the number of weekly therapy sessions.

7.1 Quantitative Review of IPT Studies

In order to evaluate the effectiveness of IPT, a meta-analysis was conducted (Mueller, Roder, & Brenner, 2007; Roder, Mueller, Mueser et al., 2006). A first step included all 35 independent IPT studies. The mean effect sizes (*ES*), defined as the average values of all assessed outcome variables, are presented in Figure 7.2 (for further information about the calculation and interpretation of *ES*, see Chapter 2). The resulting mean *ES* within the IPT groups is .52, indicating a significant improvement of IPT patients during therapy, whereas the *ES* of the placebo-condition is .23. Nevertheless, a small placebo effect could be shown, a result that is consistent with other meta-analyses (e.g., Lambert & Bergin, 1994). Standard care groups, on the other hand, obtained only a very small *ES* of .08. The IPT effects were

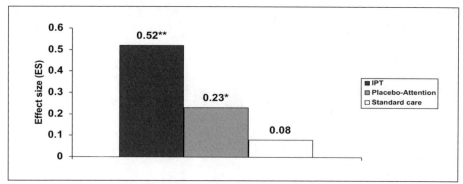

Figure 7.2 Weighted mean effect sizes of the 35 independent IPT studies.

maintained over a follow-up period of 8.1 months, which supports the evidence of generalization of IPT intervention over time. The analysis of 8 high-quality studies with high methodological rigor (randomized patient allocation, blind ratings, controlled medication) supports the results of the total meta-analysis sample of 35 studies (for details compare Roder, Mueller, Mueser et al., 2006).

7.2 Robust IPT Effects

The IPT effects are robust and independent of setting (similar effects for both inpatients and outpatients), stage of illness (similar effects for postacute and stabilized patients), and contextual conditions (no significant differences for academic and nonacademic sites). Nevertheless, the effects were influenced by the duration of illness: The longer an illness lasts, the smaller the obtainable treatment effects. It has to be critically mentioned that the duration of therapy (M = 16.6 weeks) seems to be too short for severely chronically ill patients, and clinically we observed many changes in these patients when IPT was supplied over longer periods of time (for a minimum of 6 months). Other patient characteristics such as age, sex, and daily dose of medication were not correlated with the treatment effects achieved through IPT. Age, however, did have an impact on changes in the two control conditions: Younger control patients showed a small ES, whereas middle-aged patients showed absolutely no changes in the control conditions. This points out the importance of offering integrated therapies such as IPT more broadly to middle-aged and elderly schizophrenia patients (Mueller & Roder, 2006).

7.3 Effects in Functional Levels and Symptom Reduction

IPT includes subprograms concerning neurocognition, social cognition, and social functioning, so that effects in these areas of functioning and possible symptom reduction are of special interest. Figure 7.3 summarizes the effects in these areas. The sig-

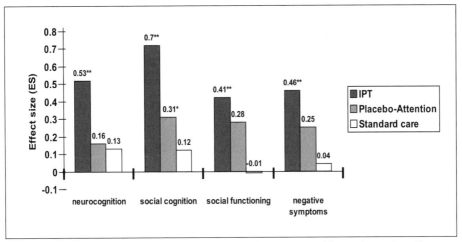

Figure 7.3 Effect sizes in the domains of neurocognition, social cognition, social functioning, and negative symptoms.

nificant *ES* in neurocognition, social cognition, and social functioning support evidence of IPT effects in proximal outcomes. Additionally, a significant reduction of negative symptoms was observed. The largest *ES* of IPT were addressed toward social cognition (*ES* = .72) and neurocognition (*ES* = .52). With respect to variables like patient characteristics and therapy setting, the only effect observed was the influence of the duration of therapy on the IPT outcome in social functioning, although an impact on symptoms or cognitive functions was not shown. Here again, the placebo-attention conditions showed larger effects compared to standard treatment with the exception of the effects in neurocognitive functions. Consequently, unspecific therapy had no additional effect compared to mere standard care in this area. This points to the recommendation that neurocognitive remediation is necessary to reduce rate-limiting neurocognitive deficits in schizophrenia patients.

7.4 IPT Subprograms: What Works?

A further analysis compared the effects of the different IPT subprograms and a combination of subprograms with each other (Mueller & Roder, 2008). An intervention based only on the neurocognitive subprogram ("Cognitive Differentiation") leads to a significant proximal outcome (*ES* = .49) but not to significant effects regarding functions of distal outcome. Yet, the combination of neurocognitive and social cognitive IPT subprograms ("Cognitive Differentiation" and "Social Perception") showed significant improvements in neurocognition (*ES* = .74), social cognition (*ES* = .82), as well as in social functioning (*ES* = .40). Additionally, the dropout rate during therapy was half as high in the combined intervention group (11.8%) as in the neurocognitive intervention group (22.2%). Studies in both IPT conditions offered an equal number of sessions, and both led to a significant symptom reduction. Therapy motivation may have worked as an unspecific mediator on the outcome. This assumption is supported by our own as well as other researchers' empirical results (Medalia & Richardson, 2005; Roder, Mueller, & Zorn, 2006). Furthermore, general outcome at follow-up as well as social functioning were strongly associated with the level of integrated IPT subprograms: The complete IPT including all five subprograms showed the largest effects in social functioning, additionally improving general therapy outcome at follow-up measurement compared to single subprograms (Mueller & Roder, 2008; Roder, Mueller, Mueser et al., 2006).

7.5 Efficacy and Effectiveness of the IPT

Several independent and well-controlled studies on IPT using strong methodological rigor demonstrated the efficacy of IPT treatment in schizophrenia patients concerning proximal as well as more distal outcomes. Patients' benefits after therapy could be maintained during a follow-up period. Additionally, IPT has been successfully evaluated in various settings and context conditions. A well-documented example was conducted in Canada: Since 2001 the IPT program has been broadly implemented into the Quebec Health Care system as part of the standard medical therapy. The research team used a slightly modified version of IPT, also including an emotional management subprogram developed by our research team as well as in vivo and booster sessions (Briand et al., 2005). By 2006, more than 100 mental health professionals in Quebec in more than 25 different clinical institutions had been trained to conduct IPT (Briand et al., 2006). The outcome of the resulting field study was included in our meta-analysis, and it strongly supports the effectiveness of IPT. Furthermore, the Quebec study proved a decrease in the outpatients' use of health-care resources (number of visits of psychiatrists and emergency departments, rehospitalization) and the related costs during patients' IPT participation compared to the year preceding commencement of IPT.

Additionally, the fact that studies in rehabilitation conditions close to the patients' daily life showed the same outcome as rigorously controlled laboratory-based studies supports strong evidence of the effectiveness of IPT. In accordance with McGurk, Twamley, and colleagues' (2007) findings, an integrated intervention based on neurocognitive, social cognitive, and social intervention areas as represented in IPT seems to be necessary in order to achieve sufficient generalization effects.

B7: Empirical Results

Part C
Further Development of IPT

8 Introduction

The IPT concept was expanded and modified in our laboratory in Bern in order to focus on advances made in intervention technology and therapy topics associated with an improved understanding of schizophrenia functioning. In two research projects supported by the Swiss National Foundation, our research group developed and evaluated two new therapy approaches for schizophrenia patients: the three cognitive social skills programs for residential, vocational, and recreational topics (WAF*; Grant No: 32–45577.95, Roder et al.) and Integrated Neurocognitive Therapy (INT; Grant No. 3200 B0–108133, Roder et al.). The efficacy and feasibility of WAF and INT were extensively evaluated in international multisite studies. Both newly developed interventions are autonomous therapy programs, not to be integrated into the IPT structure because of their conceptual differences (see Figure 8.1).

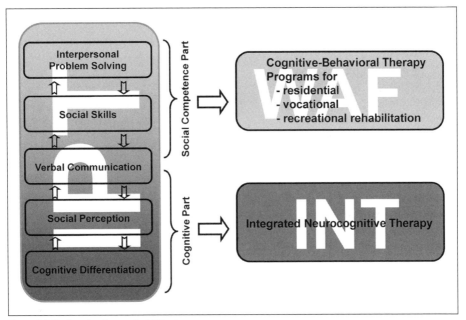

Figure 8.1 Further development of IPT subprograms.

---

* We use the German abbreviation for "**W**ohnen, **A**rbeit, **F**reizeit."

8.1 Cognitive Subprograms: INT – Integrated Neurocognitive Therapy

Some years ago, our research group revised the basic IPT subprograms Cognitive Differentiation and Social Perception and designed Integrated Neurocognitive Therapy (INT) (Mueller & Roder, 2010; Roder & Mueller, 2006). An empirically based starting point for the development of INT resulted from the evaluation of IPT and WAF: A combination of the neurocognitive and social cognitive IPT subprograms yielded superior effects in proximal and distal outcomes compared to mere neurocognitive remediation (Mueller & Roder, 2008). Furthermore, intrinsic motivation represented a strong mediator of improved functional outcome in WAF procedure (Mueller & Roder, 2005; Roder et al., 2002; Roder, Mueller, & Zorn, 2006), which is in line with data derived from other studies (Medalia & Lim, 2004; Medalia & Richardson, 2005; Nakagami et al., 2008). Finally, clinical experience and intervention research focusing on social competence strongly suggest considering patients' daily life in the therapeutic procedure in order to support the generalization and transfer of proximal therapy outcomes. The social cognitive subprograms of IPT as well as the WAF programs refer to this recommendation, which is generally left out in cognitive remediation. Against this background, and following the IPT technology, the primary aim of the development of INT was to integrate neurocognitive and social cognitive exercises using group processes as therapeutic instruments. Therefore, INT as well as IPT decisively differ from traditional lab-based cognitive remediation approaches. Another aim is the consequent focus on patients' individual resources, rather than on their deficits, for building up good compliance. INT also places a strong emphasis on patients' intrinsic motivation and considers their experiences of their own (cognitive) functioning in daily living.

8.1.1 Treatment Concept of INT

Based on the theoretical and empirical state of neurocognitive and social cognitive research described in Chapter 1 in this book, we developed a cognitive-behavioral group therapy approach. For this purpose, the original IPT model was modified. Conceptually, INT is built upon the definitions of the NIMH MATRICS initiative (Measurement and Treatment Research to Improve Cognition in Schizophrenia [Green et al., 2005; Nuchterlein et al., 2004]). Following the recommendations of this task force, six neurocognitive domains and five social cognitive domains were operationalized for therapeutic intervention. These 11 cognitive domains are integrated into four therapy subprograms (modules), each of which includes different functional domains of neurocognitive and social cognition. A schematic presentation of the INT is given in Figure 8.2.

The sequence of the four INT modules addresses incremental steps based on an increase of cognitive complexity and emotional strain (beginning with simple, basic cognitive tasks with no emotional impact) and a decrease in therapeutic structuring. The emotional relevance and the personal reference to reality may be more pronounced in the social cognitive part of each module, but it is supported by the didactic structure in the neurocognitive part as well.

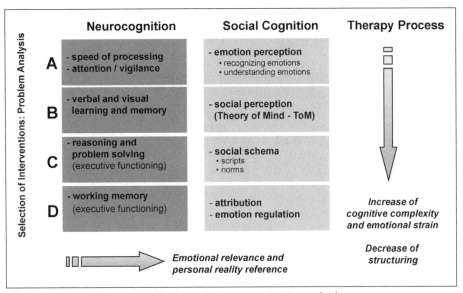

Figure 8.2 Schematic presentation of the Integrated Neurocognitive Therapy (INT).

INT is designed as a cognitive-behavioral group therapy in outpatient settings. A team of one primary therapist and one cotherapist leads a group of six to eight patients. The roles and functions of the therapy team are the same as for the IPT procedure. Our evaluation study (Roder & Mueller, 2009) included a total of 30 sessions, which took place biweekly, each lasting 90 minutes including a short break. INT also includes computer-based exercises; in the evaluation study, the CogPack computer-program distributed by Marker Software was used (Marker Software, 2009). Therefore, therapy procedure requires a computer room in addition to the standard group intervention room. During a therapy session of 90 minutes, PC-based exercises are limited to a maximum of 45 minutes. Because of the outpatient setting, exercises and therapy content are designed to place higher demands on patients' capacity and competence in a group setting compared to the cognitive subprograms of IPT. A unpublished manual for use in a multicenter research project is available (Roder & Mueller, 2006). This manual includes a broad scope of interventions in neurocognitive and social cognitive domains helping therapists to compose exercises according to the participants' needs.

Each of the four INT modules includes the same didactic therapy components (Table 8.1). Each module starts with introductory sessions using educational tools to support patients' understanding of the focused cognitive domain and its relevance in daily life. A precondition to bridging the gap between the experiences in the laboratory during therapy and the daily life context outside the lab is establishing the patients' awareness of their own resources and enhancing their insight into their deficits in cognitive functions and their corresponding limitations in coping with everyday problems. For this purpose, prototypical case vignettes (short stories) were designed for each cognitive domain. Furthermore, teaching patients about cognitive functions and their relevance in real-life situations within a vulnerability-stress-coping framework of schizophrenia

Table 8.1 Therapy components of each of the four INT modules

Each Treatment Area (A-D) of INT Comprises:

- Introduction sessions
  a) Perception of own resources and possibilities to optimize them in daily life
  b) Education in the focused therapy area (→ "insight" in problems / deficits)
     ↓ use of case vignettes
- Consecutive sessions
  a) Compensation: looking for coping strategies
  b) Restitution: practicing exercises (rehearsal)
     ↓ partly computer-based

For all therapy components: in-vivo exercises and homework assignments to promote transfer and generalization.

enhances patients' insight into their individual cognitive capacity and fosters their intrinsic therapy motivation.

In the consecutive sessions in each INT module, individual coping strategies are elaborated in the group setting. These exercises compensate for cognitive deficits and optimize individual resources for managing the demands of daily life associated with cognitive functioning. In addition to this strategy learning approach, the INT procedure includes repeated training sessions that are partially PC-based. In this rehearsal approach, a large body of exercises is group-based, using group processes and interactions to activate patients, and to simulate real-life situations. Also, during a computer session, therapists largely support group processes. Finally, in vivo exercises and homework assignments are used to promote the transfer of the learned cognitive skills into practice, to support generalization of the effects to other functions, and to maintain the effects after therapy.

8.1.2 Evaluation of INT

A randomized multicenter study included nine centers in Switzerland, Germany, and Austria, the sample comprising a total of 168 patients. In this project, the feedback given by therapists and patients was very good. The low dropout rate of only 11% and the relatively high rate of over 80% of voluntary session participation indicate a high acceptance of the INT procedure among patients. Initial study results showed a superior proximal outcome in the cognitive area compared to treatment as usual. Additionally, these favorable effects could be generalized to the more distal outcomes of social functioning and negative symptoms. The therapy effects could be maintained during a follow-up of 1 year (Roder & Mueller, 2009). INT represents a new and promising cognitive remediation approach that seems to be both feasible and effective.

8.2 Social Skills Subprograms: WAF – Vocational, Residential, and Recreational Skills

First initiated by the review of the Schizophrenia Patient Outcomes Research Team (PORT) (Lehman & Steinwachs, 1994, 2003), the treatment of schizophrenia patients with rather unspecific, standard psychological, social-competence approaches of the 1970s and 1980s (second developmental stage of social competence approaches, see Chapter 2.3) had some limitations: There was strong empirically based evidence supporting the acquisition and maintenance of social skills; but moderate evidence had been recorded for generalization and social adjustment, and only weak evidence for psychopathology. However, research has shown that taking specific social rehabilitation topics of patients' daily life into consideration improves their ability to transfer the acquired skills into practice in individual life. Residential, vocational, and recreational activities are identified as some of the key topics within social functioning (see Chapter 1 and 2). Additionally, empirical results support the evidence that booster sessions can increase the generalization and transfer of the learned skills after the end of treatment. Against this background, the scope of the IPT subprograms Social Skills and Interpersonal Problem Solving was extended in the 1990s by developing three cognitive social skills programs for residential, vocational, and recreational topics (Roder et al., 2000, 2002; Roder, Zorn et al., 2001). These three WAF programs introduce rehabilitation topics that are particularly relevant for schizophrenia patients. WAF represents cognitive and behavioral interventions to improve social competence in specific functional areas of patients' daily lives. Also, WAF comprises aftercare treatment, which starts after the end of an intensive therapy consisting of group and individually administered sessions.

8.2.1 Treatment Concept of WAF

Patients are treated with only one WAF therapy program depending on the indication. As with IPT, groups usually comprise five to eight participants guided by one therapist and one cotherapist. Each of the three WAF programs focuses on (1) sensitizing the patients to their needs, options, and skills (cognitive and emotional skills training), (2) helping them to make a decision in any one of these three areas, (3) providing support in putting the decision into action (practical implementation of skills), and (4) teaching them how to anticipate difficulties and to solve concrete problems.

All three programs have the same structure and include the same cognitive and behavioral intervention techniques. As an example of the WAF therapy procedure, Table 8.2 summarizes the contents and intervention topics of the vocational therapy program.

The goal of the vocational therapy program is to activate and to support patients in making use of rehabilitation offers in competitive or noncompetitive employment. An unusual aspect for a social competence approach is that it implements a large body of standard cognitive and behavioral methods. The program structure allows for flexible

C: Further Development

Table 8.2 Contents and intervention topics of the vocational therapy program

Stages	Intervention topics	Methods
(1) Cognitive orientation	Experience with both previous jobs and vocational rehabilitation efforts	– Positive connotation – Cognitive restructuring
(2) Individual goal attainment	– Collecting information on different jobs – Decision on the goal of the vocational rehabilitation	– Decision training – Cognitive probe – Positive reinforcement
(3) Training specific social skills for implementation of the established goals	– Getting information on job openings (by writing, by phone) – Composing a CV and letters of application – Applying for a job; job interview – Understanding employment contracts – The disorder as a discussion topic in the work environment – The effects of being employed on several personal living situations	– Model learning – Role-playing – Coaching – Positive reinforcement
(4) Coping with difficulties	– Perception of stress symptoms and early warning signs – Developing a crisis strategy for early warning signs – Difficulties in finding a job and starting work – Difficulties at the workplace caused by disorder-related symptoms – Difficulties at the workplace causing job-related stress – Interpersonal or emotional difficulties at the workplace	– Stress inoculation training – Self-control – Self-verbalization – Self-reinforcement – Self-management – Relaxation training – Communication training – Problem solving – Brainstorming – Model learning – Role-playing – Cognitive restructuring

behavior and problem analysis, thereby taking individual experience and needs as well as motivational aspects into consideration. The goal of all three WAF programs is to activate the patients and to support independent living. As can be seen in Table 8.2, in the vocational program patients initially learn to reflect on their own experiences, options, and skills related to previous jobs and vocational rehabilitation efforts. Establishing their skills to find, to get, and to perform a job follows an individual realistic goal attainment. Finally, optional and experienced difficulties associated with work are analyzed and individual stress-reducing coping skills are trained following a vulnerability-stress-coping model.

Four different types of therapeutic interventions are implemented in all three WAF programs: group therapy, individual therapy, in vivo exercises, and homework assignments. Detailed and highly standardized therapy manuals are available for all three WAF programs (Roder, Zorn et al., 2008).

8.2.2 Evaluation of WAF

The WAF was evaluated in an international multicenter study in three countries, Switzerland, Germany and Austria, which included 143 schizophrenia patients. Results suggest additional effects of the WAF compared to traditional social skills therapy concerning the global therapy effect (mean of all assessed variables). Both of the social competence approaches that were compared obtained similar successful improvements in general social skills. In distal outcome assessment, patients following the WAF programs showed neurocognitive improvements comparable to patients participating in the control group. However, only WAF patients showed a significant symptom reduction from stress-inoculation training. The symptom reduction was associated with a reduction in relapse demonstrated through a 1-year follow-up (Roder et al., 2000, 2002; Roder, Zorn et al., 2001).

Three subsequent evaluation studies – one each for the three WAF programs – using the same design (Keppeler-Derendinger, 2008; Mueller & Roder, 2005; Mueller et al., 2007; Roder, Mueller, & Zorn, 2006), collected data on the program's specific proximal outcome. Objective data provided evidence for a superior improvement in proximal outcome of the WAF vocational program compared to standard social competence therapy (Figure 8.3): Significantly more participants of the vocational program found a job during therapy compared to controls – even though the vocational program does not include active job placement. This superior effect was maintained over a follow-up period of 1 year. Furthermore, the outcome effect was strongly associated with a higher treatment motivation of WAF patients compared to those of the control condition (Roder, Mueller, & Zorn, 2006).

In another study focusing on the WAF recreational program, leisure-time activities addressing proximal outcome were significantly improved in WAF patients compared to controls, especially during the 1-year follow-up period (Mueller & Roder, 2005). In a final study including the WAF residential program, the effectivity of WAF was evident in the percentage of patients who changed to less-structured housing offers, with

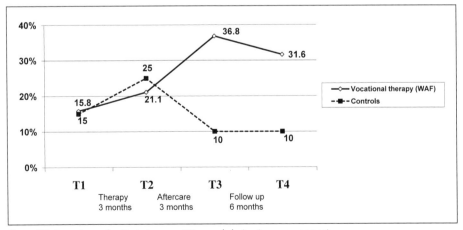

Figure 8.3 Percentage of patients in competitive work during 1-year assessment.

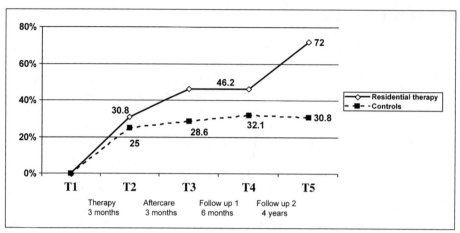

Figure 8.4 Percentage of patients changing residential status to a less structured offer during 5-year assessment.

less care during a follow-up period of 5 years (Keppeler-Derendinger, 2008; Mueller et al., 2007) (Figure 8.4). Again, the WAF program did not include active residential placements.

All in all, the WAF programs, as well as INT, are very promising and effective new therapy approaches for their rehabilitation topics. Based on IPT technology, both treatment approaches can be an appropriate part within a multimodal rehabilitation effort for people suffering from schizophrenia.

Appendix

Therapy Materials and Questionnaires (Worksheets)

Worksheet 1   Cognitive Differentiation: Step 1 – Card-Sorting Exercises

Worksheet 2   Cognitive Differentiation: Step 2 – Verbal Concept Exercises

Worksheet 3   Cognitive Differentiation – Examples for Conceptual Hierarchies

Worksheet 4   Social Perception – The Slides

Worksheet 5   Social Perception – Ratings of the Slides' Cognitive Complexity

Worksheet 6a   Social Perception – Ratings of the Slides' Emotional Load

Worksheet 6b   Social Perception – Judgments of Emotions Expressed in the Slides

Worksheet 7   Social Perception – List of Slides' Titles

Worksheet 8   Verbal Communication: Step 1 – Literal Repetition Exercise

Worksheet 9   Verbal Communication: Step 2 – Paraphrasing Exercise

Worksheet 10   Verbal Communication: Step 3 – W-Questions

Worksheet 11   Social Skills – Low Risk Situations

Worksheet 12   Social Skills – Higher Risk Situations

Worksheet 13   Social Skills – Complex Situations

Worksheet 14   Interpersonal Problem Solving – "Activities Outside the Clinic and Skills in Everyday Life"

Worksheet 15   Interpersonal Problem Solving – "Searching for an Apartment"

Worksheet 16   Interpersonal Problem Solving – "Furnishing the Apartment"

Worksheet 17   Interpersonal Problem Solving – "Living and Working in a Community"

Worksheet 18   Interpersonal Problem Solving – "Moving"

Worksheet 19   Description of the Rating Scales Used for Self-Assessment and Assessment by Others

Worksheet 20   Behavior in the Therapy Group (BT) – Assessment by Others

Worksheet 21   Household and Maintenance (HM) – Assessment by Others

Worksheet 22   Movement Therapy (MT) – Assessment by Others

Worksheet 23   Work Therapy (WT) – Assessment by Others

Worksheet 24   Planned Group Activities (GA) – Assessment by Others

Worksheet 25   Cookery Group (CG) – Assessment by Others

Worksheet 26   Hygiene and Grooming (HG) – Assessment by Others

Worksheet 27   Self-Assessment P1

Worksheet 28   Self-Assessment P2

Worksheet 29   Evaluation of Self-Assessment Questionnaires P1 and P2

Worksheet 30   Rehab Evaluation 1

Worksheet 31   Rehab Evaluation 2

Worksheet 32   Summary of Rehab Evaluation 1

Worksheet 33   Summary of Rehab Evaluation 2

Worksheet 1

Cognitive Differentiation: Step 1 – Card-Sorting Exercises*

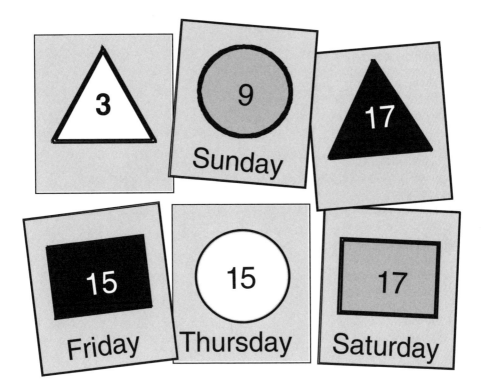

* The cards can be ordered from the first author

Worksheet 2

Cognitive Differentiation: Step 2 – Verbal Concept Exercises

A. Conceptual Hierarchies Exercise

Emotionally Neutral

1. Clothing
2. Means of Transportation
3. Cooking
4. Weather
5. Fruit
6. Summer
7. Seasons
8. Vegetables
9. Packing Bags for a Camping Trip

Emotionally Loaded

1. Hygiene
2. Jobs
3. Therapy Leave
4. Moving
5. Psychiatry
6. Medication
7. Therapies/Treatment on the Ward
8. Handicaps
9. Feelings

B. Synonyms Exercise

Emotionally Neutral

1. Group: Company, gathering, society, collection, gang, bunch, clique
2. Conversation: Talk, discussion, chat
3. Decision: Resolution, judgment
4. Walk: Step, tread, stroll, march, saunter, hike
5. Ask: Examine, query, question, inquire

Emotionally Loaded

1. Happiness: Bliss, joy, lightheartedness
2. Anger: Fury, ire, wrath, rage, madness, indignation

3. Love: Affection, care, sympathy, devotion, fondness
4. Fear: Alarm, dismay, fright, horror, terror
5. Pain: Ache, suffering, hurt
6. Courage: Bravery, audacity, valor
7. Fatigue: Exhaustion, tiredness, weariness, weakness
8. Arrogance: Pride, haughtiness, boasting
9. Hectic: Stress, tension, pressure
10. Politeness: Courtesy, good manners, civility
11. Hope: Confidence, reliance, optimism, faith
12. Fright: Shock, terror, alarm, panic
13. Friendliness: Kindness, amiability, gentleness
14. Harmony: Agreement, balance
15. Misfortune: Adversity, bad luck, disaster, tragedy
16. Quarrel: Dispute, fight, squabble, argument
17. Nervousness: Tension, uneasiness, anxiety
18. Sadness: Dejection, gloom, unhappiness, tearfulness, melancholy
19. Friend: Acquaintance, buddy, pal, mate
20. Medicine: Remedy, cure, drug, pharmaceutical
21. Laugh: Chuckle, giggle, grin
22. Cry: Sob, weep, blubber, wail
23. Exhausted: Worn out, tired, run down, weary

C. Antonyms Exercise

Emotionally Neutral

1. Short – Long
2. Beginning – End
3. Day – Night
4. Expert – Amateur
5. Man – Woman
6. Quiet – Loud
7. Rain – Sunshine
8. Precision – Inaccuracy
9. Win – Lose
10. Sweet – Sour
11. Hot – Cold
12. Above – Below
13. Back – Front
14. Slow – Fast
15. Hungry – Full
16. Active – Passive
17. Clean – Dirty
18. Fat – Thin

19. Closed – Open
20. Narrow – Wide
21. Wet – Dry
22. Modern – Old-Fashioned
23. Liquid – Solid
24. Yesterday – Tomorrow
25. Left – Right

Emotionally Loaded

1. Love – Hate
2. Lucky – Unlucky
3. Sad – Happy
4. Dream – Reality
5. Work – Play
6. Praise – Criticize
7. Healthy – Sick
8. Ugly – Pretty
9. Intelligent – Stupid
10. Boring – Exciting
11. Nervous – Relaxed
12. Moody – Calm
13. Cry – Laugh
14. Despair – Hope

D. Word Definitions Exercise

Emotionally Neutral

(objects)

1. Door
   – Material: wood, plastic, metal, glass
   – Shape: rectangular
   – Location: a large opening in the wall
   – Function: means of entry and exit for a building or a room
2. Heating
   – Material: metal
   – Shape: rib like
   – Location: most of the time below windows in living space
     etc.
3. Mirror
4. Book
5. Sink

6. Curtain
7. Window
8. Telephone
9. Shelf
10. Bed
11. Car

(abstract concepts)

12. Summer: warm season, from June through September
13. Hunger: basic need for food
14. Thirst: basic need for liquid
15. Group: (small) number (of people)
16. Air: transparent essential mixture of gas
17. Wind: air movement of varying strength
18. Time: progress of events, difference between "now" and "later," as well as "before"
19. Hobby: enjoyable and relaxing leisure activity
20. Light: visible source of energy, natural or artificial
21. Weather: Interaction of energies in the form of light, water, and air

Emotionally Loaded

1. Work: Productive activity to support oneself
2. Vacation: Leisure time, for relaxing and resting
3. Education: Preparation for an occupation/job

E. Word Clue Exercise

The two words printed on the word cards are followed by examples for clue words.

Emotionally Neutral

1. *Pen* – Pencil (Ink)
2. Lighter – *Match* (Book)
3. *Giraffe* – Monkey (Neck)
4. Shirt – *Pants* (Leg)
5. Water – *Soap* (Bubbles)
6. *Snow* – Ice (Flake)
7. *Fish* – Frog (Gills)
8. *Bed* – Couch (Night)
9. *Ocean* – Lake (Salt)
10. Boots – *Sandals* (Summer)
11. *Candle* – Lamp (Flame)
12. Paper – *Pen* (Swan)

13. Tool – *Hammer* (Nail)
14. Summer – *Winter* (Snow)
15. *Window* – Frame (Glass)
16. Plate – *Bowl* (Soup)
17. Dollar – *Coin* (Metal)
18. *Knife* – Spoon (Meat)
19. *Sleep* – Rest (Dream)
20. Bread – *Butter* (Milk)
21. *Breakfast* – Supper (Morning)
22. *Rain* – Sun (Water)

Emotionally Loaded

1. *Laughing* – Anger (Happiness)
2. *Optimism* – Despair (Hope)
3. Anger – *Sadness* (Gloom)
4. *Crying* – Laughing (Tears)
5. *Fear* – Happiness (Anxiety)
6. *Jealousy* – Love (Envy)
7. Hate – *Love* (Affection)
8. *Boredom* – Relaxation (Monotony)
9. Good Luck – *Bad Luck* (Misfortune)
10. Harmony – *Disagreement* (Fight)
11. *Stressed* – Relaxed (Tension)

F. Context-Dependent Words Exercise

1. Bulb: Light, flower
2. Leaf: Tree, table
3. Pen: Fountain, pig, swan
4. Chain: Jewelry, bicycle, store
5. Scale: Weight, sheath of a plant, rating
6. Bowl: Fish, fruit, sport
7. Buck: Male deer, dollar
8. Glasses: Drinking, eyes
9. Bridge: Card game, construction, dental work
10. Bar: Steel, pub
11. Bank: River, money
12. Nail: Construction, finger
13. Ball: Toy, dance
14. Ring: Finger, boxing
15. Stool: Foot, toilet
16. Pass: Ticket, sports throw, mountain

17. Beam: Wood, light
18. Fork: Eating utensil, road crossing
19. Tank: Water, military
20. Duck: Animal, crouch down
21. Horn: Animal, car, musical instrument

Worksheet 3

Cognitive Differentiation – Examples for Conceptual Hierarchies

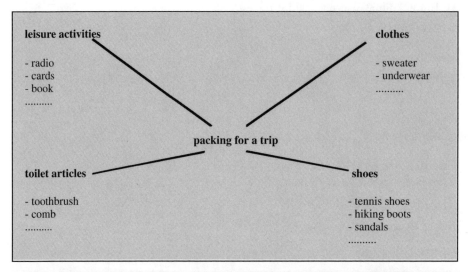

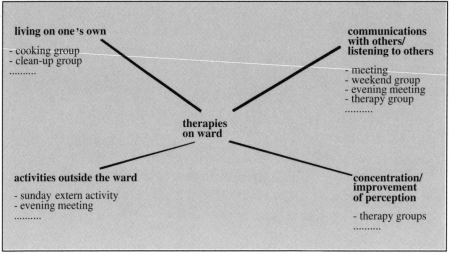

Worksheet 4

Social Perception – The Slides

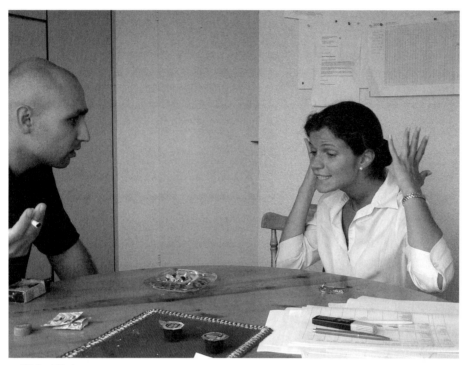

Slide 35: Argument

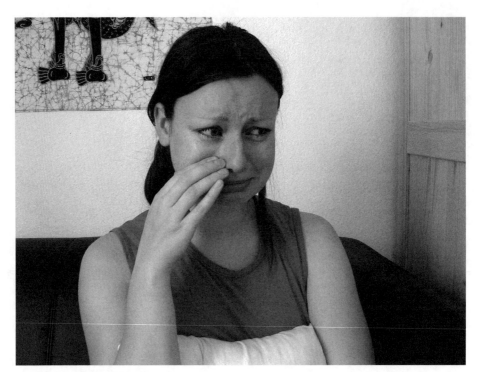

Slide 40: Crying Woman

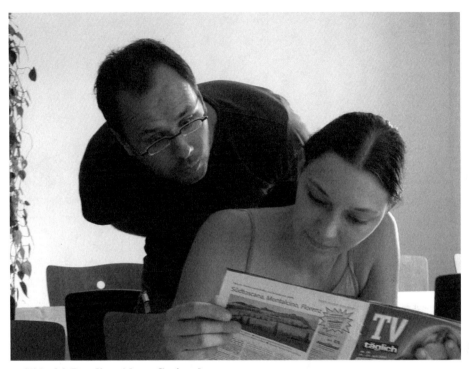

Slide 36: Reading Along Curiously

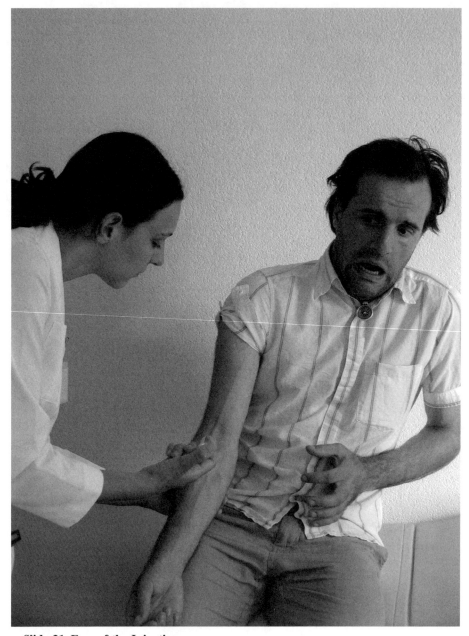

Slide 21: Fear of the Injection

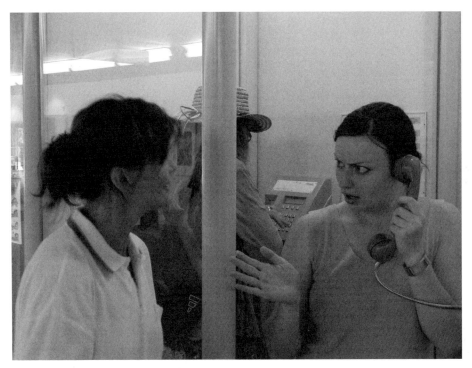

Slide 03: Dispute About the Phone

Worksheet 5

Social Perception – Ratings of the Cognitive Complexity of the Slides

Slide	Low cognitive complexity (in %)	Moderate cognitive complexity (in %)	High cognitive complexity (in %)
1	18	31	**51**
2	**63**	26	11
3	4	38	**58**
4	**48**	39	13
5	21	**46**	33
6	3	16	**81**
7	33	**46**	21
8	**58**	33	9
9	1	15	**84**
10	11	43	**46**
11	**40**	31	29
12	38	**45**	17
13	**48**	34	18
14	25	**45**	30
15	**45**	41	14
16	15	**56**	29
17	9	36	**55**
18	7	44	**49**
19	2	19	**79**
20	3	19	**78**
21	**53**	33	14
22	33	**51**	16
23	10	34	**56**
24	41	**45**	14
25	11	31	**58**
26	34	**45**	21
27	14	36	**50**
28	24	**46**	30
29	9	30	**61**
30	**50**	39	11
31	10	30	**60**
32	25	**56**	19
33	6	33	**61**
34	6	45	**49**
35	16	**50**	34
36	**45**	34	21
37	0	31	**69**
38	**40**	39	21
39	3	8	**89**
40	**60**	31	9

Percentage in **bold** = highest value for this slide.

Worksheet 6a

Social Perception – Ratings of the Emotional Load of the Slides

Slide	Not/barely emotionally loaded (%)	Somewhat emotionally loaded (%)	High emotionally loaded (%)
1	18	**48**	34
2	23	**39**	38
3	24	38	**38**
4	30	**36**	34
5	20	37	**43**
6	25	**46**	29
7	18	39	**43**
8	**38**	31	31
9	24	**44**	32
10	**41**	31	28
11	**48**	33	19
12	14	26	**60**
13	21	36	**43**
14	27	**38**	35
15	**64**	26	10
16	33	**40**	27
17	**40**	36	24
18	35	**40**	25
19	**52**	33	15
20	17	**50**	33
21	23	26	**51**
22	9	25	**66**
23	33	**38**	29
24	**37**	35	28
25	7	20	**73**
26	26	**44**	30
27	30	35	**35**
28	**43**	24	33
29	10	34	**56**
30	32	**39**	29
31	**36**	29	35
32	**36**	31	33
33	25	35	**40**
34	21	**44**	35
35	30	**48**	22
36	**60**	25	15
37	**43**	38	19
38	25	33	**42**
39	19	**46**	35
40	13	29	**58**

Percentage in **bold** = highest value for this slide.

Worksheet 6b

Social Perception – Judgments of Emotions Expressed in the Slides

Slide	Happiness (%)	Surprise (%)	Anger (%)	Sadness (%)	Fear (%)
1	**94**	6			
2	6	**70**	1	3	20
3		21	**74**	4	1
4	3		4	**90**	3
5			2	**98**	
6	**98**	1	1		
7		45	1	**54**	
8	5	**71**		24	
9	**99**	1			
10	1	**55**	18	13	13
11	20	**74**	1		5
12	8	1		**90**	1
13	3	1		**96**	
14	1			**78**	21
15	23	**66**	11		
16	4	3	11	24	**58**
17	1	4	**93**		3
18	8	**78**			14
19	25	**53**	11	8	3
20	**96**	1	3		
21	1	5			**94**
22	3	**94**		3	
23	6	34	**55**	4	1
24	39	**61**			
25		3		4	**93**
26	**99**				1
27	**99**	1			
28	46	**51**	3		
29	2	**98**			
30			1	**95**	4
31	**94**	5	1		
32		**91**	3		6
33	**88**	11		1	
34	2	11	13		**74**
35	3	9	**88**	1	
36	15	**83**	1	1	
37	5	43	**47**	4	1
38			**77**	19	4
39	**96**	1	3		
40	1			**96**	3

Percentage in **bold** = highest value for this slide.

Worksheet 7

Social Perception – List of the Titles of the Slides*

Slide no.	Title
1	Conversation in a train
2	Surprise
3	Dispute about the phone
4	Sad train ride
5	Sad news
6	Amusement on a merry-go-round
7	Accident in front of the window
8	Nasty surprise
9	Stroll around town
10	Demonstration
11	Fake astonishment
12	Moving farewell
13	Supporting a friend
14	Comfort and despair
15	Astonished radio host
16	Yuck! Spiders!
17	Threat
18	Watch out for the ball!
19	Sales talk
20	Demonstrations are fun
21	Fear of the injection
22	Misfortune
23	Fighting couple
24	For me?
25	Great danger/threat
26	Fun, joy with friends
27	Break in summer
28	Oh, watch!
29	Funeral
30	Comfort
31	Happiness
32	Dear me! Look at this!
33	Gift giving at Christmas
34	Aggression and defense
35	Argument
36	Reading along curiously
37	Fight about the bill
38	Protest
39	Fun school trip
40	Crying woman

*The slides can be ordered from the first author.

Worksheet 8

Verbal Communication – Step 1: Literal Repetition Exercise

Emotionally Neutral

5–10-word sentences

1. On Saturday we are going shopping in town. (8)
2. This weekend I am going to visit a friend. (9)
3. My sister gave birth to her baby yesterday. (8)
4. The restaurant is closed on Mondays. (6)
5. My roommate needs to go to the hospital on Tuesday. (10)
6. Our cooking group is making pizza and a salad today. (10)
7. The bulb of my bedside lamp is burned out. (9)
8. Tomorrow evening I would like to go the movies. (9)
9. The bus was very crowded today. (6)
10. Yesterday there was a flea market in town. (8)
11. On weekends I often take walks to nearby villages. (9)
12. Marianne bought herself a new pair of jeans. (8)
13. Later on, I will go and pay my phone bill. (10)

11–15-word sentences

1. Today I have an important appointment at 2 p.m. so I can't go to therapy. (15)
2. Give me the empty bottles; I am passing the bottle bank anyway. (12)
3. While Eric was cleaning the dining room yesterday, he knocked over a vase. (13)
4. Although it is June, the lake is still too cold for swimming. (12)
5. Yesterday I took my radio to get it fixed because the antenna was broken. (14)
6. Once you're done cleaning your room, you need to help me in the kitchen. (15)
7. Linda's new bicycle is equipped with a special mirror and a speedometer on the handlebar. (15)
8. When we go to the theater, I will put on my new dress. (13)
9. I don't know which book to give Jim for his birthday. (11)
10. This morning when I got to the bus stop, the bus had already left. (14)
11. If the weather stays warm, we can go swimming later today. (11)
12. Last Monday Cindy went to the beauty shop and got her hair washed and cut. (15)

16–20-word sentences

1. In the Sunday cooking group we made a cereal mix that contained oatmeal, nuts, bananas, apples, and raisins. (18)
2. The entire hospital is being renovated, and the work is scheduled to be finished in 2010. (16)

3. The ivy plant on the window ledge in my room is very dry because I forgot to water it yesterday. (20)
4. Since the post office closes at 5 p.m., you will have to hurry to get your package there. (18)
5. From this fall on, the high school has new rules about leaving the school grounds during lunch. (17)
6. The lake rose 10 feet within a single week, and some of the docks were flooded. (16)
7. When I take my next vacation, I must not forget my passport like I did last time. (17)
8. Anna, a friend of mine from the workshop, has invited me to go for coffee at the canteen. (18)

Emotionally Loaded

5–10-word sentences

1. Please stop criticizing everything I do! (6)
2. It's nice you could come see me. (7)
3. Please just leave! I can't stand you any longer. (9)
4. Thank you for helping with kitchen duty! (7)
5. Tomorrow I'll start working in the woodwork shop. (8)
6. My father is in the hospital for surgery. (8)
7. The group leader was very pleased with my work today. (10)
8. Please be so kind as to leave me alone! (9)
9. I hope my sister gets home O.K. in this snow! (10)
10. Why do you always blame me for everything? (8)
11. I am looking forward to seeing you tomorrow. (8)

11–15-word sentences

1. Your mother called today and asked me to tell you she can't come. (13)
2. I really don't feel like doing the dishes and cleaning up the kitchen right now. (15)
3. You're coming tonight, aren't you? We can take a walk together. (11)
4. Why do you always have to correct me? I know when I am wrong. (14)
5. I am really looking forward to going to the circus with you. (12)
6. I'm having trouble concentrating today because I didn't sleep well last night. (12)
7. Why can't you be on time for once? You always keep me waiting. (13)
8. How nice of you to stop by. I'm so glad to see you again. (14)
9. I was so surprised to find out my roommate was sick and had a fever. (15)
10. I hope the weather is good; otherwise we won't be able to go cycling. (14)
11. Can't you walk with me? I'm afraid to go home alone after dark. (13)

16–20-word sentences

1. I am really upset you didn't meet me at the movie theater like you said you would. (17)
2. Please tell me what is wrong with you. You've been grumpy and have hardly spoken all day long! (18)
3. You are always telling me how sloppy I am, but you are sloppy about how you keep your room too! (20)
4. Why can't you be a little more considerate? When I want to sleep, you always turn up the music! (19)
5. I'm sorry I was so unfriendly to you yesterday. I was just in a bad mood. (16)
6. Why did it have to rain on day we wanted to take a trip to the park! (17)

Worksheet 9

Verbal Communication: Step 2 – Paraphrasing Exercise

Emotionally Neutral

1. Car
2. Summer
3. Sports
4. Weather
5. Shoes
6. Pants
7. Hand
8. Train
9. Restaurant
10. Shower
11. Aftershave
12. Porter
13. Mail
14. Radio
15. Hairdresser
16. Breakfast
17. Newspaper
18. Mirror
19. Soap
20. Flowers
21. Bicycle
22. Room
23. Ballpoint pen
24. Boat
25. Lake
26. Towel
27. Wind
28. Lighter
29. Wallet
30. Stone
31. Cooking – Vegetables
32. Winter – Heating
33. Hiking – Backpack
34. House – Door
35. Bank – Check

Emotionally Loaded

1. Joyful
2. Happy
3. Sad
4. Suffer
5. Angry
6. Aggressive
7. Relaxed
8. Love (verb)
9. Uncertainty
10. Afraid
11. Friendship
12. Criticize
13. Praise
14. Impress
15. Likable
16. Pleasant
17. Shock
18. Hope
19. Family
20. Handicap
21. Love (noun)
22. Medication
23. Happiness
24. Luck
25. Content
26. Tenderness
27. Psychiatry
28. Laugh
29. Forgiveness
30. Worry
31. Date – Happiness
32. Problems – Headache
33. Work – Appreciation
34. Accident – Luck
35. Husband – Jealousy

Worksheet 10
Verbal Communication – Step 3: W-Questions

Lower Level of Difficulty

1. What?
2. Why?
3. How?
4. When?
5. Who?
6. Where?

Higher Level of Difficulty

1. What?
2. Where to?
3. Why?
4. When?
5. How?
6. With what?
7. How far?
8. Who?
9. Whose?
10. Which?
11. To whom?
12. Where?
13. How much?

Worksheet 11
Social Skills – Low-Risk Situations

A. Thanking

1. A fellow resident sewed two buttons on a shirt for you. Now he is returning the shirt. You are very pleased. You thank him and promise you will do him a favor in return.
2. A fellow resident, without being asked, helped you do the dishes. He has dried all the plates and saved you a lot of work. Now everything is done. You want to thank him and let him know how pleased you were to have his help.
3. During occupational therapy a fellow resident tells you there is a good movie on television in the evening. You thank him for the information.
4. Your friend has just offered you a very nice book for your birthday. You go see her and thank her for the present.
5. One evening you are late for dinner. When you arrive you see that the others are nearly finished with the meal but they have kept your portion warm. You thank them for keeping your meal warm.
6. An old friend stops to visit you. You take a walk together and talk. Your friend invites you for coffee and cake at a café nearby. When your friend is leaving you want to thank him for the visit and for the coffee and cake.

B. Giving a Compliment

1. A fellow resident who is on kitchen duty today has cooked an excellent meal. You talk to him and tell him how much you enjoyed the meal he cooked.
2. A fellow resident who does oil paintings is hanging up one of his pictures in the common room. You like the picture very much. You tell him how much you like the painting.
3. A fellow resident has made a clay vase. You like the vase. You talk to her and tell her you like the vase.
4. A resident has just cleaned the living room. It looks so nice you really enjoy being in the room. You decide to tell him what a good job of cleaning he did.
5. A resident has just bought a new dress. You think it fits her very well and she looks good in it. You decide to tell her how nice the dress looks on her.
6. A friend has helped you finish a piece of work. Thanks to him you are finished an hour earlier than you thought you would. You think your friend has done a very good job. You tell him what a good job he did and how much you appreciate his help.

C. Gathering Information

1. You have forgotten what time your doctor appointment is on Friday. You call his assistant and inquire about the exact time of the appointment.
2. You want to speak to your psychologist but you can't find her office telephone number. You decide to ask the ward staff for her number. You knock on the door and are asked what it is you need.
3. There is a miniature golf course on the hospital grounds. You would like to play but don't know where to get the ball and club. You ask a fellow resident.
4. You are visiting the hospital's cafeteria for the first time. Since you've only been at the hospital for a few days, you don't know your way around very well. You aren't sure if the tables are waited or if it is self-serve. You ask someone at a neighboring table for information.
5. You would like to go to the movies but don't know which films are being shown that day. You call a friend who gets a daily newspaper to find out what movies are playing and what time they start.
6. You go to a store to buy an alarm-clock. You ask the salesperson for a simple, inexpensive model. The salesperson shows you several different models. You can't decide which one to take so you thank the salesperson and leave the store.

D. Assertive Refusal of a Request

1. A fellow resident who never seems to have cigarettes of his own asks you for the third time if he can have one of yours. Since you don't have much money yourself, you say no in a friendly but clear manner.
2. A fellow resident who frequently doesn't do his share of the household chores asks you to do the dishes for him. Since you've done favors for him many times, you deny his request.
3. A resident from another ward asks you detailed questions about matters you consider very personal. You don't want to talk to him about it. You explain that you don't like his questions and are not going to answer them. You change the subject.
4. A staff member mistakenly claims it is your turn to clean up the recreation room. Since you know you're not on clean-up duty, you refuse to clean the room. You explain the reason why you are not going to clean the area as asked.
5. Someone selling magazine subscriptions comes to your apartment door. He wants to sell you a subscription to a new magazine. Since you're not interested, you deny in a friendly but clear manner and say good-bye to him.
6. You've had a very hard day and you are tired. Your boss comes in for the third time this month and asks you to stay overtime. Since you would really like to go home this evening, you deny this request.

Worksheet 12

Social Skills – Higher Risk Situations

A. Making a Request

1. You ask a fellow resident to bring you a chocolate bar from the store. He agrees to do so.
2. You ask a fellow resident to help you put the tablecloth on the table. She agrees.
3. Your desk in occupational therapy is near a very loud machine. The noise bothers you and makes it difficult for you to concentrate on your work. You speak to the therapist and ask for a different desk. The therapist says he will try to find a different place for you. That answer is good enough for the moment.
4. You enter the ward office and ask a staff member for an extension on your community pass. After agreeing on an exact time when you will be back, the staff member grants your request.
5. You're worried about the side effects of a new medication you are taking. You want to talk to the doctor about your concerns. You call her up to make an appointment. The receptionist arranges an appointment with you.
6. It's 6 p.m. and you are standing at the busstop nearby an older man. There is no store or moneychanger close by and you don't have the exact change for the bus fare. You ask the man if he has change for a dollar. He does and gives you the change.

B. Making an Apology

1. You borrow a magazine from a fellow resident and accidentally spill juice on it, making a few pages sticky and dirty. You explain the accident and say you are sorry for what happened. The resident accepts your apology.
2. You forgot that you were supposed to set the table together with another resident. The other resident has set the table all by himself. You apologize to him. He is angry at first but after you explain why you forgot he accepts your apology.
3. You come very late to group and the group needs to stop in the middle of an activity so the therapist can give the instructions again, which you missed by being late. You apologize to the therapist and the group for being late and for the interruption. They accept your apology.
4. You've missed your appointment with your therapist. You call him, apologize, and request a new appointment. The therapist accepts your apology and gives you a new appointment.
5. While shopping you accidentally step on the foot of another shopper who reacts with a little scream. You tell her you are sorry for stepping on her foot. She accepts the apology.

6. It is just before midnight and you're listening to your favorite record. Suddenly some-one knocks on your door. It is your neighbor who complains about the music being too loud. You apologize to the neighbor and promise to turn the music down. The neighbor accepts your apology.

C. Behavior Change Requests

1. Your roommate is listening to very loud music. The loud music irritates you and you ask your roommate to turn the radio off. Your roommate first wants to know the reason. You explain the reason and he turns the radio down.
2. You are supposed to wash the dishes together with a fellow resident but she is smoking a cigarette and talking to another resident. Since you want to get done quickly, you are impatient to begin. You tell her you would like to get the dishes done soon and ask her to postpone her conversation and help you with the dishes. She agrees.
3. A resident from another ward has said he would meet you at 8 a.m. to do aerobics. You are on time but your fellow resident arrives half an hour late. You tell him you do not appreciate his being late. Then both of you do your exercises.
4. You have bought a fellow resident a pack of cigarettes but they are the wrong brand and she criticizes you for not remembering the right brand and insults you. You state you are sorry for the error but do not appreciate being criticized and insulted over such an unimportant matter. You turn and walk away.
5. You are in a store and you have just paid for an item you bought. The cashier gives you the wrong change. You point out the error to her and request the right amount of change. She counts the money again and gives you the missing amount.
6. A sweater you've just bought has a hole in it and you return it immediately to the store. You show the salesperson the hole in the sweater and request an exchange. After seeing the receipt, the salesperson exchanges the sweater for you.

D. Starting a Conversation

1. You've just moved to another unit and would like to get to know your new fellow residents. You walk up to the man whose room is next to yours, introduce yourself and ask him a few questions. He answers your questions and then you say good-bye.
2. There is a new resident on the ward today. After lunch he sits down in one of the lounge chairs outside. Since you want to get a bit of sun yourself, you take the chair next to him and start a conversation.
3. There is a new therapist on your ward. Since you don't know her yet, you decide to introduce yourself. When she comes out of her office, you speak to her. A short conversation follows.
4. You have received information from a social worker about an emotional support group. You are attending the group today for the first time. Someone you have seen

before at the hospital is sitting at a table drinking a soda. You go up and ask him to tell you about the group. He tells you what you want to know.

5. You are taking the bus to work, as you do every morning. A person your age, whom you often see on the bus, is sitting across from you. The person seems to recognize you too and greets you with a nod. You start up a conversation with the person and chat for a while.

6. You meet your new neighbor in the hallway. You have never seen him before, but he seems nice. You would like to get to know him better. You greet him and begin a conversation. Your neighbor is glad to talk to you.

E. Initiating an Activity with Others

1. You need to go to the laboratory for the first time to have a blood sample taken. Since you're new on the ward, you don't know the way. You go to the ward office and ask a staff member to accompany you. After having explained your situation, the staff member agrees.

2. One evening you are sitting with other residents in the recreation room. You've read the paper already and would like to play a game. You ask a fellow resident if he would like to play a game with you. He joins you in the game.

3. After occupational therapy you would like to take a walk. You ask a fellow resident whether he would like to come along. After a moment's hesitation, he agrees to join you.

4. You would like to go to the movies to see a new film that's playing. Since you don't want to go alone, you ask a fellow resident if he would like to join you. He wants to know more details about the film first, but then agrees.

5. You've arranged a trip with some friends who are visiting you. Since they don't know the area very well, you suggest a place to go to. They agree.

6. You live in a community with three roommates and you have all decided to invite friends over for dinner. You go up to your friends and arrange a time. They are very pleased and thank you for the invitation.

Worksheet 13

Social Skills – Complex Situations

Behavior in Complex Situations

1. You are sitting in your favorite restaurant and would like to pay the bill. As you are about to pull out your wallet, you realize that you have left it at home. There is no one in the restaurant you know. You motion to the waitress, whom you've seen before, and tell her your situation.
2. A friend of yours is in the hospital with a minor illness. He will have to have a small operation. Today you go and visit him at the hospital. Although he is still somewhat weak, you have a short conversation with him.
3. You would like to be accepted to live at a residential care home. They invite you to come for an interview. First, the interviewer asks why you want to live at the residential care home. Then you ask questions about the home.
4. You see an ad for an apartment in the paper you call the number listed in the ad and inquire about the apartment. You ask a number of questions about it.
5. You call a company to inquire about a job offer you saw in the newspaper.
6. You are visiting a job center because you are looking for a job. The person in charge asks you where you last worked. You tell him about your illness and that you are completely recovered. You tell him that he may get a verification of this from the physician treating you at the hospital.

Worksheet 14

Interpersonal Problem Solving – "Activities Outside the Clinic and Skills in Everyday Life"

These problem areas are usually dealt with quite early and in parallel to the course of rehabilitation. The methods used are mainly classically socio-therapeutic.

A. Hygiene and Grooming

- **Actual State:** Poor independent grooming skills
- **Target State (goal):** A socially acceptable standard of personal grooming

B. Room Care or Household Responsibilities

- **Actual State:** Insufficient order and cleanliness in personal space
- **Target State (goal):** Tidying and cleaning according to norms on the ward

C. Money Management and Shopping Skills

- **Actual State:** Inadequate consumer behavior and bad handling of small amounts of money
- **Target State (goal):** Correct calculations, knowing the approximate prices of important consumer goods. Development of a consumer behavior adapted to needs and possibilities

D. Cooking

- **Actual State:** Insufficient or inexistent cooking skills
- **Target State (goal):** Basic knowledge about and skills in cooking

Worksheet 15

Interpersonal Problem Solving – "Searching for an Apartment"

A. Financial Limitations

– **Actual State:** Unclear financial possibilities of different patients
– **Target State (goal):** Candidates for a living community know their financial limitations and can set their desired rent accordingly.

B. Determining Desired Characteristics of an Apartment

– **Actual State:** Vagueness of the desired characteristics
– **Target State (goal):** Definition of characteristics, such as "location," "size," "number of rooms," etc

C. Resources for Locating an Apartment

– **Actual State:** Insufficient knowledge about finding apartments as well as skills in carrying out searches.
– **Target State (goal):** Sufficient knowledge about possibilities of finding apartments (e.g., through posting or finding ads, black-boards, social workers) as well as basic skills of realizing them.

D. Needed Actions to Locate an Apartment

– **Actual State:** Patients haven't undertaken any steps toward finding an apartment
– **Target State (goal):** Own contribution toward finding an apartment (e.g., posting an ad, replying to ads, calling in)

For legal as well as for practical reasons, important steps, such as "actually contacting the future landlord," "first visit to the apartment," or "closing a contract" are carried out without the patient concerned.

Worksheet 16

Interpersonal Problem Solving – "Furnishing the Apartment"

A. Characteristics of the Apartment

- **Present State:** Lack of knowledge about important characteristics of the apartment
- **Target State (goal):** Exact knowledge about the location (street, house number, floor), the spatial situation, the furnishings as well as the layout of the rooms

B. Needed Furniture

- **Present State:** Uncertainty about available and needed furniture
- **Target State (goal):** Exact idea about available and needed furniture

C. Financing

- **Present State:** Uncertainty about individual financial possibilities
- **Target State (goal):** Clear knowledge about individual financial possibilities

D. Where to Shop for Furniture

- **Present State:** Uncertainty about possibilities of shopping for needed furniture
- **Target State (goal):** Clear knowledge about possibilities of finding furniture

Worksheet 17

Interpersonal Problem Solving – "Living and Working in a Community"

A. Duties/Responsibilities of Living in a Community

- **Present State:** Lack of knowledge about the work and duties accumulating in living communities that need dealing with
- **Target State (goal):** Concrete, detailed definition of household duties, exact knowledge about tasks that need to be carried out alone and independently

B. Organizing the Household

- **Present State:** No clarity about possibilities of carrying out the previously defined housework together
- **Target State (goal):** Distribution of tasks; exact definition of individual duties (e.g., cooking, cleaning, shopping); arranging for "professional" aid in the beginning

C. Arranging a Daily Schedule

- **Present State:** Lack of knowledge about possibilities of scheduling individual duties
- **Target State (goal):** Exact individual daily schedule with clearly defined points in time when the different roommates are to carry out their household duties

D. Integration into the Community

- **Present State:** Renter's lack of knowledge about rights and duties of the renter toward the owner and the community
- **Target State (goal):** Clear definition of rights and duties in the sense of rules of the house and the flat

Worksheet 18

Interpersonal Problem Solving – "Moving"

A. Individual Duties

– **Present State:** Uncertainty about individual duties in the context of moving
– **Target State (goal):** Clear definition of individual tasks (e.g., who is responsible for packing up which items?)

B. Transport

– **Present State:** Uncertainty about which items are to be transported by which means of transport
– **Target State (goal):** Clear decision about means of transport according to individual needs

C. Developing a Schedule

– **Present State:** Uncertainty about the timing of moving
– **Target State (goal):** Concrete schedule

D. Evaluating the Quality and Practicality of the Schedule

– **Present State:** Uncertainty about the quality and the practicality of the schedule
– **Target State (goal):** Raising the certainty (e.g., by going through the plan) and closing eventual gaps in planning

Worksheet 19

Description of the Rating Scales – Used for Self-Assessment and Assessment by Others

- All Rehab score sheets are based on a 2-week period, the only exception being the FP Questionnaire, which is based on a single session.
- Rehab evaluation takes place every other week.
- Two different therapists should always complete all questionnaires.

Rating Scales

1. Attendance:

1 = Patient is present, i.e., for at least 70% of the therapy duration
0 = Patient is not present or is absent or is present less than 70% of the therapy duration

2. Punctuality

1 = Patient is punctual for therapy session
0 = Patient needs to be prompted to attend therapy or is escorted there after not having appeared independently within 5 minutes

3. Proactivity

1 = Patient attends therapy without staff prompting or supervision
0 = Patient needs to be prompted to attend therapy or is escorted there after not having appeared independently within 5 minutes

4. Behavior in the Therapy Group (BT)

- The primary therapist fills in the BT Questionnaire together with the cotherapist immediately after each IPT session

5. Personal Functioning

- Three different questionnaires evaluate skills of looking after oneself:
  HM (Household Maintenance)

HG (Hygiene and Grooming)
GP (Food Preparation)
– HM: The household duties are reassigned once a week during the morning confer-
ence
– Each patient is always assigned to do his RM (Room Maintenance)
– A patient is either in charge of KM (Kitchen Maintenance), WM (Ward Mainte-
nance), or is off duty

RM includes:

– Making one's own bed
– Changing the bedding once every 2 weeks
– Dusting
– Vacuuming
– Tidying up clothes and other items
– Keeping one's closet tidy

KM includes:

– Setting the table
– Getting meals from the elevator
– Preparing meals, also keeping food warm for patients who might not make it in time
– Bringing leftovers back to the elevator
– Washing, drying, and putting away dishes
– Cleaning the kitchen
– Mopping the kitchen floor on Thursdays

WM includes:

– Airing out the living room (smoking and dining room)
– Emptying ashtrays and garbage cans
– Vacuuming
– Dusting
– For KM and WM, groups of 3–4 people are in charge at a time
– Group members decide each day who is responsible for which task or area, i.e.:
Patient A: Kitchen area
Patient B: Table and food area
Each area is then evaluated individually
– If jobs are assigned after mealtimes (breakfast, lunch, dinner), only this point in time
is evaluated. The remainder is subtracted from the patient's score, i.e., morning: 4
points; noon: . . .; evening: . . .
– KM is always evaluated after meals, and WM and RM are evaluated at 9:30 a.m.
and 11:00 a.m. on weekends.

6. Self-Evaluation Questionnaire

–   Each patient completes the Self-Evaluation Questionnaire once every other week, in the presence of a staff member
–   There are two parallel forms that should be handed out to the patients alternately to ensure that the questionnaire is not filled out the same way each time. Both forms are to be evaluated with the same scoring sheet
–   The Self-Evaluation Questionnaire can also be rated without the scoring sheets, by means of the Self-Evaluation Questionnaires P1 and P2
–   It is only necessary for the patients to complete the questions that have been assessed by the observers as well, i.e., if the food preparation group's meeting has been cancelled, no self-evaluation is required
–   If therapy sessions have been cancelled or a patient was sick, on holiday, or on weekend leave, the unattended activities or tasks that have not been executed are not included in the final score

7. Rehab Scoring

–   The target state (goal) is determined by taking into account available therapy activities, performance in household maintenance (HM), as well as any absence due to illness or vacation
–   The present individual scores are listed in the Rehab Scoring Sheet 1
–   The relationship between the present state recorded and the potential target state for each skill area is expressed as a percentage in the Rehab Scoring Sheet 2

An average percentage rate is computed for each designated interval (2-week intervals) by adding up the different percentage rates and dividing the sum by the number of rating scales administered (maximum of 6)
–   The percentage rates of the individual content areas are presented graphically on curves depicting the course of therapy in the Rehab Questionnaire Summary 1
–   The Rehab Questionnaire Summary 2 compares the mean average rates based on observer evaluation with the average rates based on the patient's self-evaluation (the patient's ability to appropriately interpret and deal with reality)

Worksheet 20

Behavior in the Therapy Group (BT) – Assessment by Others

Unit _____ Patient _____
Therapy Group _____ Period of Observation _____

			BT (Behavior in the Therapy Group)	
			Session 1	Session 2
			Date	Date
– Attendance:	1 = yes	0 = no	1 0	1 0
– Punctuality:	1 = punctual	0 = not on time	1 0	1 0
– Proactivity:	1 = independent	0 = requires prompting and supervision	1 0	1 0

Content Evaluation
0 = never / 1 = occasionally / 2 = sometimes / 3 = frequently / 4 = mostly / 5 = always

1) Eye Contact:

   Frequency of eye contact is rated, not direction (patients or therapists)   543210   543210
   (5 = Patient always has eye contact during therapy)

2) Participation in Group Discussions:

   Spontaneous task-oriented participation is rated, not responses given when directly   543210   543210
   addressed (5 = Patient always actively participates in the discussion)

3) Content of Speech:

a) Theme-oriented responses are rated (Remark is always related to the topic discussed)   543210   543210

b) The ability to appraise what is being discussed and to apply it according to other con-   543210   543210
   versation topics is rated (5 = Patient always succeeds in detaching himself/herself
   from a concrete situation and generalizing to other areas)

4) Formal Aspects of Speech:

a) The ability to formulate complete sentences is rated, vocabulary and presentation   543210   543210
   techniques are not (5 = Patient always makes complete sentences)

b) Clarity and volume of speech are rated, slurred speech due to extrapyramidal side ef-   543210   543210
   fects produced by neuroleptics are not (5 = Patient always speaks loudly)

5) Interactional Skills (Ability to Participate in a Group)

a) The ability to verbally communicate with *all* group members – patients and therapists   543210   543210
   alike – is rated (5 = Patient always relates to fellow patients and therapists alike)

b) Constructive participation during the therapy session is rated (5 = Patient always con-   543210   543210
   structively participates in the therapy session)

6) Posture / Facial Expression

a) The patient's peace of mind is rated, as compared to, say, tension or fatigue. Side ef-   543210   543210
   fects of neuroleptics (e.g., akathisia) are not rated (5 = Patient always seems relaxed
   and well-balanced)

b) Adequate or appropriate behavior is rated, as opposed to e.g., pretense or mannerisms   543210   543210
   (5 = Patient always behaves adequately)

$\Sigma_{1+2} =$ $\Sigma_1 =$ $\Sigma_2 =$

Worksheet 21

Household and Maintenance (HM) – Assessment by Others

Patient: . . . . Therapy Group: . . . .
Period of observation: . . . .

HM (Household Maintenance)

Date	Kitchen Maintenance						Ward Maintenance		Room Maintenance	
	Morning	S	Noon	S	Evening	S		S		S
Mon										
Tues										
Wed										
Thur										
Fri										
Sat										
Sun										
Mon										
Tues										
Wed										
Thur										
Fri										
Sat										
Sun										
1st week	KM: Σ =		S: Σ =				WM: Σ =	S: Σ =	RM: Σ =	S: Σ =
2nd week	KM: Σ =		S: Σ =				WM: Σ =	S: Σ =	RM: Σ =	S: Σ =

RATING SCALES:

- For Kitchen Maintenance (KM), Ward Maintenance (WM) and Room Maintenance (RM):

  5 = Excellent
  4 = Good
  3 = Satisfactory
  2 = Unsatisfactory
  1 = Very unsatisfactory
  0 = No work done at all

- For Self-Reliance (S):

  1 = Patient works without prompting or supervision
  0 = Patient requires prompting or supervision

1st week
Σ KM + WM + RM =

2nd week
Σ KM + WM + RM =

Worksheet 22

Movement Therapy (MT) – Assessment by Others

Patient:.......................... Therapy Group.......

Period of observation:..........

MT (Movement Therapy)

Date	Attendance	Punctuality	Self-reliance	
Mon				1st Week
Tues				Σ A =
Wed				Σ P =
Thur				Σ S =
Fri				
Sat Sun				
Mon				2nd Week
Tues				Σ A =
Wed				Σ P =
Thur				Σ S =
Fri				
Sat Sun				

Attendance   1 = Yes   Punctuality   1 = punctual   Self-reliance   1 = comes without prompting
           0 = No   0 = not on time   0 = requires prompting

Worksheet 23

Work Therapy (WT) – Assessment by Others

WT (Work Therapy)

Patient: . . . . Therapy Group . . . .

Period of observation: . . . .

Work Therapist: . . . .

Date	Attendance	Punctuality	Weekly Performance Level (as compared to healthy people who are not hospitalized)		
Mon			quantitative ☐	4 = 100–80% 3 = 80–60% 2 = 60–40% 1 = 40–20% 0 = <20%	1st Week: Σ A = Σ P =
Tues					
Wed			qualitative ☐	4 = excellent 3 = good 2 = average 1 = below average 0 = unsatisfactory	
Thur					
Fri					
Sat Sun					
Mon			quantitative ☐	4 = 100–80% 3 = 80–60% 2 = 60–40% 1 = 40–20% 0 = <20%	2nd Week: Σ A = Σ P =
Tues					
Wed			qualitative ☐	4 = excellent 3 = good 2 = average 1 = below average 0 = unsatisfactory	
Thur					
Fri					
Sat Sun					
Attendance: 1 = yes 0 = no	Punctuality	1 = punctual 0 = not on time	Particular problems:		

Worksheet 24

Planned Group Activities (GA) – Assessment by Others

GA (Planned Group Activities)

Patient: . . . . Therapy Group . . . .
Period of observation: . . . .

Date	CE (Communal Evening)			M I (Meeting I)			M II (Meeting II)			SA (Sunday Activity)		
	Attendance	Punctuality	Self-reliance	Attendance	Punctuality	Self-reliance	Attendance	Punctuality	Self-reliance	Attendance	Punctuality	Self-reliance
Mon												
Tues												
Wed												
Thur												
Fri												
Sat												
Sun												
Mon												
Tues												
Wed												
Thur												
Fri												
Sat												
Sun												

Attendance	Punctuality	Self-reliance
1 = yes	1 = punctual	1 = comes without prompting
0 = no	0 = not on time	0 = requires prompting

CE: $\Sigma T =$
$\Sigma P =$
$\Sigma S =$

M: $\Sigma T =$
$\Sigma P =$
$\Sigma S =$

$\Sigma T =$
$\Sigma P =$
$\Sigma S =$

SA: $\Sigma T =$
$\Sigma P =$
$\Sigma S =$

Worksheet 25

Cookery Group (CG) – Assessment by Others

Patient: . . . . Therapy Group . . . . . Date (1st cooking experience):	**FP** (Food Preparation)

Attendance:	1 = yes	0 = no	1 0
Self-reliance:	1 = independent	0 = requires prompting	1 0

1. Head Chef (in charge of cooking)		2. Assistant cook (in charge of all preparatory tasks and of assisting the head chef)	
1) How well is the menu planned? (i. e., making the shopping-list, making use of available financial resources). (5 = Patient masters the situation)	0 = not at all 1 = very poor 2 = unsatisfactory 3 = satisfactory 4 = good 5 = excellent 0 1 2 3 4 5	1) How well is the menu planned? (i. e. making the shopping-list, making use of available financial resources). (5 = Patient masters the situation)	0 = not at all 1 = very poor 2 = unsatisfactory 3 = satisfactory 4 = good 5 = excellent 0 1 2 3 4 5
2) How well are the steps involved in cooking a meal carried out without supervision? (5 = Patient performs all the steps without prompting or supervision)	0 = never 1 = occasionally 2 = sometimes 3 = frequently 4 = mostly 5 = always 0 1 2 3 4 5	2) How self-reliant is the patient when doing the shopping? (5 = Patient always does the shopping him/herself)	0 = never 1 = occasionally 2 = sometimes 3 = frequently 4 = mostly 5 = always 0 1 2 3 4 5
3) How good is the meal? (5 = Meal is excellent)	0 = not at all 1 = very poor 2 = unsatisfactory 3 = satisfactory 4 = good 5 = excellent 0 1 2 3 4 5	3) How well does the patient help the head chef (without taking over the lead from him/her or sinking into passivity? (5 = Patient always fulfils the chores assigned to the head chef's assistant)	0 = never 1 = occasionally 2 = sometimes 3 = frequently 4 = mostly 5 = always 0 1 2 3 4 5
4) Does the patient clean up the kitchen before he/she goes? (5 = Kitchen has been cleaned up very well)	0 = not at all 1 = very poor 2 = unsatisfactory 3 = satisfactory 4 = good 5 = excellent 0 1 2 3 4 5	4) Does the patient clean up the kitchen before he/she goes? (5 = Kitchen is cleaned up very well)	0 = not at all 1 = very poor 2 = unsatisfactory 3 = satisfactory 4 = good 5 = excellent 0 1 2 3 4 5
$\Sigma\ 1 + 2 + 3 + 4 =$		$\Sigma\ 1 + 2 + 3 + 4 =$	

Worksheet 26

Hygiene and Grooming (HG) – Assessment by Others

Patient: . . . . Therapy Group . . . .

Period of observation: . . . .

HG (Hygiene and Grooming)

1) How well is the patient groomed? How well does he/she attend to personal hygiene? (This includes washing, manicure, etc., while use of make-up, nail-polish, etc., are not considered in this rating.)
(5 = Patient always takes an interst in his/her personal hygiene and is always well-groomed)

0 = never
1 = occasionally
2 = sometimes
3 = frequently
4 = mostly
5 = always

0 1 2 3 4 5

2) How well does the patient attend to his/her clothing? (This includes cleanliness, is his/her clothing torn, ragged, etc., while aspects of fashion are not considered in the rating).
(5 = His/her clothing is in very good condition)

0 = never
1 = occasionally
2 = sometimes
3 = frequently
4 = mostly
5 = always

0 1 2 3 4 5

3) Does the patient take care of points 1) and 2) without having to be constantly reminded to do so?
5 = Patient always keeps him/herself clean and takes care of his/her own clothes)

0 = never
1 = occasionally
2 = sometimes
3 = frequently
4 = mostly
5 = always

0 1 2 3 4 5

Worksheet 27

Self-Assessment P1

Patient: . . . . Therapy Group	**P1**
Period of observation:.	

SELF-EVALUATION

The following statements relate to **your behavior during the last two weeks.** Try to decide if these statements apply to you or not. Then mark the column that best applies to you.

1) Whatever I had to say in the therapy group (A or B) during the last two weeks was always to the point.

☐ False	☐ Partially true	☐ Almost always true	☐ True

2) I always felt relaxed and at ease in the therapy group (rather than tired or tense).

☐ True	☐ Almost always true	☐ Partially true	☐ False

3) I participated actively and spontaneously in therapeutic group discussions.

☐ False	☐ Partially true	☐ Almost always true	☐ True

4) I attended all therapy activities (work therapy, therapy group, movement therapy, etc.) during the last two weeks.

☐ True	☐ Almost always true	☐ Partially true	☐ False

5) I always arrived on time for all therapy activities organized (therapy group, work therapy, movement therapy, etc.).

☐ True	☐ Almost always true	☐ Partially true	☐ False

6) I always came to the therapy activities on my own initiative without having to be told to come by the staff.

☐ False	☐ Partially true	☐ Almost always true	☐ True

7) I always saw to it that my personal appearance was impeccable (personal hygiene, grooming, condition of clothes) during the last two weeks.

☐ True	☐ Almost always true	☐ Partially true	☐ False

8) I carried out well all the work assigned to the food preparation group.

☐ False	☐ Partially true	☐ Almost always true	☐ True

9) I fulfilled all my household responsibilities (on the ward as well as in my own room).

☐ True	☐ Almost always true	☐ Partially true	☐ False

10) I worked very quickly and efficiently in work therapy during the last two weeks.

☐ True	☐ Almost always true	☐ Partially true	☐ False

11) The work I did in work therapy during the last two weeks was of highest quality.

☐ False	☐ Partially true	☐ Almost always true	☐ True

REMARKS

Worksheet 28

Self-Assessment P2

<table>
<tr><td colspan="4">Patient: .... Therapy Group .....

Period of observation:. ....   **P2**</td></tr>
<tr><td colspan="4" align="center">**SELF-EVALUATION**</td></tr>
<tr><td colspan="4">The following statements relate to **your behavior during the last two weeks.** Try to decide if these statements apply to you or not. Then mark the column that best applies to you.</td></tr>
<tr><td colspan="4">1) I have performed my household responsibilities well and kept my room very clean during the last two weeks.</td></tr>
<tr><td>☐ False</td><td>☐ Partially true</td><td>☐ Almost always true</td><td>☐ True</td></tr>
<tr><td colspan="4">2) I have always been well-groomed and have taken excellent care of my clothing during the last two weeks.</td></tr>
<tr><td>☐ True</td><td>☐ Almost always true</td><td>☐ Partially true</td><td>☐ False</td></tr>
<tr><td colspan="4">3) I was able to carry out all the steps involved in food preparation.</td></tr>
<tr><td>☐ False</td><td>☐ Partially true</td><td>☐ Almost always true</td><td>☐ True</td></tr>
<tr><td colspan="4">4) I always made it to the therapy activities without prompting, i. e. the staff did not have to tell me to go.</td></tr>
<tr><td>☐ True</td><td>☐ Almost always true</td><td>☐ Partially true</td><td>☐ False</td></tr>
<tr><td colspan="4">5) I attended all of the therapy activities planned during the last two weeks (work therapy, group therapy, movement therapy, etc.).</td></tr>
<tr><td>☐ True</td><td>☐ Almost always true</td><td>☐ Partially true</td><td>☐ False</td></tr>
<tr><td colspan="4">6) I was always on time for all therapy activities (work therapy, movement therapy, group therapy, etc.).</td></tr>
<tr><td>☐ False</td><td>☐ Partially true</td><td>☐ Almost always true</td><td>☐ True</td></tr>
<tr><td colspan="4">7) I always spontaneously took part in group therapy.</td></tr>
<tr><td>☐ True</td><td>☐ Almost always true</td><td>☐ Partially true</td><td>☐ False</td></tr>
<tr><td colspan="4">8) Whatever I said in group therapy (A or B) during the last two weeks was always to the point.</td></tr>
<tr><td>☐ False</td><td>☐ Partially true</td><td>☐ Almost always true</td><td>☐ True</td></tr>
<tr><td colspan="4">9) I was always relaxed rather than tense or tired in group therapy.</td></tr>
<tr><td>☐ True</td><td>☐ Almost always true</td><td>☐ Partially true</td><td>☐ False</td></tr>
<tr><td colspan="4">10) I did high-quality work during the last two weeks of work therapy.</td></tr>
<tr><td>☐ True</td><td>☐ Almost always true</td><td>☐ Partially true</td><td>☐ False</td></tr>
<tr><td colspan="4">11) I worked fast enough during the last two weeks of work therapy.</td></tr>
<tr><td>☐ False</td><td>☐ Partially true</td><td>☐ Almost always true</td><td>☐ True</td></tr>
<tr><td colspan="4">REMARKS

</td></tr>
</table>

Worksheet 29

Evaluation of Self-Assessment Questionnaires P1 and P2

Potential Scores/Area:

Area	Potential Score	P1 Question No.	P2 Question No.
Therapy Areas	6	1	8
	6	2	9
	6	3	7
Total	18		
Attendance	18	4	5
Punctuality	18	5	6
Self-Reliance	18	6	4
Personal Functioning	6 (HG)	7	2
	6 (FP)	8	3
	6 (HM)	9	1
Total	18		
Work	9 (quant.)	10	11
	9 (qual.)	11	10
Total	18		
Max. Potential Score	108 points		

Worksheet 30

Rehab Evaluation 1

Patient: . . . . Therapy Group . . . . . .

Period of observation: . . . .

REHA — SCORING SHEET 1 (Individual Actual Scores)

	Attendance									Punctuality								Self-Reliance									Therapy Areas		Work			Personal Functioning			
	FP	WT	CE	MI	MII	SA	BT	MT	Σ*	WT	CE	MI	MII	SA	BT	MT	Σ*	FP	CE	MI	MII	SA	BT	MT	HM	Σ*	BT	Σ*	quant	qual	Σ*	HM	FP	HG	Σ*
1st week																																			
2nd week																																			
Σ																																			
3rd week																																			
4th week																																			
Σ																																			
5th week																																			
6th week																																			
Σ																																			
7th week																																			
8th week																																			
Σ																																			
9th week																																			
10th week																																			
Σ																																			
11th week																																			
12th week																																			
Σ																																			

* Current scores

Worksheet 31

Rehab Evaluation 2

Patient: . . . . Therapy Group . . . .

Period of observation: . . . .

REHA — SCORING SHEET 2 (Individual Actual and Potential Scores; Percentage)

	2 weeks Max. Score (Potential score) (W. 100%)	1st + 2nd week Σ Current Score	%	3rd + 4th week Σ Current Score	%	5th + 6th week Σ Current Score	%	7th + 8th week Σ Current Score	%	9th + 10th week Σ Current Score	%	11th + 12th week Σ Current Score	%
Attendance	1 FP/Session 10 WT 4 BT 7 GA 4 MT } 26												
Indiv. Potential Score													
Punctuality	10 AT 4 BT 7 GA 4 MT } 26												
Indiv. Potential Score													
Self-Reliance	1 FP 42 KM 7 GA 14 WM 4 BT 14 RM 4 MT												
Indiv. Potential Score													
Therapy Areas	200												
Indiv. Potential Score													
Work	8 quantitative 8 qualitative } 16												
Indiv. Potential Score													
Personal Functioning	15 HG 70 WM 20 FP 70 RM 210 KM												
Indiv. Potential Score													
Σ Total	S % : 6 = Ø %												
Self-Evaluation	90												
Indiv. Potential Score													

Worksheet 32

Summary of Rehab Evaluation 1

Patient: . . . . Therapy Group . . . . .

Period of observation:. . . . .

REHA QUESTIONNAIRE SUMMARY 1

Attendance (red)
Punctuality (blue)
Self-reliance (black)

Therapy areas (green)
Work (orange)
Personal functioning (brown)

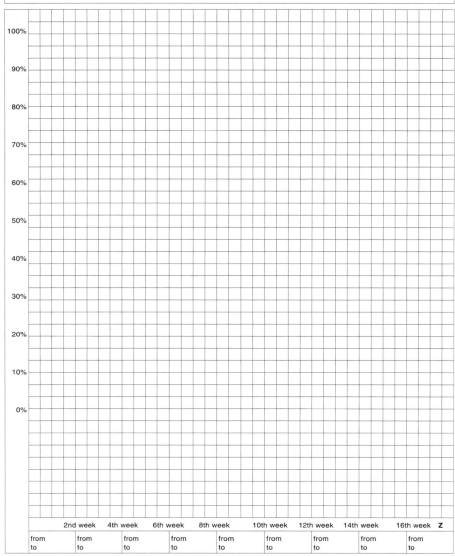

Worksheet 33

Summary of Rehab Evaluation 2

Patient: . . . . Therapy Group . . . . .

Period of observation:. . . . .

REHA QUESTIONNAIRE SUMMARY 2

Total curve (red)
Self-evaluation curve (black)

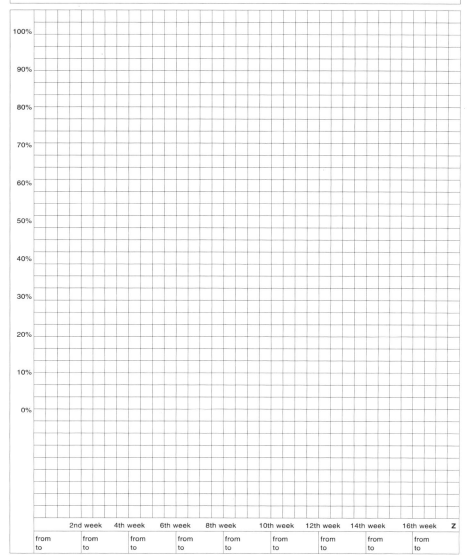

Bibliography

Addington, J., & Addington, D. (1999). Neurocognitive and social functioning in schizophrenia. *Schizophrenia Bulletin, 25*, 173–182.

Addington, J., & Addington, D. (2008). Social and cognitive functioning in psychosis. *Schizophrenia Research, 99*, 176–181.

Addington, J., Saeedi, H., & Addington, D. (2006a). Influence of social perception and social knowledge on cognitive and social functioning in early psychosis. *British Journal of Psychiatry, 189*, 373–378.

Addington, J., Saeedi, H., & Addington, D. (2006b). Facial affect recognition: A mediator between cognitive and social functioning in psychosis? *Schizophrenia Research, 85*, 142–150.

Aleman, A., Agrawal, N., Morgan, K. D., & Davis, A. S. (2006). Insight in psychosis and neuropsychological function. *British Journal of Psychiatry, 189*, 204–212.

Aleman, A., Hijman, R., deHaan, E. H. F., & Kahn, R. S. (1999). Memory impairment in schizophrenia: A meta-analysis. *American Journal of Psychiatry, 156*, 1358–1366.

Alguero, V. M. (2006). *Intervención cognitivo-conductual basada en la terapia psicológica integrada en pacientes con diagnostico de esquizofrenia tipo paranoide en fase de remisión parcial. Tesis presentada como uno de los requisitos para pbtener el grado de magister en psicologia clinica.* Panamá: Universidad de Panamá.

Allen, D. N., Strauss, G. P., Donohue, B., & van Kammen, D. P. (2007). Factor analytic support for social cognition as a separable cognitive domain in schizophrenia. *Schizophrenia Research, 93*, 325–333.

Amering, M., & Schmolke, M. (2007). *Recovery: Das Ende der Unheilbarkeit.* Bonn, Germany: Psychiatrie-Verlag.

Andreasen, N. C. (1983). *Scale for the Assessment of Negative Symptoms (SANS).* Iowa City: The University of Iowa.

Andreasen, N. C. (1984). *Scale for the Assessment of Positive Symptoms (SAPS).* Iowa City: The University of Iowa.

Andreasen, N. C. (1987). Creativity and mental illness: Prevalence rates in writers and their first-degree relatives. *American Journal of Psychiatry, 144*, 1288–1292.

Andreasen, N. C., Carpenter, W.T. J., Kane, J. M., Lasser, R. A., Marder, S. R., & Weinberger, D. R. (2005). Remission in schizophrenia: Proposed criteria and rationale for consensus. *American Journal of Psychiatry, 162*, 441–449.

Andreasen, N. C., Grove, W. M., Shapiro, R. W., Keller, M. B., Hirschfeld, R. M. A., & McDonald-Scott, P. (1981). Reliability of lifetime diagnosis: A multicenter collaborative perspective. *Archives of General Psychiatry, 38*, 400–405.

Andreasen, N. C., Paradiso, S., & O'Leary, D. S. (1998). "Cognitive dysmetria" as an integrative theory of schizophrenia: A dysfunction in cortical-subcortical-cerebellar circuitry? *Schizophrenia Bulletin, 24*, 203–218.

Anthony, W. (1993). Recovery from mental illness: The guiding vision of the mental health service system in the 1990s. *Psychosocial Rehabilitation Journal, 16*, 11–23.

Anthony, W. A. (1979). *Principles of psychiatric rehabilitation*. Baltimore, MD: University Park Press.

Antons, K. (2000). *Praxis der Gruppendynamik* (8. Aufl.). Göttingen: Hogrefe.

APA task force. (2009). *Training grid outlining best practices for recovery and improved outcomes for people with serious mental illness*. Retrieved from http://www.apa.org/practice/grid.html

Argyle, M. (1988). *Bodily communication* (2nd ed.). London: Methuen & Co.

Asarnow, R. F., Steffy, R. A., MacCrimmon, D. J., & Cleghorn, J. M. (1978). An attentional assessment of foster children at risk for schizophrenia. In L. C. Wynne, R. L. Cromwell & S. Matthysse (Eds.), *The nature of schizophrenia: New approaches to research and treatment* (pp. 339–358). New York: Wiley.

Aubin, G., Stip, E., Gelinas, I., Rainvill, C., & Chapparo, C. (2009). Daily activity, cognition and community functioning in persons with schizophrenia. *Schizophrenia Research, 107*, 313–318.

Bandura, A. (1977). *Social learning theory*. Englewood Cliffs, NJ: Prentice-Hall.

Barch, D., & Carter, C. (2005). Amphetamine improves cognitive function in medicated individuals with schizophrenia and in healthy volunteers. *Schizophrenia Research, 77*, 43–58.

Bäuml, J., Kissling, W., Meurer, C., Wais, A., & Lauter, H. (1991). Informationszentrierte Angehörigengruppen zur Complianceverbesserung bei schizophrenen Patienten. *Psychiatrische Praxis, 18*, 48–54.

Baxter, R. D., & Liddle, P. F. (1998). Neuropsychological deficits associated with schizophrenic syndromes. *Schizophrenia Research, 30*, 239–249.

Bebbington, P. E., Bhugra, D., Brugha, T., Singleton, N., Farrell, M., Jenkins, R., … Meltzer, H. (2004). Psychosis, victimization and childhood disadvantage: evidence from the second British National Survey of Psychiatric Morbidity. *British Journal of Psychiatry, 185*, 220–226.

Bebbington, P., Wilkins, S., Jones, P., Foerster, A., Murray, R., Toone, B., & Lewis, S. (1993). Life events and psychosis. Initial results from the Camberwell Collaborative Psychosis Study. *The British Journal of Psychiatry, 162*, 72–79.

Bechard-Evans, L., Schmitz, N., Abadi, S., Joober, R., King, S., Malla, A. (2007). Determinants of help-seeking and system related components of delay in the treatment of first-episode psychosis. *Schizophrenia Research, 96*, 206–214.

Beck, A. (1970). Cognitive therapy: Nature and relation to behavior therapy. *Behavior Therapy, 1*, 184–200.

Beck, A. T., & Rector, N. A. (2000). Cognitive therapy of schizophrenia: A new therapy for the new millennium. *American Journal of Psychotherapy, 54*, 291–300.

Beck, A. T., Rush, A. J., Shaw, B. F., & Emery, G. (1979). *Cognitive therapy of depression*. New York: Guilford.

Bell, M., Bryson, G., Greig, T., Corcoran, C., & Wexler, B. E. (2001). Neurocognitive enhancement therapy with work therapy. *Archives of General Psychiatry, 58*, 763–768.

Bell, M., Bryson, G., & Lysaker, P. (1997). Positive and negative affect recognition in schizophrenia: A comparison with substance abuse and normal control subjects. *Psychiatry Research, 73*, 73–82.

Bell, M., Tsang, H. W. H., Greig, T. C., & Bryson, G. J. (2008). Neurocognition, social cognition, perceived social discomfort, and vocational outcomes in schizophrenia. *Schizophrenia Bulletin, 35*, 738–747.

Bell, M., Zito, W., Greig, T., & Wexler, B. E. (2008). Neurocognitive enhancement therapy and competitive employment in schizophrenia: Effects on clients with poor community functioning. *American Journal of Psychiatric Rehabilitation, 11*, 109–122.

Bellack, A. S. (2004). Skills training for people with severe mental illness. *Psychiatric Rehabilitation Journal, 27*, 375–391.

Bellack, A. S. (2006). Scientific and consumer models of recovery in schizophrenia: Concordance, contrasts, and implications. *Schizophrenia Bulletin, 32*, 432–442.

Bellack, A. S., Green, M. F., Cook, J. A., Fenton, W., Harvey, P. W., Heaton, R. K., ... Wykes, T. (2007). Assessment of community functioning in people with schizophrenia and other severe mental illnesses: A white paper based on an NIMH-sponsored workshop. *Schizophrenia Bulletin, 33*, 805–822.

Bellack, A. S., Morrison, R., & Mueser, K. (1989). Social problem solving in schizophrenia. *Schizophrenia Bulletin, 15*, 101–116.

Bellack, A. S., Morrison, R. L., Wixted, J. T., & Mueser, K. T. (1990). An analysis of social competence in schizophrenia. *British Journal of Psychiatry, 156*, 809–818.

Bellack, A. S., Mueser, K. T., Gingerich, S., & Agresta, J. (1997). *Social skills training for schizophrenia.* New York: Guilford.

Bellack, A. S., Mueser, K. T., Gingerich, S., & Agresta, J. (2004). *Social skills training for schizophrenia. A step-by step guide* (2nd ed.). New York: Guilford.

Bellack, A. S., Sayers, M., Mueser, K. T., & Bennett, M. (1994). Evaluation of a social problem solving in schizophrenia. *Journal of Abnormal Psychology, 103*, 371–378.

Bellucci, D. M., Glaberman, K., & Haslam, N. (2002). Computer-assisted cognitive rehabilitation reduces negative symptoms in the severely mentally ill. *Schizophrenia Research, 59*, 225–232.

Ben-Yishay, Y., Piasetsky, E. B., & Rattok, J. (1985). A systematic method for ameliorating disorders in basic attention. In M. J. Meir, A. L. Benton, & L. Diller (Eds.), *Neuropsychological Rehabilitation* (pp. 165–181). New York: Guilford.

Bender, W., Gerz, L., John, K., Mohr, F., Vaitl, P., & Wagener, U. (1987). Kognitive Therapieprogramme bei Patienten mit schizophrener Residualsymptomatik. Untersuchungen über Wirksamkeit und klinische Erfahrungen. *Neuropsychiatrie, 2*, 212–217.

Benedict, R. H. B., Harris, H., Markow, T., McGormick, J. A., Nuechterlein, K. H., & Asarnow, R. F. (1994). Effects of attention training on information processing in schizophrenia. *Schizophrenia Bulletin, 20*, 537–546.

Bigelow, N. O., Paradiso, S., Adolphs, R., Moser, D. J., Arndt, S., Heberlein, A., ... Andreasen, N. C. (2006). Perception of socially relevant stimuli in schizophrenia. *Schizophrenia Research, 83*, 257–267.

Bilder, R., Ventura, J., & Cienfuegos, A. (2003). *Clinical Global Impression of Cognition in Schizophrenia (CGI-CogS) manual and rating sheet.* Los Angeles, CA: UCLA Department of Psychiatry.

Blakemore, S.-J., & Frith, S. D. (2000). Functional neuroimaging studies of schizophrenia. In J. C. Mazziotta, A. W. Toga, & R. S. J. Frackowiak (Eds.), *Brain mapping: The disorders* (pp. 523–544). San Diego, CA: Academic Press.

Bleuler, E. (1911). *Dementia Praecox oder die Gruppe der Schizophrenien.* Leipzig, Germany: Deuticke.

Blumenthal, S., Bell, V., Schüttler, R., & Vogel, R. (1993). Ausprägung und Entwicklung von Basissymptomen bei schizophrenen Patienten nach einem kognitiven Therapieprogramm. *Schizophrenie, 8*, 20–28.

Boden, R., Sundström, J., Lindström, E., & Lindström, L. (2009). Association between symptomatic remission and functional outcome in first-episode schizophrenia. *Schizophrenia Research, 107*, 232–237.

Bowen, L., Wallace, C., Glynn, S., Nuechterlein, K., Lutzger, J., & Kuehnel, T. (1994). Schizophrenics' cognitive functioning and performance in interpersonal interactions and skills training procedures. *Journal of Psychiatry Research 28*, 289–301.

Bowie, C. R., & Harvey, P. D. (2005). Cognition in schizophrenia: Impairments, determinants, and functional importance. *Psychiatric Clinics North America, 28*, 613–633.

Bowie, C. R., Reichenberg, A., McClure, M. M., Leung, W. L., & Harvey, P. D. (2008). Age-associated differences in cognitive performance in older community dwelling schizophrenia patients: Differential sensitivity of clinical neuropsychological and experimental information processing tests. *Schizophrenia Research, 106*, 50–58.

Bowie, C. R., Reichenberg, A., Patterson, T. L., Heaton, B. K., & Havey, P. D. (2006). Determinants of real-world functional performance in schizophrenia subjects: Correlations with cognition, functional capacity, and symptoms. *American Journal of Psychiatry, 163*, 418–425.

Bracy, O. (1995). *CogRehab Software*. Indianapolis, IN: Psychological Software Services.

Brekke, J., Kay, D. D., Lee, K. S., & Green, M. F. (2005). Biosocial pathways to functional outcome in schizophrenia. *Schizophrenia Research, 80*, 213–225.

Brekke, J., & Nakagami, E. (2010). The relevance of neurocognition and social cognition for outcome and recovery in schizophrenia. In V. Roder & A. Medalia (Eds.), *Neurocognition and social cognition in schizophrenia patients. Comprehension and treatment* (pp. 23–36). Basel, Switzerland: Karger.

Brenner, H. D. (1986). Zur Bedeutung von Basisstörungen für Behandlung und Rehabilitation. In W. Böker & H. D. Brenner (Eds.), *Bewältigung der Schizophrenie* (pp. 142–158). Bern, Switzerland: Huber.

Brenner, H. D. (1987, March). *Treatment of basic cognitive dysfunctions and their pervasive effect on overt behavior in schizophrenia*. International Congress on Schizophrenia Research, Belleview-Biltmore, Clearwater, FL.

Brenner, H. D., Böker, W., Hodel, B., & Wyss, H. (1989). Cognitive treatment of basic pervasive dysfunctions in schizophrenia. In S. C. Schulz & C. A. Tamminga (Eds.), *Schizophrenia: Scientific progress* (pp. 358–367). New York: Oxford University Press.

Brenner, H. D., Hodel, B., Kube, G., & Roder, V. (1987). Kognitive Therapie bei Schizophrenen: Problemanalyse und empirische Ergebnisse. *Nervenarzt, 58*(2), 72–83.

Brenner, H. D., Hodel, R., Roder, V., & Corrigan, P. (1992). Treatment of cognitive dysfunctions and behavioral deficits in schizophrenia. *Schizophrenia Bulletin, 18*, 21–25.

Brenner, H. D., Roder, V., Hodel, B., Kienzle, N., Reed, D., & Liberman, R. P. (1994). *Integrated Psychological Therapy for schizophrenic patients*. Seattle, WA: Hogrefe & Huber.

Brenner, H. D., Stramke, W. G., Hodel, B., & Rui, C. (1982). Untersuchungen zur Effizienz und Indikation eines psychologischen Therapieprogrammes bei schizophrenen Basisstörungen. In F. Reimer (Hg.), *Verhaltenstherapie in der Psychiatrie* (pp. 73–98). Weinsberg, Germany: Weissenhof.

Brenner, H. D., Stramke, W. G., Mewes, J., Liese, F., & Seeger, G. (1980). Erfahrungen mit einem spezifischen Therapieprogramm zum Training kognitiver und kommunikativer Fähigkeiten in der Rehabilitation chronisch schizophrener Patienten. *Nervenarzt, 51*, 106–112.

Briand, C., Bélanger, R., Hamel, V., Nicole, L., Stip, E., Reinharz, D., ... Lesage, A. (2005). Implementation of the multi-site Integrated Psychological Treatment (IPT) program for people with schizophrenia. Elaboration of renewed version. *Sante Mental au Quebec, 30*(1), 73–95.

Briand, C., Vasiliadis, H. M., Lesage, A., Lalonde, P., Stip, E., Nicole, L., ... Villeneuve, K. (2006). Including Integrated Psychological Treatment as part of standard medical therapy for patients with schizophrenia. *Journal of Nervous and Mental Disease, 194*, 463–470.

Bronfenbrenner, U. (1979). *The ecology of human development: Experiments by nature and design*. Cambridge, MA: Harvard University Press.

Broome, M. R., Wooley, J. B., Tabraham, P., Johns, L. C., Bramon, E., Murray, G. K., ... Murray, R. M. (2005). What causes the onset of psychosis? *Schizophrenia Research, 79*, 23–34.

Brown, G. W., Birley, J. L., & Wing, J. K. (1972). Influence of family life on the course of schizophrenic disorders: A replication. *British Journal of Psychiatry, 121*, 241–258.

Brüne, M. (2005). Emotion recognition, "Theory of Mind," and social behavior in schizophrenia. *Psychiatry Research, 133*, 135–147.

Brüne, M., Abdel-Hamid, M., Lehmkämper, C., & Sonntag, C. (2007). Mental state attribution, neurocognitive functioning, and psychopathology: What predicts poor social competence in schizophrenia best? *Schizophrenia Research, 92*, 151–159.

Buchanan, R. W., & Carpenter, W. T. (1997). The neuroanatomies of schizophrenia. *Schizophrenia Bulletin, 23*, 367–372.

Buchkremer, G., Klingberg, S., Holle, R., Schulze Mönking, H., & Hornung, W. P. (1997). Psychoeducational psychotherapy for schizophrenic patients and their key relatives or care-givers: Results of a 2-year follow-up. *Acta Psychiatrica Scandinavica, 96*, 483–491.

Buckley, L., & Pettit, T. (2007). Supportive therapy for schizophrenia. *Schizophrenia Bulletin, 33*, 859–860.

Bustillo, J. R., Lauriello, J., Horan, W. P., & Keith, S. J. (2001). The psychosocial treatment of schizophrenia: An update. *American Journal of Psychiatry, 158*, 163–175.

Butzlaff, R. L., & Hooley, J. M. (1998). Expressed emotion and psychiatric relapse: A meta-analysis. *Archives of General Psychiatry, 55*, 547–552.

Camchong, J., Dyckman, K. A., Chapman, C. E., Yanasak, N. E., & McDowell, J. E. (2006). Basal ganglia – thalamocortical circuitry disruptions in schizophrenia during delayed response tasks. *Biological Psychiatry, 60*, 235–241.

Chadwick, P., Birchwood, M., & Trower, P. (1996). *Cognitive therapy for delusions, voices and paranoia*. Chichester, UK: Wiley.

Chen, E. Y., Hui, C. L., Dunn, E. L., Miao, M. Y., Yeung, W. S., Wong, C. K., . . . Tang, W. N. (2005). A prospective 3-year longitudinal study of cognitive predictors of relapse in first-episode schizophrenic patients. *Schizophrenia Research, 77*, 99–104.

Choi, K. H., & Kwon, J. H. (2006). Social cognition enhancement training for schizophrenia: A preliminary randomized controlled trial. *Community Mental Health Journal, 42*, 177–187.

Chua, S. E., & McKenna, P. J. (1995). Schizophrenia – A brain disease? *British Journal of Psychiatry, 166*, 563–582.

Cochrane Collaboration. (2009). Retrieved from http://www.cochrane.org

Cohen, A. S., Forbes, C. B., Mann, M. C., & Blanchard, J. J. (2006). Specific cognitive deficits and differential domains of social functioning in schizophrenia. *Schizophrenia Research, 81*, 227–238.

Cohen A. S., Leung, W. W., Saperstein, A. M., & Blanchard, J. J. (2006). Neuropsychological functioning and social anhedonia: Results from a community high-risk study. *Schizophrenia Research, 85*, 132–141.

Cohen, C. I. (1993). Poverty and the course of schizophrenia: Implications for research and policy. *Hospital and Community Psychiatry, 44*, 951–958.

Cohen, J. (1988). *Statistical power analysis for the behavioral sciences*. Hillsdale, NJ: Erlbaum.

Cohen, R., Florin, I., Grusche, A., Meyer-Osterkamp, S., & Sell, H. (1973). Dreijährige Erfahrung mit einem Münzsystem auf einer Station für extrem inaktive, chronisch schizophrene Patienten. *Zeitschrift für Klinische Psychologie, 2*, 243–277.

Combs, D. R., Adams, S. D., Penn, D. L., Roberts, D., Tiegreen, J., & Stern, P. (2007). Social Cognition and Interaction Training (SCIT) for inpatients with schizophrenia spectrum disorders: preliminary findings. *Schizophrenia Research, 91*, 112–116.

Combs, D. R., Penn, D. L., Wicher, M., & Waldheter, E. (2007). The ambiguous intentions hostility questionnaire (AIHQ): A new measure for evaluating hostile social-cognitive biases in paranoia. *Cognitive Neuropsychiatry, 12*, 128–143.

Combs, D. R., Tosheva, A., Wanner, J., & Basso, M. R. (2006). Remediation of emotion perception deficits in schizophrenia: The use of attentional prompts. *Schizophrenia Research, 87*, 340–341.

Conley, R. R., Ascher-Svanum, H., Zhu, B., Faries, D. E., & Kinon, B. J. (2007). The burden of depressive symptoms in the long-term treatment of patients with schizophrenia. *Schizophrenia Research, 90*, 186–197.

Corcoran, R., Mercer, G., & Frith, C. D. (1995). Schizophrenia, symptomatology and social inference: Investigating "theory of mind" in people with schizophrenia. *Schizophrenia Research, 17*, 5–13.

Cornblatt, B., Lenzenweger, M., Dworkin, R., & Erlenmeyer-Kimling, L. (1992). Childhood attentional dysfunctions predict social deficits in unaffected adults at risk for schizophrenia. *British Journal of Psychiatry, 161*(Suppl. 18), 59–64.

Corrigan, P. W. (2006). Recovery from schizophrenia and the role of evidence-based psychosocial interventions. *Expert Review Neurotherapeutics, 6*, 993–1004.

Corrigan, P. W., & Addis, I. B. (1995). The effects of cognitive complexity on a social sequencing task in schizophrenia. *Schizophrenia Research, 16*, 137–144.

Corrigan, P. W., & Green, M. F. (1993). The situational feature recognition test: A measure of schema comprehension for schizophrenia. *International Journal of Methods in Psychiatric Research, 3*, 29–36.

Corrigan, P. W., Hirschbeck, J. N., & Wolfe, M. (1995). Memory and vigilance training to improve social perception in schizophrenia. *Schizophrenia Research, 17*, 257–265.

Corrigan, P. W., & Penn, D. L. (2001). *Social cognition in schizophrenia*. Washington, DC: American Psychological Association.

Couture, S. M., Penn, D. L., & Roberts, D. L. (2006). The functional significance of social cognition in schizophrenia: A review. *Schizophrenia Bulletin, 32*(Suppl. 1), 44–63.

Crespo-Facorro, B., Roiz-Santiañes, R., Pelayo-Terán, J. M., Pérez-Iglesias, R., Carrasco-Marín, E., Mata, I., ... Vázquez-Barquero, J. L. (2007). Low-activity allele of cathechol-o-methyltransferase (COM^TL) is associated with increased lateral ventricles in patients with first episode non-affective psychosis. *Progress in Neuro-Psychopharmacology and Biological Psychiatry, 31*, 1514–1518.

Cromwell, R. L., & Spaulding, W. (1978). How schizophrenics handle information. In W. E. Fann, I. Karacan, A. D. Pokorny, & R. L. Williams (Eds.), *The phenomenology and treatment of schizophrenia* (pp. 127–162). New York: Spectrum.

Crumlish, N., Whitty, P., Clarke, M., Browne, S., Kamali, M., Gervin, M., ... O'Callaghan, E. (2009). Beyond the critical period: Longitudinal study of 8-year outcome in first-episode non-affective psychosis. *British Journal of Psychiatry, 194*, 18–24.

Davidson, L., O'Connell, M., Tondora, J., Lawless, M., & Evans, A. (2005). Recovery in serious mental illness: A new wine or just a new bottle? *Professional Psychology: Research and Practice, 36*, 480–487.

Davies, L. M., Lewis, S., Jones, P. B., Barnes, T. R. E., Gaughran, F., Hayhurst, K., ... Lloyd, H., on behalf of the CUtLASS team. (2007). Cost-effectiveness of first- v. second-generation antipsychotic drugs: Results from a randomized controlled trial in schizophrenia responding poorly to previous therapy. *British Journal of Psychiatry, 191*, 14–22.

Davis, J. M., Chen, N., & Glick, I. D. (2003). A meta-analysis of the efficacy of second-generation antipsychotics. *Archives of General Psychiatry, 60*, 553–564.

Day, R. (1989). Schizophrenia. In G. W. Brown & T. O.Harris (Eds.), *Life events and illness* (pp. 113–138). New York: Guilford.

DeAmicis, L., & Cromwell, R. (1979). Reaction time crossover in process schizophrenics, their relatives and control subjects. *Journal of Nervous and Mental Disease, 167*, 593–600.

Deegan, P. (1988). Recovery: The lived experience of rehabilitation. *Psychosocial Rehabilitation Journal, 11*, 11–19.

Delahunty, A., & Morice, R. (1993). A training programme for the remediation of cognitive deficits in schizophrenia: Preliminary results. *Psychological Medicine, 23*, 221–227.

Derogatis, L. R. (1977). *SCL-90-R, administration, scoring & procedures manual-I for the revised version*. Baltimore, MD: Clinical Psychometric Research.

Derogatis, L. R. (1993). *BSI, administration, scoring & procedures manual-3rd edition*. Minneapolis, MN: National Computer Systems.

Derogatis, L. R. (1994). *SCL-90-R, administration, scoring & procedures manual*. Minneapolis, MN: National Computer Systems.

Dibben, C. R. M., Rice, C., Laws, K., & McKenna, P. J. (2009). Is executive impairment associated with schizophrenic syndromes? A meta-analysis. *Psychological Medicine, 39*, 381–392.

Dickerson, F., Boronow, J., Ringel, N., & Parente, F. (1999). Social functioning and neurocognitive deficits in outpatients with schizophrenia: A 2-year follow-up. *Schizophrenia Research, 37*, 13–20.

Dohrenwend, B. P., Shrout, P. E., Link, B. G., Skodol, A. E., & Stueve, A. (1995). Life events and other possible psychosocial risk factors for episodes of schizophrenia and major depression: A case-control study. In C. M. Mazure (Ed.), *Does stress cause psychiatric illness?* (pp. 34–65). Washington, DC: American Psychiatric Press.

Donahoe, C., Carter, M., Bloom, W., Hirsch, G., Laasi, N., & Wallace, C. (1990). Assessment of interpersonal problem solving skills. *Psychiatry, 53*, 329–339.

Drake, J. R. (2008). Insight into illness: Impact on diagnosis and outcome of nonaffective psychosis. *Current Psychiatry Reports, 10*, 210–216.

Drake, R. J., & Lewis, S. W. (2003). Insight and neurocognition in schizophrenia. *Schizophrenia Research, 62*, 165–173.

Ekman, P. (2009). *Official site*. Retrieved from http://www.paulekman.com/.

Ekman, P., & Friesen, M. V. (1976). *Pictures of facial affect*. Palo Alto, CA: Consulting Psychologists Press.

Ekman, P., Friesen, W. V., & Ellsworth, P. (1972). *Emotion in the human face: Guidelines for research and an integration of findings*. New York: Pergamon.

Ellis, A. (1957). Rational psychotherapy and individual psychology. *Journal of Individual Psychology, 13*, 38–44.

Erlenmeyer-Kimling, L., & Cornblatt, B. (1978). Attentional measures in a study of children at high-risk for schizophrenia. In L. C. Wynne, R. L. Cromwell, & S. Matthysse (Eds.), *The nature of schizophrenia: New approaches to research and treatment* (pp. 359–365). New York: Wiley.

Erlenmeyer-Kimling, L., Rock, D., Roberts, S. A., Janal, M., Kestenbaum, C., Cornblatt, B., ... Gottesman, I. I. (2000). Attention, memory, and motor skills as childhood predictors of schizophrenia-related psychoses: The New York High-Risk Project. *American Journal of Psychiatry, 157*, 1416–1422.

Falloon, I. R. H., Boyd, J. L., & McGill, C. W. (1984). *Family care of schizophrenia*. New York: Guilford.

Feuerstein, R. (1980). *Instrumental enrichment*. Baltimore, MD: University Park Press.

Filbey, F. M., Toulopoulou, T., Morris, R. G., McDonald, C., Bramon, E., Walshe, M., & Murray, R. M. (2008). Selective attention deficits reflect increased genetic vulnerability to schizophrenia. *Schizophrenia Research, 101*, 169–175.

First, M. B., Spitzer, R. L., Gibbon, M., & Williams, J. B. W. (2002). *Structured Clinical Interview for DSM-IV-TR Axis I disorders, research version, patient edition. (SCID-I/P)*. New York: Biometrics Research, New York State Psychiatric Institute.

Fiszdon, M. J., Choi, J., Goulet, J., & Bell, M. D. (2008). Temporal relationship between change in cognition and change in functioning in schizophrenia. *Schizophrenia Research, 105*, 105–113.

Fowler, D., Garety, P., & Kuipers, E. (1995). *Cognitive behaviour therapy for psychosis. Theory and practice*. Chichester, UK: Wiley.

Frese, F. J., Stanley, J., Kress, K., & Vogel-Scibilia, S. (2001). Integrating evidence-based practices and the recovery model. *Psychiatry Service, 52*, 1462–1468.

Frith, C. (1992). *The cognitive neuropsychologie of schizophrenia*. Hove, UK: Lawrence.

Frith, C. D. (2004). Schizophrenia and theory of mind. *Psychological Medicine, 34*, 385–389.

Frommann, N., Streit, M., & Wölwer, W. (2003). Remediation of facial affect recognition impairments in patients with schizophrenia: A new training program. *Psychiatry Research, 117*, 281–284.

Fu, C. H. Y., Suckling, J., Williams, S. C. R., Andrew, C. M., Vythelingum, G. N., & McGuire, P. K. (2005). Effects of psychotic state and task demand on prefrontal function in schizophrenia: An fMRI study of overt verbal fluency. *American Journal of Psychiatry, 162*, 485–494.

Fuentes, I., Garcia, S., Ruiz, J. C., Soler, M. J., & Roder, V. (2007). Social perception training in schizophrenia: A pilot study. *International Journal of Psychology and Psychological Therapy, 7*, 1–12.

Funke, B., Reinecker, H., & Commichau, A. (1989). Grenzen kognitiver Therapiemethoden bei schizophrenen Langzeitpatienten. *Nervenarzt, 60*, 750–756.

Garcia, S., Fuentes, I., Gallach, E., Ruiz, J. C., & Roder, V. (2003). An application of IPT in a Spanish sample: Empirical study of the social perception programme. *International Journal of Psychology and Psychological Therapy, 3*, 299–310.

Garety, P. A., Bebbington, P., Fowler, D., Freeman, D., & Kuipers, E. (2007). Implications for neurobiological research of cognitive models of psychosis: A theoretical paper. *Psychological Medicine, 37*, 1377–1391.

Gil Sanz, D., Lorenzo, D. M., Seco, R. B., Rodríguez, M. A., Martínez, I. L., Sánchez Calleja, R., & Álvarez Soltero, A. (2009). Efficacy of a social cognition training program for schizophrenic patients: A pilot study. *The Spanish Journal of Psychology, 12*, 184–191.

Glynn, S. M., Marder, S. R., Liberman, R. P., Blair, K., Wirshing, W. C., Wirshing, D. A., … Mintz, J. (2002). Supplementing clinic-based skills training with manual-based community support sessions: Effects on social adjustment of patients with schizophrenia. *American Journal of Psychiatry, 159*, 829–837.

Gottesman, I. I., & Shields, J. A. (1982). *Schizophrenia: The epigenetic puzzle*. Cambridge, UK: Cambridge University Press.

Gray, J. A., & Roth, B. L. (2007). Molecular targets for treating cognitive dysfunction in schizophrenia. *Schizophrenia Bulletin, 33*, 1100 – 1119.

Green, M. (1997). *Schizophrenia from a neurocognitive perspective: Probing the impenetrable darkness:* . New York: Allyn & Bacon.

Green, M. (1998). *Schizophrenia as a neurocognitive disorder*. Boston: Ayllon & Bacon.

Green, M. F. (1996). What are the functional consequences of neurocognitive deficits in schizophrenia? *American Journal of Psychiatry, 153*, 321–330.

Green, M. F. (2007). Cognition, drug treatment, and functional outcome in schizophrenia: A tale of two transitions. *American Journal of Psychiatry, 164*, 992–994.

Green, M. F., Kern, R. S., Braf, D. L., & Mintz, J. (2000). Neurocognitive deficits and functional outcome in schizophrenia: Are we measuring the "right stuff"? *Schizophrenia Bulletin, 26*, 119–136.

Green, M. F., Kern, R. S., & Heaton, R. K., (2004) Longitudinal studies of cognition and functional outcome in schizophrenia: Implication for MATRICS. *Schizophrenia Research, 72*, 41–51.

Green, M. F., & Nuechterlein, K. H. (1999). Should schizophrenia be treated as a neurocognitive disorder? *Schizophrenia Bulletin, 25*, 309–319.

Green, M. F., & Nuechterlein, K. H. (2004). The MATRICS initiative: Developing a consensus cognitive battery for clinical trials. *Schizophrenia Research, 72*, 1–3.

Green, M. F., Nuechterlein, K. H., Kern, R. S., Baade, L. E., Fenton, W. S., Gold, J. M., …

Marder, S. R. (2008). Functional co-primary measures for clinical trials in schizophrenia: results from the MATRICS psychometric and standardization study. *American Journal of Psychiatry, 165*, 221–228.

Green, M. F., Olivier, B., Crawley, J. N., Penn, D. L., & Silverstein, S. (2005). Social cognition in schizophrenia: Recommendations from the measurement and treatment research to improve cognition in schizophrenia new approaches conference. *Schizophrenia Research, 31*, 882–887.

Green, M. F., Penn, D. L., Bentall, R., Carpenter, W. T., Gaebel, W., Gur, R. C., ... Heinssen, R. (2008). Social cognition in schizophrenia: an NIMH workshop on definition, assessment, and research opportunities. *Schizophrenia Bulletin, 34*, 1211–1220.

Greenwood, K. E., Landau, S., & Wykes, T. (2005). Negative symptoms and specific cognitive impairments as combined targets for improved functional outcome with cognitive remediation therapy. *Schizophrenia Bulletin, 31*, 910–921.

Häfner, H., Löffler, W., Maurer, K., Riecher-Rössler, A., & Stein, A. (2003). *IRAOS – Interview for the Retrospective Assessment of the Onset and Course of Schizophrenia and other psychoses*. Göttingen, Germany: Hogrefe & Huber.

Harvey, P., & Keefe, R. (2001). Studies of cognitive change in patients with schizophrenia following novel antipsychotic treatment. *American Journal of Psychiatry, 158*, 176–184.

Harvey, P. D., Koren, D., Reichenberg, A., & Bowie, C. R. (2006). Negative symptoms and cognitive deficits: What is the nature of their relationship? *Schizophrenia Bulletin, 32*, 250–258.

Harvey, P. D., Patterson, T. L., Potter, L. S., Zhong, K., & Brecher, M. (2006). Improvement in social competence with short-term atypical antipsychotic treatment: A randomized, double-blind comparison of quetiapine versus risperidone for social competence, social cognition and neuropsychological functioning. *American Journal of Psychiatry, 163*, 1918–1925.

Heaton, R. K. (1981). *Wisconsin Card Sorting Test manual*. Odessa, Ukraine: Psychological Assessment Resources.

Heaton, R. K., Marcotte, T. D., Rivera-Mindt, M., Sadek, J., Moore, D. J., Bentley, H., ... HNRC Group. (2004). The impact of HIV-associated neuropsychological impairment on everyday functioning. *Journal of the International Neuropsychological Society, 10*, 317–331.

Heim, M., Wolf, S., Göthe, U., & Kretschmar, J. (1989). Kognitives Training bei schizophrenen Erkrankungen. *Psychiatrie, Neurologie und medizinische Psychologie, 41*, 367–375.

Heinrichs, R. (2001). *In search of madness: Schizophrenia and neuroscience*. Oxford, UK: Oxford University Press.

Heinrichs, R. W., Ammari, N., Miles, A. A., & McDermid Vaz, S. (2008). Cognitive performance and functional competence as predictors of community independence in schizophrenia. *Schizophrenia Bulletin*, doi:10.1093/schbul/sbn095

Heinrichs, R. W., Statucka, M., Goldberg, J. O., & McDermid Vaz, S., (2006). The University of California Performance Skills Assessment (UPSA) in schizophrenia. *Schizophrenia Research, 88*, 135–141.

Helldin, L., Kane, J. M., Karilampi, U., Norlander, T., & Archer, T. (2007). Remission in prognosis of functional outcome: A new dimension in the treatment of patients with psychotic disorder. *Schizophrenia Research, 93*, 160–168.

Hermanutz, M., & Gestrich, J. (1987). Kognitives Training mit Schizophrenen. *Nervenarzt, 58*, 91–96.

Hodel, B. (1994). Reaktionsdefizite und ihre Wirkungen auf den Therapieerfolg bei schizophrenen Erkrankten. *Schizophrenie, 9*(1), 31–38.

Hodel, B., & Brenner, H. D. (1996). Ein Trainingsprogramm zur Bewältigung von maladaptiven Emotionen bei schizophren Erkrankten. Erste Ergebnisse und Erfahrungen. *Nervenarzt, 67*, 564–571.

Hodel, B., & Brenner, H. D. (1988, February). *Die Wirkung kognitiver Interventionen auf die*

Verhaltensebene bei Schizophrenen. Paper presented at The Congress for Clinical Psychology and Psychotherapy, Berlin, Germany.

Hodel, B., Brenner, H. D., Merlo, M. C. G., & Teuber, J. F. (1998). Emotional management therapy in early psychosis. *British Journal of Psychiatry, 172*(Suppl. 33), 128–133.

Hodel, B., Kern, R. S., & Brenner, H. D. (2004). Emotion management training (EMT) in persons with treatment-resistant schizophrenia: First results. *Psychiatry Research, 68*, 107–108.

Hofer, A., Baumgartner, S., Bodner, T., Edlinger, M., Hummer, M., Kemmler, G. et al. (2005). Patient outcomes in schizophrenia II: The impact of cognition. *European Psychiatry, 20*, 395–402.

Hogarty, G. E., & Anderson, C. (1986). Eine kontrollierte Studie über Familientherapie, Training sozialer Fertigkeiten und unterstützende Chemotherapie in der Nachbehandlung Schizophrener: Vorläufige Effekte auf Rezidive und Expressed Emotion nach einem Jahr. In W. Böker & H. D. Brenner (Eds.), *Die Bewältigung der Schizophrenie* (pp. 72–86). Bern: Huber.

Hogarty, G. E., & Flesher, S. (1999a). Practice principles of Cognitive Enhancement Therapy for schizophrenia. *Schizophrenia Bulletin, 25*, 693–708.

Hogarty, G. E., & Flesher, S. (1999b). Developmental theory for a Cognitive Enhancement Therapy of schizophrenia. *Schizophrenia Bulletin, 25*, 677–692.

Hogarty, G. E., Flesher, S., Ulrich, R., Carter, M., Greenwald, D., Pogue-Geile, M., . . . Zoretich, R. (2004). Cognitive enhancement therapy for schizophrenia: Effects of a 2-year randomized trial on cognition and behavior. *Archives of General Psychiatry, 61*, 866–876.

Hogarty, G. E., Greenwald, D. P., & Eack, S. M. (2006). Durability and mechanism of effects of cognitive enhancement therapy. *Psychiatric Services, 57*, 1751–1757.

Honigfeld, G., Gillis, R. O., & Klett, J. C. (1966). NOSIE-30: A treatment-sensitive ward behavior scale. *Psychological Reports, 19*, 180–182.

Hooley, J. M. (2007). Expressed emotion and relapse of psychopathology. *Annual Reviews of Clinical Psychology, 3*, 329–352.

Horan, W. P., Kern, R. S., & Green, M. F. (2008). Social cognition training for individuals with schizophrenia: Emerging evidence. *American Journal of Psychiatric Rehabilitation, 11*, 205–252.

Horan, W. P., Kern, R. S., Shokat-Fadai, K., Sergi, M. J., Wynn, J. K., & Green, M. F. (2009). Social cognitive skills training in schizophrenia: An initial efficacy study of stabilized outpatients. *Schizophrenia Research, 107*, 47–54.

Horan, W. P., Nuechterlein, K. H., Wynn, J. K., Lee, J., Castelli, F., & Green, M. F. (2009). Disturbances in the spontaneous attribution of social meaning in schizophrenia. *Psychological Medicine, 39*, 635–643.

Hori, H., Noguchi, H., Hashimoto, R., Nakabayashi, T., Omori, M., Takahshi, M., . . . Kunugi, H. (2006). Antipsychotic medication and cognitive function in schizophrenia. *Schizophrenia Research, 86*, 138–146.

Howes, O. M., Asselin, M. C., Murray, R. M., McGuire, P., & Grasby, P. M. (2006). The pre-synaptic dopaminergic system before and after the onset of psychosis: Initial results from an ongoing 18F-fluoroDOPA PET study. *Schizophrenia Research, 81*, 14.

Hubmann, W., John, K., Mohr, F., Kreuzer, S., & Bender, W. (1991). Soziales Verhaltenstraining mit chronisch schizophrenen Patienten. In R. Schüttler (Hrsg.), *Theorie und Praxis kognitiver Therapieverfahren bei schizophrenen Patienten* (S. 118–128). Munich, Germany: Zuckschwerdt.

Hunter, R. H., Wilkniss, S., Gardner, W., & Silverstein, S. M. (2008). The Multimodal Functional Model – Advancing case formulation beyond the "diagnose and treat" paradigm: Improving outcomes and reducing aggression and the use of control procedures in psychiatric care. *Psychological Services, 5*, 11–25.

Iqbal, Z., Birchwood, M., Chadwick, P., & Trower, P. (2000). Cognitive approach to depression

Iqbal, Z., Birchwood, M., Chadwick, P., & Trower, P. (2000). Cognitive approach to depression and suicidal thinking in psychosis. 2. Testing the validity of a social ranking model. *British Journal of Psychiatry, 177*, 522–528.

Jackson, H., McGorry, P., Edwards, J., Hulbert, C., Henry, L., Francey, S., ... Dudgeon, P. (1998). Cognitively-oriented psychotherapy for early psychosis (COPE). *British Journal of Psychiatry, 172*, 93–100.

James, A. C., James, S., Smith, D. M., & Javaloyes, A. (2004). Cerebellar, prefrontal cortex, and thalamic volumes over two time points in adolescent-onset schizophrenia. *American Journal of Psychiatry, 161*, 1023–1029.

Janssen, I., Krabbendam, L., Bak, M., Hanssen, M., Vollebergh, W., de Graaf, R., & van Os, J. (2004). Childhood abuse as a risk factor for psychotic experiences. *Acta Psychiatrica Scandinavica, 109*, 38–45.

Jeppesen, P., Petersen, L., Thorup, A., Abel, M. B., Ohlenschlaeger, J., Christensen, T. O., ... Nordentoft, M. (2008). The association between pre-morbid adjustment, duration of untreated psychosis and outcome in first-episode psychosis. *Psychological Medicine, 38*, 1157–1166.

Jeste, S. D., Patterson, T. I., Palmer, B. W., Dolder, C. R., & Jeste, D. V. (2003). Cognitive predictors of medication adherence among middle-aged and older outpatients with schizophrenia. *Schizophrenia Research, 63*, 49–58.

Jones, P. B., Barnes, T. R., Davies, L., Dunn, G., Lloyd, H., Hayhurst, K. P., ... Lewis, S. W. (2006). Randomized controlled trial of the effect on quality of life of second- vs first-generation antipsychotic drugs in schizophrenia: Cost Utility of the Latest Antipsychotic Drugs in Schizophrenia Study (CUtLASS 1). *Archives of General Psychiatry, 63*, 1079–1087.

Kanfer, F. H., Reinecker, H., & Schmelzer, D. (2000). *Selbstmanagement-Therapie: Ein Lehrbuch für die klinische Praxis* (3rd ed.). Berlin, Germany: Springer.

Kapur, S., Mizrahi, R., & Li, M. (2005). From dopamine to salience to psychosis – linking biology, pharmacology and phenomenology of psychosis. *Schizophrenia Research, 79*, 59–68.

Karow, A., Pajonk, F. G., Reimer, J., Hirdes, F., Osterwald, C., Naber, D., & Moritz, S. (2008). The dilemma of insight into illness in schizophrenia: Self- and expert-rated insight and quality of life. *European Archives of Psychiatry and Clinical Neuroscience, 258*, 152–159.

Kay, R. S. (1991). *Positive and negative syndromes in schizophrenia*. New York: Brunner/Mazel.

Kay, S. R., Opler, L. A., & Lindenmayer, J.-P. (1989). The Positive and Negative Syndrome Scale (PANSS): Rationale and standardisation. *British Journal of Psychiatry, 155*(Suppl. 7), 59–65.

Kayser, N., Sarfati, Y., Besche, C., & Hardy-Baylé, M. C. (2006). Elaboration of a rehabilitation method based on a pathogenetic hypothesis of "theory of mind" impairment in schizophrenia. *Neuropsychological rehabilitation, 16*, 83–95.

Kee, K. S., Green, M. F., Mintz, J., & Brekke, J. S. (2003). Is emotion processing a predictor of functional outcome in schizophrenia? *Schizophrenia Bulletin, 29*, 487–497.

Kee, K. S., Horan, W. P., Salovey, P., Kern, R. S., Sergi, M. J., Fiske, A. P., ... Green, M. F. (2009). Emotional intelligence in schizophrenia. *Schizophrenia Research, 107*, 61–68.

Keefe, R. S. E. (2007). Cognitive deficits in patients with schizophrenia: Effects and treatment. *Journal of Clinical Psychiatry, 14*(Suppl. 14), 8–13.

Keefe, R. S. E. (2008). Should cognitive impairment be included in the diagnostic criteria for schizophrenia? *World Psychiatry, 7*, 22–28.

Keefe, R. S. E., Bilder, R. M., Davis, S. M., Harvey, P. D., Palmer, B. W., Gold, J. M., ... for the CATIE Investigators and the Neurocognitive Working Group. (2007). Neurocognitive effects of antipsychotic medications in patients with chronic schizophrenia in the CATIE trial. *Archives of General Psychiatry, 64*, 633–647.

Keefe, R. S. E., & Fenton, W. S. (2007). How should DSM-V criteria for schizophrenia include cognitive impairment? *Schizophrenia Bulletin, 33*, 912–920.

Keefe, R. S. E., Poe, M., Walker, T., Kang, J., & Harvey, P. (2006). The schizophrenia cognition rating scale: An interview-based assessment and its relationship to cognition, real-world functioning, and functional capacity. *American Journal of Psychiatry, 163,* 426–432.

Keefe, R. S. E., Sweeney, J. A., Gu, H., Hamer, R. M., Perkins, D. O., McEvoy, J. P., & Lieberman, J. A. (2007). Effects of olanzapine, quetiapine, and risperidone on neurocognitive function in early psychosis: A randomized, double-blind 52-week comparison. *American Journal of Psychiatry, 164,* 1061–1071.

Kelly, J. A., & Lamparski, D. M. (1985). Outpatient treatment of schizophrenia, social skills and problem-solving training. In M. Hersen & A. S. Bellack (Eds.), *Handbook of Clinical Behavior Therapy with Adults* (pp. 485–506). New York: Plenum.

Kendler, K. S., McGuire, M., Gruenberg, A. M., O'Hare, A., Spellman, M., & Walsh, D. (1993). The Roscommon family study. 1. Methods, diagnosis of probands, and risk of schizophrenia in relatives. *Archives of General Psychiatry, 50,* 527–540.

Keppeler-Derendinger, U. (2008). *Gruppentherapieprogramm zur Rehabilitation von schizophren Erkrankten im Wohnbereich.* (Unpublished doctoral dissertation). University of Fribourg, Switzerland.

Kern, R. S., Glynn, S. M., Horan, W. P., & Marder, S. R. (2009). Psychosocial treatments to promote functional recovery in schizophrenia. *Schizophrenia Bulletin, 35,* 347–361.

Kern, R. S., Green, M. F., Mintz, J., & Liberman, R. P. (2003). Does "errorless learning" compensate for neurocognitive impairments in the work rehabilitation of persons with schizophrenia? *Psychological Medicine, 33,* 433–442.

Kern, R. S., Green, M. F., Mitchell, S., Kopelowicz, A., Mintz, J., & Liberman, R. P. (2005). Extensions of errorless learning for social problem-solving deficits in schizophrenia. *American Journal of Psychiatry, 162,* 513–519.

Kern, R. S., & Horan, W. P. (2010). Definition and measurement of neurocognition and social cognition. In V. Roder & A. Medalia (Eds.), *Neurocognition and social cognition in schizophrenia patients. Comprehension and treatment* (pp. 1–22). Basel, Switzerland: Karger.

Kern, R. S., Liberman, R. P., Becker, R., Drake, R. E., Sugar, C. A., & Green, M. F. (2009). Errorless learning for training individuals with schizophrenia at a community mental health setting providing work experience. *Schizophrenia Bulletin, 35,* 807–815.

Kern, R. S., Liberman, R. P., Kopelowicz, A., Mintz, J., & Green, M. F. (2002). Applications of errorless learning for improving work performance in persons with schizophrenia. *American Journal of Psychiatry, 159,* 1921–1926.

Kern, R. S., Nuechterlein, K. H., Green, M. F., Baade, L. E., Fenton, W. S., Gold, J. M., . . . Marder, S. R. (2008). The MATRICS consensus cognitive battery, part 2: Co-norming and standardization. *American Journal of Psychiatry, 165,* 214–220.

Kerr, S. L., & Neale, J. M. (1993). Emotion perception in schizophrenia: Specific deficit or further evidence of generalized poor performance? *Journal of Abnormal Psychology, 102,* 312–318.

Kile, S. J. (2007). Neuropsychiatric update: Neuroimaging schizophrenia. *Psychopharmacological Bulletin, 40,* 156–167.

Kingdon, A., & Turkington, D. (2005). *Cognitive therapy of schizophrenia.* New York: Guilford.

Kingsep, P., Nathan, P., & Castle, D. (2003). Cognitive behavioural group treatment for social anxiety in schizophrenia. *Schizophrenia Research, 63,* 121–129.

Kirkbride, J. B., Morgan, C., Fearon, P., Dazzan, P., Murray, R. M., & Jones, P. B. (2007). Neighborhood-level effects on psychoses: Re-examining the role of context. *Psychological Medicine, 37,* 1413–1425.

Kolb, B., & Nonneman, A. J. (1976). Functional development of the prefrontal cortex continues into adolescence. *Science, 193,* 335–336.

Kopelowicz, A., Liberman, R. P., & Zarate, R. (2006). Recent advances in social skills training for schizophrenia. *Schizophrenia Bulletin, 32*(Suppl. 1), 12–23.

Krabbendam, L., & Aleman, A. (2003). Cognitive rehabilitation in schizophrenia: A quantitative analysis of controlled studies. *Psychopharmacology, 169*, 376–382.

Kraemer, S., Sulz, K. H. B., Schmid, R., & Lässle, R. (1987). Kognitive Therapie bei standard-versorgten schizophrenen Patienten. *Der Nervenarzt, 58,* 84–90.

Kraemer, S., Zinner, H. J., Riehl, T., Gehringer, M., & Möller, H. J. (1990). Kognitive Therapie und Verhaltenstraining zur Förderung sozialer Kompetenz für chronisch schizophrene Patienten. In G. E. Kühne, H. D. Brenner, & G. Huber (Eds.), *Kognitive Therapie bei Schizophrenen* (pp. 73–82). Jena, Germany: Gustav Fischer.

Kurtz, M. M. (2003). Neurocognitive rehabilitation for schizophrenia. *Current Psychiatry Reports, 5*, 303–310.

Kurtz, M. M. (2005). Neurocognitive impairments across the lifespan in schizophrenia: An update. *Schizophrenia Research, 74*, 15–26.

Kurtz, M. M., Moberg, P. J., Mozley, L. H., Swanson, C. L., Gur, R. C., & Gur, R. E. (2001). Effectiveness of an attention and memory training program on neuropsychological defficits in schizophrenia. *Neurorehabilitation and Neural Repair, 15*, 23–28.

Kurtz, M. M., & Mueser, K. T. (2008). A meta-analysis of controlled research on social skills training for schizophrenia. *Journal of Consulting and Clinical Psychology, 76*, 491–504.

Kurtz, M. M., Seltzer, J. C., Shagan, D. S., Thime, W. R., & Wexler, B. E. (2007). Computer-assisted cognitive remediation in schizophrenia: What is the active ingredient? *Schizophrenia Research, 89*, 251–260.

Lambert, M. J., & Bergin, A. E. (1994). *The effectiveness of psychotherapy. Handbook of psychotherapy and behavior change* (4th ed.). Oxford, UK: Wiley.

Lee, K. H., Brown, W. H., Egleston, P. N., Green, R. D. J., Farrow, T. F. D., Hunter, M. D., ... Woodruff, P. W. R. (2006). A functional magnetic resonance imaging study of social cognition in schizophrenia during an acute episode and after recovery. *American Journal of Psychiatry, 163*, 1926–1933.

Leeson, V. C., Barnes, T. R. E., Hutton, S. B., Ron, M. A., & Joyce, E. M. (2009). IQ as a predictor of functional outcome in schizophrenia: A longitudinal, four-year study of first episode psychosis. *Schizophrenia Research, 107*, 55–60.

Leff, J., Berkowitz, N., Shavit, A., Strachan, I., Glass, I., & Vaughn, C. (1989). A trial of family therapy v. a relatives group for schizophrenia. *British Journal of Psychiatry, 154*, 58–66.

Leff, J., Kuipers, L., Berkowitz, R., Eberlein-Vries, R., & Sturgeon, D. (1982). A controlled trial of social intervention in the families of schizophrenic patients. *British Journal of Psychiatry, 141*, 121–134.

Leff, J. P., & Vaughn, C. (1985). *Expressed emotion in families.* New York: Guilford.

Lehman, A. F., & Steinwachs, D. M. (1994). *Literature review: Treatment approaches for schizophrenia.* Baltimore: Schizophrenia Patient Outcomes Research Team (PORT), University of Maryland.

Lehman, A. F., & Steinwachs, D. M. (2003). Evidence-based psychological treatment practices in schizophrenia: Lessons from the Patient Outcomes Research Team (PORT) project. *Journal of the American Academy of Psychoanalysis and Dynamic Psychiatry, 31*, 141–154.

Leichsenring, F., Rabung, S., & Leibing, E. (2004). The efficacy of short-term psychodynamic psychotherapy in specific psychiatric disorders. A meta-analysis. *Archives of General Psychiatry, 61*, 1208–1216.

Leucht, S., & Lasser, R. (2006). The concepts of remission and recovery in schizophrenia. *Pharmacopsychiatry, 39*, 161–170.

Lewis, L., Unkefer, E. P., O'Neal, S. K., Crith, C. J., & Fultz, J. (2003). Cognitive rehabilitation with patients having persistent, severe psychiatric disabilities. *Psychiatric Rehabilitation Journal, 26*, 325–331.

Liberman, R. P. (2008). *Recovery from disability: Manual of psychiatric rehabilitation*. Washington, DC: American Psychiatric Press.

Liberman, R. P., Jacobs, H. E., Boone, S. E., Foy, D. W., Donahoe, C. P., Falloon, I. R. H., ... Wallace, C. J. (1986). Fertigkeitentraining zur Anpassung Schizophrener an die Gemeinschaft. In W. Böker & H. D. Brenner (Eds.), *Bewältigung der Schizophrenie* (pp. 96–112). Bern: Huber.

Liberman, R. P., & Kopelowicz, A. (2005). Recovery from schizophrenia: A concept in search of research. *Psychiatric Services, 56*, 735–742.

Liberman, R. P., Kopelowicz, A., Venture, J., & Gutkind, D. (2002). Operational criteria and factors related to recovery from schizophrenia. *International Review of Psychiatry, 14*, 256–272.

Liberman, R. P., Wallace, C. J., Blackwell, G., Eckman, T. A., Vaccaro, J. V., & Kuehnel, T. G. (1993). Innovations in skills training for the seriously mentally ill: The UCLA social and independent living skills modules. *Innovations and Research, 2*, 43–60.

Liddle, P. F. (2000). Cognitive impairment in schizophrenia: Its impact on social functioning. *Acta Psychiatrica Scandinavica, 101*, 11–16.

Lieberman, J. A., Drake, R. E., Sederer, L. I., Begler, A., Keefe, R., Perkins, D., & Stroup, S. (2008). Science and recovery in schizophrenia. *Psychiatric Services, 59*, 487–496.

Lieberman, J. A., Stroup, T. S., McEvoy, J. P., Swartz, M. S., Rosenheck, R. A., Perkins, D. O., ... Hsiao, J. K. (2005). Effectiveness of antipsychotic drugs in patients with chronic schizophrenia. *New England Journal of Medicine, 353*, 1209–1223.

Lincoln, T. (2006). *Kognitive Verhaltenstherapie der Schizophrenie. Ein individuenzentrierter Ansatz zu Veränderung von Wahn, Halluzinationen und Negativsymptomatik*. Göttingen: Hogrefe.

Lincoln, T. M., Suttner, C., & Nestoriuc, Y. (2008). Wirksamkeit kognitiver Interventionen für Schizophrenie. Eine Meta-Analyse. *Psychologische Rundschau, 59*, 217–232.

Lincoln, T. M., Wilhelm, K., & Nestoriuc, Y. (2007). Effectiveness of psychoeducation for relapse, symptoms, knowledge, adherence and functioning in psychotic disorder: A meta-analysis. *Schizophrenia Research, 96*, 232–245.

Lindenmayer, J. P., McGurk, S. R., Mueser, K. T., Kahn, A., Wance, D., Hoffman, L., ... Xie, H. (2008). A randomized controlled trial of cognitive remediation among inpatients with persistent mental illness. *Psychiatric Services, 59*, 241–247.

Lombardo-Ferrari, M. C., Kimura, L., Nita, L. M., & Elkis, H. (2006). Structural brain abnormalities in early-onset schizophrenia. *Arquivos de neuro-psiquiatria, 64*(3-B), 741–746.

Loong, J. W. K. (1989). *Wisconsin Card Sorting Test (WCST)*. La Luna Court, San Luis Obispo, CA: Wang Neuropsychological Laboratory.

Lopez-Luengo, B., & Vasquez, C. (2003). Effects on attention process training on cognitive functioning of schizophrenia patients. *Psychiatry Research, 119*, 41–53.

Lysaker, P. H., Bryson, G. J., Lancaster, R. S., Evans, J. D., & Bell, M. D. (2002). Insight in schizophrenia: Associations with executive function and coping style. *Schizophrenia Research, 59*, 41–47.

Lysaker, P. H., Lancaster, R. S., Nees, M. A., & Davis, L. W. (2004). Attributional style and symptoms as predictors of social function in schizophrenia. *Journal of Rehabilitation Research and Development, 41*, 225–232.

Lysaker, P. H., Roe, D., & Yanos, P. T. (2007). Toward understanding the insight paradox: Internalized stigma moderates the association between insight and social functioning, hope, and self-esteem among people with schizophrenia spectrum disorder. *Schizophrenia Bulletin, 33*, 192–199.

MacDonald, A. W. 3rd, Carter, C. S., Kerns, J. G., Ursu, S., Barch, D. M., Holmes, A. J., ... Cohen, J. D. (2005). Specificity of prefrontal dysfunction and context processing deficits to schizophrenia in never-medicated patients with first-episode psychosis. *American Journal of Psychiatry, 162*, 475–484.

Malla, A., Norman, R., Schmitz, N., Manchanda, R., Bechard-Evans, L., Takhar, J., & Haricharan, R. (2006). Predictors of rate and time to remission in first episode psychosis: A two-year outcome study. *Psychological Medicine, 36*, 649–658.

Malla, A., & Payne, J. (2005). First-episode psychosis: Psychopathology, quality of life, and functional outcome. *Schizophrenia Bulletin, 31*, 650–71.

Maples, N. J., & Velligan, D. I. (2008). Cognitive adaption training: Establishing environmental supports to bypass cognitive deficits and improve functional outcomes. *American Journal of Psychiatric Rehabilitation, 11*, 164–180.·

Marker Software (2009). *Cogpack.* Retrieved from http://www.markersoftware.com

Mass, R. (2001). *Eppendorfer Schizophrenie-Inventar (ESI).* Göttingen: Hogrefe.

MATRICS. (2009). *Measurement And Treatment Research to Improve Cognition in Schizophrenia.* Official Site retrieved from http://www.markersoftware.com

MATRICS Assessment, Inc. (2006). *Matrics consensus cognitive battery (MCCB).* Retrieved from http://www.matricsinc.org/MCCB.htm#1

Matza, L. S., Buchanan, R., Purdon, S., Brewster-Jordan, J., Zhao, Y., & Revicki, D. A. (2006). Measuring changes in functional status among patients with schizophrenia: The link with cognitive impairments. *Schizophrenia Bulletin, 32*, 666–678.

Mausbach, B. T., Moore, R., Bowie, C., Cardenas, V., & Patterson, T. L. (2009). A review of instruments for measuring functional recovery in those diagnosed with psychosis. *Schizophrenia Bulletin, 35*, 307–318.

Mayer, J. D., Salovey, P., & Caruso, D. (2000). Competing models of emotional intelligence. In R. Sternberg (Ed.), *Handbook of human intelligence* (pp. 396–420). New York: Cambridge.

McDonald, S., Flanagan, S., Rollino, J., & Kinch, J. (2003). TASIT: A new clinical tool for assessing social perception after traumatic brain injury. *Journal of Head Trauma Rehabilitation, 18*, 219–238.

McEvoy, J. P. (2008). Functional outcomes in schizophrenia. *Journal of Clinical Psychiatry, 69*(Suppl. 3), 20–24.

McFarlane, W. R., Lukens, E., Link, B., Dushay, R., Deakins, S. A., Newmark, M., . . . Toran, J. (1995). Multiple-family groups and psychoeducation in the treatment of schizophrenia. *Archives of General Psychiatry, 52*, 679–687.

McGrath, J. (2005). Myths and plain truths about schizophrenia epidemiology: The NAPE lecture 2004. *Acta Psychiatrica Scandinavica, 111*, 4–11.

McGrath, J. J. (2006). Variations in the incidence of schizophrenia: Data versus dogma. *Schizophrenia Bulletin, 32*, 195–197.

McGurk, S. R., & Mueser, K. T. (2004). Cognitive functioning, symptoms and work in supported employment: A review and heuristic model. *Schizophrenia Research, 72*, 147–173.

McGurk, S. R., Mueser, K. T., Feldman, K., Wolfe, R., & Pascaris, A. (2007). Cognitive training for supported employment: 2–3 year outcomes of a randomized controlled trial. *American Journal of Psychiatry, 164*, 437–441.

McGurk, S. R., Mueser, K. T., & Pascaris, A. (2005). Cognitive training and supported employment for persons with severe mental illness: One-year results from a randomized controlled trial. *Schizophrenia Bulletin, 31*, 898–909.

McGurk, S. R., Twamley, E. W., Sitzer, D. I., McHugo, G. J., & Mueser, K. T. (2007). A meta-analysis of cognitive remediation in schizophrenia. *American Journal of Psychiatry, 164*, 1791–1802.

McKibbin, C. L., Brekke, J. S., Sires, D., Jeste, D. V., & Patterson, T. L. (2004). Direct assessment of functional abilities: Relevance to persons with schizophrenia. *Schizophrenia Research, 72*, 53–67.

McMonagle, T., & Sultana, A. (2000). *Token economy for schizophrenia*. Oxford, UK: The Cochrane Library.

Medalia, A., & Freilich, B. (2008). The neuropsychological educational approach to cognitive remediation (NEAR) model: Practice principles and outcome studies. *American Journal of Psychiatric Rehabilitation, 11*, 123–143.

Medalia, A., & Lim, R. W. (2004). Self-awareness of cognitive functioning in schizophrenia. *Schizophrenia Research, 71*, 331–338.

Medalia, A., Revheim, N., & Casey, M. (2000). Remediation of memory disorders in schizophrenia. *Psychological Medicine, 30*, 1451–1459.

Medalia, A., Revheim, N., & Casey, M. (2001). The remediation of problem-solving skills in schizophrenia. *Schizophrenia Bulletin, 27*, 259–267.

Medalia, A., Revheim, N., & Casey, M. (2002). Remediation of problem-solving skills in schizophrenia: Evidence of a persistent effect. *Schizophrenia Research, 57*, 165–171.

Medalia, A., Revheim, N., & Herlands, T. (2002). *Remediation of cognitive deficits in psychiatric outpatients: A clinician's manual*. New York: Montefire Medical Center Press.

Medalia, A., & Richardson, R. (2005). What predicts a good response to cognitive remediation interventions? *Schizophrenia Bulletin, 31*, 942–953.

Medalia, A., & Thysen, J. (2008). Insight into neurocognitive dysfunction in schizophrenia. *Schizophrenia Bulletin, 24*, 1221–1230.

Medalia, A., Thysen, J., & Freilich, B. (2008). Do people with schizophrenia who have objective cognitive impairments identify cognitive deficits on a self report measure? *Schizophrenia Research, 105*, 156–164.

Menditto, A., Wallace, C., Liberman, R., Vander Wal, J., Jones, N., & Stuve, P. (1999). Functional assessment of independent living skills. *Psychiatric Rehabilitation Skills, 3*, 200–219.

Milev, P., Ho, B. C., Arndt, S., & Andreasen, N. C. (2005). Predictive values of neurocognition and negative symptoms on functional outcome in schizophrenia: A longitudinal first-episode study with 7-year follow-up. *American Journal of Psychiatry, 162*, 495–506.

Mintz, A. R., Dobson, K. S., & Romney, D. M. (2003). Insight in schizophrenia: A meta-analysis. *Schizophrenia Research, 61*, 75–88.

Mohamed, S., Fleming, S., Penn, D., & Spaulding, W. (1999). Insight in schizophrenia: Its relationship to measures of executive functions. *Journal of Nervous and Mental Disease, 187*, 525–531.

Moriarty, P. J., Lieber, D., Bennett, A., White, L., Parrella, M., Harvey, P. D., & Davis, K. L. (2001). Gender differences in poor outcome patients with lifelong schizophrenia. *Schizophrenia Bulletin, 27*, 103–13.

Moritz, S., Ferahli, S., & Naber, D. (2004). Memory and attention performance in psychiatric patients: Lack of correspondence between clinical-rated and patient-rated function with neuropsychological test results. *Journal of International Neuropsychological Society, 10*, 623–633.

Moritz, S., & Woodward, T. S. (2007a). Metacognitive Training for schizophrenia patients (MCT): A pilot study on feasibility, treatment adherence, and subjective efficacy. *German Journal of Psychiatry, 10*, 69–78.

Moritz, S., & Woodward, T. S. (2007b). Metacognitive Training in schizophrenia: From basic research to knowledge translation and intervention. *Current Opinion in Psychiatry, 20*, 619–625.

Moritz, S., Woodward, T. S., Stevens, C., Hauschildt, M., & Metacognition Study Group. (2009). *Metacognitive Training for patients with schizophrenia (MCT). British version*. Hamburg, Germany: VanHam Campus Verlag.

Mueller, D. R., Keppeler, U., & Roder, V. (2007). Effektivität der Therapie spezifischer sozialer

Fertigkeiten im Wohnbereich für schizophren Erkrankte: eine kontrollierte Studie über fünf Jahre. *Nervenarzt, 78(*Suppl. 2), 67.

Mueller, D. R., Pfammatter, M., Roder, V., & Brenner, H. D. (2006). Kognitiv-verhaltenstherapeutische Ansätze in der Behandlung schizophren Erkrankter. In H. J. Möller (Ed.), *Therapie psychischer Erkrankungen* (pp. 296–309). Stuttgart, Germany: Thieme.

Mueller, D. R., & Roder, V. (2005). Social skills training in recreational rehabilitation of schizophrenia patients. *American Journal of Recreational Therapy, 4*(3), 11–19.

Mueller, D. R., & Roder, V. (2006). Efficacy of cognitive behavioural group therapy with young and middle-aged schizophrenia inpatients: Are the effects affected by the age of the patients? *Actas Espanolas de Psyquiatria, 34*(Suppl. 1), 84–84.

Mueller, D. R., & Roder, V. (2007). Integrated Psychological Therapy for schizophrenia patients. *Expert Review of Neurotherapeutics, 7*(1), 1–3.

Mueller, D. R., & Roder, V. (2008). Empirical evidence for group therapy addressing social perception in schizophrenia. In J. B. Teiford (Ed.), *Social perception: 21st century issues and challenges* (pp. 51–80). New York: Nova Science Publishers.

Mueller, D. R., & Roder, V. (2010). Integrated Psychological Therapy and Integrated Neurocognitive Therapy. In V. Roder & A. Medalia (Eds.), *Neurocognition and social cognition in schizophrenia patients. Comprehension and treatment* (pp. 118–144). Basel, Switzerland: Karger.

Mueller, D. R., Roder, V., & Heuberger, A. (2009). Efficacy of social cognitive remediation in schizophrenia patients: A meta-analysis. *Schizophrenia Bulletin, 35*(Suppl. 1), 346–347.

Müller, D. R., Roder, V., & Brenner, H. D. (2007). Effektivität des Integrierten Psychologischen Therapieprogramms (IPT). Eine Meta-Analyse über 28 unabhängige Studien. *Nervenarzt, 78*, 62–73.

Mueser, K. T., Bellack, A. S., Morrison, R. L., & Wixted, J. T. (1990). Social competence in schizophrenia: Premorbid adjustment, social skills, and domains of functioning. *Journal of Psychiatric Research, 24*, 51–63.

Mueser, K. T., & McGurk, S. R. (2004). Schizophrenia. *The Lancet, 363*, 2063–2072.

Mueser, K. T., Wallace, C. J., & Liberman, R. P. (1995). New developments in social skills training. *Behavior Change, 12*, 31–40.

Murray, G. K., Cheng, F., Clark, L., Barnett, J. H., Blackwell, A. D., & Jones, P. B. (2008). Reinforcement and reversal learning in first-episode psychosis. *Schizophrenia Bulletin, 34*, 848–855.

Mutsatsa, S. H., Joyce, E. M., Hutton, S. B., & Barnes, T. R. E. (2006). Relationship between insight, cognitive function, social function and symptomatology in schizophrenia. *European Archives of Psychiatry and Clinical Neuroscience, 256*, 356–363.

Nakagami, E., Xie, B., Hoe, M., & Brekke, J. S. (2008). Intrinsic motivation, neurocognition and psychosocial functioning in schizophrenia: Testing mediator and moderator effects. *Schizophrenia research, 105*, 95–104.

Nasrallah, H. A. (2008). Meta-analysis trends in schizophrenia over three decades. *Schizophrenia Research, 108*, 1–2.

Nelson, A. L., Combs, D. R., Penn, D. L., & Basso, M. R. (2007). Subtypes of social perception deficits in schizophrenia. *Schizophrenia Research, 94*, 139–147.

Nienow, T. M., Docherty, N. M., Cohen, A. S., & Dinzeo, T. J. (2006). Attentional dysfunction, social perception, and social competence: What is the nature of the relationship? *Journal of Abnormal Psychology, 115*, 408–417.

Nopoulos, P., Flashman, L., Flaum, M., Arndt, S., & Andreasen, N. (1994). Stability of cognitive functioning early in course of schizophrenia. *Schizophrenia Research, 14*, 29–37.

Norman, R. M., Malla, A. K., Cortese, L., Cheng, S., Diaz, K., McIntosh, E., . . . Voruganti, M. D.

(1999). Symptoms and cognition as predictors of community functioning: A prospective analysis. *American Journal of Psychiatry, 156*, 400–405.

Norman, R. M. G., Malla, A. K., McLean, T. S., McIntosh, E. M., Neufeld, R. W. J., Voruganti, L. P., & Cortese, L. (2002). An evaluation of a stress management program for individuals with schizophrenia. *Schizophrenia Research, 58*, 293–303.

Nuechterlein, K. H., Barch, D. M., Gold, J. M., Goldberg, T. E., Green, M. F., & Heaton, T. E. (2004). Identification of separable cognitive factors in schizophrenia. *Schizophrenia Research, 72*, 29–39.

Nuechterlein, K. H., & Dawson, M. E. (1984a). A heuristic vulnerability/stress model of schizophrenic episodes. *Schizophrenia Bulletin, 10*, 300–312.

Nuechterlein, K. H., & Dawson, M. E. (1984b). Information processing and attentional functioning in the developmental course of schizophrenic disorders. *Schizophrenia Bulletin, 10*, 160–203.

Nuechterlein K. H., Dawson, M. E., & Green, M. F. (1994). Information-processing abnormalities as neuropsychological vulnerability indicators for schizophrenia. *Acta Psychiatrica Scandinavica/Supplementum, 384*, 71–79.

Nuechterlein, K. H., Green, M. F., Kern, R. S., Baade, L. E., Barch, D. M., Cohen, J. D., ... Marder, M. (2008). The MATRICS consensus cognitive battery, part 1: test selection, reliability, and validity. *American Journal of Psychiatry, 165*, 203–213.

Nuechterlein, K. H., & Subotnik, K. L. (1998). The cognitive origins of schizophrenia and prospects for intervention. In T. Wykes, N. Tarrier, & S. Lewis (Eds.), *Outcome and innovation in psychological treatment of schizophrenia* (pp. 17–41). Chichester, UK: Wiley.

O'Brien, M. P., Gordon, J. L., Bearden, C. E., Lopez, S. R., Kopelowicz, A., & Cannon, T. D. (2006). Positive family environment predicts improvement in symptoms and social functioning among adolescents at imminent risk for onset of psychosis. *Schizophrenia Research, 81*, 269–75.

Ochoa, S., Usall, J., Villalta-Gil, V., Vilaplana, M., Marquez, M., Valdelomar, M., & Haro, J. M. (2006). Influence of age at onset on social functioning in outpatients with schizophrenia. *European Journal of Psychiatry, 20*, 157–163.

Ohara, K., Sato, Y., Tanabu, S., Yoshida, K., & Shibuya, H. (2006). Magnetic resonance imaging study of the ventricle-brain ratio in parents of schizophrenia subjects. *Progress in Neuro-Psychopharmacology and Biological Psychiatry, 30*(1), 89–92.

Olbrich, R. (1996). Computer based psychiatric rehabilitation: Current activities in Germany. *European Psychiatry, 11*, 60–65.

Olbrich, R. (1998). Computergestützte psychiatrische Rehabilitation. *Psychiatrische Praxis, 25*(3), 103–104.

Olbrich, R. (1999). Psychologische Verfahren zur Reduktion kognitiver Defizite. Erfahrungen mit einem computergestützten Trainingsprogramm. *Fortschritte der Neurologie Psychiatrie, 67*(Suppl. 2), 74–76.

Olbrich, R., & Mussgay, L. (1990). Reduction of schizophrenic deficits by cognitive training. An evaluative study. *European Archives of Psychiatry and Neurological Sciences, 239*, 366–369.

Osborn, A. F. (1963). *Applied imagination* (3rd ed.). New York: Scribners.

Overall, J. E., & Gorham, D. R. (1976). BPRS. Brief Psychiatric Rating Scale. In W. Guy (Ed.), *ECDEU assessment manual for psychopharmacology* (pp. 157–169). Rockville, MD: National Institute of Mental Health.

Özgürdal, S., Littmann, E., Hauser, M., von Reventlow, H., Gudlowski, Y., Witthaus, H., ... Juckel, G. (2009). Neurocognitive performances in participants of at-risk mental state for schizophrenia and in first-episode patients. *Journal of clinical and experimental Neuropsychology, 31*, 392–401.

Patterson, T. L., Goldman, S., McKibbin, C. L., Hughes, T., & Jeste, D. V. (2001). UCSD performance-based skills assessment: Development of a new measure of everyday functioning for severely mentally ill adults. *Schizophrenia Bulletin, 27*, 235–245.

Paul, G. L., & Lentz, R. J. (1977). *Psychosocial treatment of chronic mental patients*. Cambridge, MA: Harvard University Press.

Peer, J. E., Rothmann, T., Penrod, R., Penn, D., & Spaulding, W. D. (2004). Social cognitive bias and neurocognitive deficit in paranoid symptoms: Evidence for an interaction effect and changes during treatment. *Schizophrenia Research, 71*, 463–471.

Peer, J. E., & Spaulding, W. D. (2007). Heterogeneity in recovery of psychosocial functioning during psychiatric rehabilitation: An exploratory study using latent growth mixture modeling. *Schizophrenia Research, 93*, 186–193.

Penadés, R., Boget, T., Catalan, R., Bernardo, M., Gasto, C., & Salamero, M. (2003). Cognitive mechanisms, psychosocial functioning, and neurocognitive rehabilitation in schizophrenia. *Schizophrenia Research, 63*, 219–227.

Penn, D., Corrigan, P., Bentall, R., & Racenstein, J. (1997). Social cognition in schizophrenia. *Psychological Bulletin, 121*, 114–132.

Penn, D., Corrigan, P., Martin, J., Ihnen, G., Racenstein, J., Nelson, D., . . . Hope, D. A. (1999). Social cognition and social skills in schizophrenia: The role of self-monitoring. *Journal of Nervous and Mental Disease, 187*, 188–190.

Penn, D. L., & Combs, D. (2000). Modification of affect deficits in schizophrenia. *Schizophrenia Research, 46*, 217–229.

Penn, D. L., Mueser, K. T., Doonan, R., & Nishith, P. (1995). Relations between social skills and ward behavior in chronic schizophrenia. *Schizophrenia Research, 16*, 225–232.

Penn, D. L., Roberts, D., Combs, D., & Sterne, A. (2007). Best practices: The development of the Social Cognition and Interaction Training program for schizophrenia spectrum disorder. *Psychiatric Services, 58*, 449–451.

Penn, D. L., Roberts, D., Munt, E. D., Silverstein, E., Jones, N., & Sheitman, B. (2005). A pilot study of Social Cognition and Interaction Training (SCIT) for schizophrenia. *Schizophrenia Research, 80*, 357–359.

Penn, D. L., Sanna, L. J., & Roberts, D. L. (2008). Social cognition in schizophrenia: An overview. *Schizophrenia Bulletin, 34*, 408–411.

Perlick, D. A., Rosenheck, R. A., Kaczynski, R., Bingham, S., & Collins, J. (2008). Association of symptomatology and cognitive deficits to functional capacity in schizophrenia. *Schizophrenia Research, 99*, 192–199.

Perris, C. (1989). *Cognitive therapy for patients with schizophrenia*. New York: Cassel.

Perris, C., Fowler, D., Skagerlind, L., Chambon, O., Henry, L., Richter, J., & Vals Blanco, J. (1998). The assessment of dysfunctional working models of self and others in severely disturbed patients: A preliminary crossnational study. In C. Perris & P. D. McGorry (Eds.), *Cognitive psychotherapy of psychotic and personality disorders: Handbook of theory and practice* (pp. 63–73). Chichester, UK: Wiley.

Perris, C., Fowler, D., Skagerlind, L., Olsson, M., & Thorson, C. (1998). Development and preliminary application of a new scale for assessing working models of self and others (DWMS) in severely disturbed patients. *Acta Psychiatrica Scandinavica, 98*, 219–223.

Peter, K., Glaser, A., & Kühne, G. E. (1989). Erste Erfahrungen mit der kognitiven Therapie Schizophrener. *Psychiatrische Neurologie und medizinische Psychologie, 41*, 485–491.

Peter, K., Kühne, G. E., Schlichter, A., Haschke, R., & Tennigkeit, M. (1992). Ergebnisse der kognitiven Therapie und der Verlauf schizophrener Psychosen im ersten und zweiten Jahr nach der Entlassung. Zur Problematik der Langzeitwirkung kognitiver Therapie. In H. D. Brenner & W. Böker (Eds.), *Verlaufsprozesse schizophrener Erkrankungen. Dynamische Wechselwirkungen relevanter Faktoren* (pp. 350–361). Bern: Huber.

Pfammatter, M., Junghan, U. M., & Brenner, H. D. (2006). Efficacy of psychological therapy in schizophrenia: Conclusions from meta-analyses. *Schizophrenia Bulletin, 32*(Suppl. 1), 64–80.

Phillips, L. J., Francey, S. M., Edwards, J., & McMurray, N. (2007). Stress and psychosis: Toward the development of new models of investigation. *Clinical Psychology Review, 27*, 307–317.

Pilling, S., Bebbington, P., Kuipers, E., Garety, P., Geddes, J., Orbach, G., & Morgan, C. (2002). Psychological treatments in schizophrenia: I. Meta-analysis of family intervention and cognitive behaviour therapy. *Psychological Medicine, 32*, 763–782.

Pinkham, A. E., & Penn, D. L. (2006). Neurocognitive and social cognitive predictors of interpersonal skill in schizophrenia. *Psychiatry Research, 143*, 167–178.

Pinkham, A. E., Penn, D. L., Perkins, D. O., Graham, K. A., & Siegel, M. (2007). Emotion perception and social skill over the course of psychosis: A comparison of individuals "at-risk" for psychosis and individuals with early and chronic schizophrenia spectrum illness. *Cognitive Neuropsychiatry, 12*, 198–212.

Pinkham, A. E., Penn, D. L., Perkins, D. O., & Lieberman, J. (2003). Implications for the neural basis of social cognition for the study of schizophrenia. *American Journal of Psychiatry, 160*, 815–824.

Portin, P., & Alanen, Y. O. (1997a). A critical review of genetic studies of schizophrenia. I. Epidemiological and brain studies. *Acta Psychiatrica Scandinavica, 95*, 1–5.

Portin, P., & Alanen, Y. O. (1997b). A critical review of genetic studies of schizophrenia. II. Molecular genetic studies. *Acta Psychiatrica Scandinavica, 95*, 73–80.

President's New Freedom Commission on Mental Health. (2004). *Report to the President*. Retrieved from http://www.mentalhealthcommission.gov/reports/reports.htm

Prouteau, A., Verdoux, H., Briand, C., Lesage, A., Lalonde, P., Nicole, L., ... Stip, E. (2005). Cognitive predictors of psychosocial functioning outcome in schizophrenia: A follow-up study of subjects participating in a rehabilitation program. *Schizophrenia Research, 77*, 343–353.

Rabinowitz, J., Levine, S. Z., Haim, R., & Häfner, H. (2007). The course of schizophrenia: Progressive deterioration, amelioration or both? *Schizophrenia Research, 91*, 254–258.

Racenstein, J. M., Harrow, M., Reed, R., Martin, E., & Penn, D. L. (2002). The relationship between positive symptoms and instrumental work functioning in schizophrenia: A 10 year follow-up study. *Schizophrenia Research, 56*, 95–103.

Ragland, J. D., Minzenberg, M. J., & Carter, C. S. (2007). Neuroimaging of cognitive disability in schizophrenia: Search for pathophysiological mechanism. *International Review of Psychiatry, 19*, 417–427.

Ralph, R. O., & Corrigan, P. W. (2005). *Recovery in mental illness: Broadening our understanding of wellness*. Washington, DC: American Psychology Association.

Rancone, R., Mazza, M., Frangou, I., De Risio, A., Ussorio, D., Tozzini, C., & Casacchia, M. (2004). Rehabilitation of theory of mind deficits in schizophrenia: A pilot study of metacognitive strategies in group treatment. *Neuropsychological Rehabilitation, 14*, 421–435.

Raz, S., & Raz, N. (1990). Structural brain abnormalities in the major psychoses: A quantitative review of the evidence from computerized imaging. *Psychological Bulletin, 108*(1), 93–108.

Read, J., van Os, J., Morrison, A. P., & Ross, C. A. (2005). Childhood trauma, psychosis and schizophrenia: A literature review with theoretical and clinical implications. *Acta Psychiatrica Scandinavica, 112*, 330–350.

Rector, N., Seeman, M. V., & Segal, Z. V. (2003). Cognitive therapy for schizophrenia: A preliminary randomized controlled trial. *Schizophrenia Research, 63*, 1–11.

Reeder, C., Smedley, N., Butt, K., Bogner, D., & Wykes, T. (2006). Cognitive predictors of social functioning improvements following cognitive remediation therapy. *Schizophrenia Bulletin, 32*(Suppl. 1), 123–131.

Reinecker, H. (1987). *Grundlagen der Verhaltenstherapie*. Munich, Germany: Urban & Schwarzenberg.

Resnick, S., Fontana, A., Lehman, A. F., & Rosenheck, R. (2005). An empirical conceptualization of the recovery orientation. *Schizophrenia Research, 75*, 119–128.

Resnick, S. G., Rosenheck, R. A., Canive, J. M., De-Souza, C., Stroup, T. S., McEvoy, J., ... Lieberman, J. (2008). Employment outcomes in a randomized trial of second-generation antipsychotics and perphenazine in the treatment of individuals with schizophrenia. *Journal of Behavioral Health Services and Research, 35*, 15–25.

Revheim, N., Schechter, I., Kim, D., Silipo, G., Allingham, B., Butler, P., & Javitt, D. C. (2006). Neurocognitive symptom correlates of daily problem-solving skills in schizophrenia. *Schizophrenia Research, 83*, 237–245.

Roberts, D., & Penn, D. L. (2009). Social Cognition and Interaction Training (SCIT) for outpatients with schizophrenia. *Psychiatry Research, 166*, 141–147.

Roberts, D., Penn, D. L., & Combs, D. (2006). *Social Cognition and Interaction Training*. Unpublished treatment manual. Chapel Hill, NC: University of North Carolina.

Roder, V. (1988). *Untersuchungen zur Effektivität kognitiver Therapieinterventionen mit schizophrenen Patienten*. Inaugural dissertation, University of Bern, Switzerland.

Roder, V. (1990). Evaluation einer kognitiven Schizophrenietherapie. In: Kühne, G. E., Brenner, H. D., Huber, G. (Eds.) *Kognitive Therapie bei Schizophrenen* (pp. 27–39). Jena, Germany: Fischer.

Roder, V., Brenner, H. D., & Kienzle, N. (2008). *Integriertes Psychologisches Therapieprogramm bei schizophren Erkrankten IPT*. Weinheim, Germany: Beltz.

Roder, V., Brenner, H. D., Kienzle, N., & Hodel, B. (1988). *Integriertes Psychologisches Therapieprogramm (IPT) für schizophrene Patienten*. Munich, Germany: Psychologie Verlags Union.

Roder, V., Brenner, H. D., Mueller, D. R., Lächler, M., Zorn, P., Reisch, T., ... Schwemmer, V. (2002). Development of specific social skills training programmes for schizophrenia patients: Results of a multicentre study. *Acta Psychiatrica Scandinavica, 105*, 363–371.

Roder, V., Brenner, H. D., Mueller, D., Reisch, T., Lächler, M., Zorn, P., ... Jenull, B. (2001). Effekte neuer kognitiv-behavioraler Therapieprogramme zur Verbesserung spezifischer sozialer Fertigkeiten bei schizophren Erkrankten: Eine kontrollierte Studie. *Nervenarzt, 72*, 709–716.

Roder, V., & Kienzle, N. (1986, October). *Ein multimodales Behandlungskonzept in der Rehabilitation and Rückfallprophylaxe schizophrener Patienten*. Vortrag, gehalten auf dem Kongreß der Deutschen Gesellschaft für Psychiatrie und Nervenheilkunde (DGPPN), Bayreuth, Germany.

Roder, V., Kienzle, N., & Studer, K. (1988, May). *Specific psychological therapy programs for treatment of cognitive and social disorders with individuals vulnerable to schizophrenia*. Paper presented at the IV. International Congress on Rehabilitation in Psychiatry, Oerebro, Sweden.

Roder, V., & Mueller, D. R. (2006). *Integrated Neurocognitive Therapy (INT) for schizophrenia patients*. Unpublished manual. Bern, Switzerland: University Psychiatric Hospital.

Roder, V., & Müller, D. R. (2009). Remediation of neuro- and social cognition: Results of an international randomized multisite study. *Schizophrenia Bulletin, 35*(Suppl. 1), 353–354.

Roder, V., Mueller, D. R., & Lächler, M. (2006). *Integrierte Neurokognitive Therapie (INT) für schizophren Erkrankte*. Unpublished manual. Bern, Switzerland: Universitäre Psychiatrische Dienste.

Roder, V., Mueller, D. R., Mueser, K. T., & Brenner, H. D. (2006). Integrated Psychological Therapy (IPT) for schizophrenia: Is it effective? *Schizophrenia Bulletin, 32*, 81–93.

Roder, V., Mueller, D. R., & Zorn, P. (2006). Therapieverfahren zu sozialen Fertigkeiten bei schizophren Erkrankten in der Arbeitsrehabilitation. Vorteile des Aufbaus arbeitsspezifischer gegenüber unspezifischer sozialer Fertigkeiten. *Zeitschrift für Klinische Psychologie und Psychotherapie, 35*, 256–266.

Roder, V., & Schmidt, S. (2009). Social cognition as a possible mediator between neuro-cognition and social functioning. *European Archives of Psychiatry and Clinical Neuroscience, 259*(Suppl. 1), 41.

Roder, V., Studer, K., &Brenner, H. D. (1987). Erfahrungen mit einem integrierten psychologischen Therapieprogramm zum Training kommunikativer und kognitiver Fähigkeiten in der Rehabilitation schwer chronisch schizophrener Patienten. *Schweizer Archiv für Neurologie und Psychiatrie, 138*, 31–44.

Roder, V., Zorn, P., & Brenner, H. D. (2000). Kognitiv-behaviorale Programme für schizophren Erkrankte zum Aufbau sozialer Kompetenzen im Wohn-, Arbeits- und Freizeitbereich: Überblick und empirische Ergebnisse. *Verhaltenstherapie und psychosoziale Praxis, 32*, 195–211.

Roder, V., Zorn, P., Mueller, D. R., & Brenner, H. D. (2001). Skills training for improving recreational, residential, and vocational outcomes in schizophrenia patients. *Psychiatric Services, 52*, 1439–1441.

Roder, V., Zorn, P., Pfammatter, M., Andres, K., Brenner, H. D., & Mueller, D. R. (2008). *Praxishandbuch zur verhaltenstherapeutischen Behandlung schizophren Erkrankter* (2nd ed.). Bern: Huber.

Rose, D., & Wykes, T. (2008). What do clients think of Cognitive Remediation Therapy?: A consumer-led investigation of satisfaction and side effects. *American Journal of Psychiatric Rehabilitation, 11*, 181–204.

Rosen, K., & Garety, P. (2005). Predicting recovery from schizophrenia: A retrospective comparison of characteristics at onset of people with single and multiple episodes. *Schizophrenia Bulletin, 31*, 735–750.

Rosenheck, R. A., Leslie, D. L., & Doshi, J. A. (2008). Second generation antipsychotics: Cost-effectiveness, policy options, and political decision making. *Psychiatry Services, 59*, 5515–520.

Rosenheck, R. A., Leslie, D. L., Sindelar, J., Miller, E. A., Lin, H., Stroup, T. S., . . . for the CATIE study investigators. (2006). Cost-effectiveness of second generation antipsychotics and perphenazine in a randomized trial of treatment for chronic schizophrenia. *American Journal of Psychiatry, 163*, 2080–2089.

Rosenthal, R., Hall, J. A., DiMatteo, M. R., Rogers, P. L., & Archer, D. (1979). *Sensitivity to non-verbal communication: the PONS test*. Baltimore, MD: John Hopkins University Press.

Rummel, C., Hansen, W. P., Helbig, A., Pitschel-Walz, G., & Kissling, W. (2005). Peer-to-peer psychoeducation in schizophrenia: A new approach. *Journal of Clinical Psychiatry, 66*, 1580–1585.

Rummel, C., Pitschel-Walz, G., & Kissling, W. (2005). "Family members inform family members" – family members as group moderators for psychoeducational groups in schizophrenia. *Psychiatrische Praxis, 32*, 87–92.

Rummel-Kluge, C., Pitschel-Walz, G., Bäuml, J., & Kissling, W. (2006). Psychoeducation in schizophrenia – results of a survey of all psychiatric institutions in Germany, Austria, and Switzerland. *Schizophrenia Bulletin, 32*, 765–75.

Rüsch, N., Spoletini, I., Wilke, M., Bria, P., Di Paola, M., Di Iulio, F., . . . Spalletta, G. (2007). Prefrontal – thalamic – cerebellar gray matter networks and executive functioning in schizophrenia. *Schizophrenia Research, 93*, 79–89.

Russell, T. A., Chu, E., & Phillips, M. L. (2006). A pilot study to investigate the effectiveness of emotion recognition remediation in schizophrenia using the micro-expression training tool. *British Journal of Clinical Psychology, 45*, 579–583.

Salovey, P., Woolery, A., & Mayer, J. D. (2001). Emotional intelligence: Conceptualization and measurement. In C.J.O. Fletcher & M.S. Clark (Eds.), *The Blackwell handbook of social psychology: Interpersonal processes* (pp. 279–307). Malden, MA: Blackwell.

San, L., Ciudad, A., Alvarez, E., Bobes, J., & Gilaberte, I. (2007). Symptomatic remission and social/vocational functioning in outpatients with schizophrenia: Prevalence and associations in a cross-sectional study. *European Psychiatry, 22,* 490–498.

Sandford, J.A., & Browne, R.J. (1988). *Captain's log cognitive system.* Richmond, VA: Brain Train.

Sarfati, Y., Passerieux, C., & Hardy-Baylé, M. (2000). Can verbalization remedy the theory of mind deficit in schizophrenia? *Psychopathology, 33,* 246–251.

Sartory, G., Zorn, C., Groetzinger, G., & Windgassen, K. (2005). Computerized cognitive remediation improves verbal learning and processing speed in schizophrenia. *Schizophrenia Research, 75,* 219–223.

Schenkel, L., Spaulding, W., DiLillo, D., & Silverstein, S. (2005). Histories of childhood maltreatment in schizophrenia: Relationships with premorbid functioning, symptomatology and cognitive deficits. *Schizophrenia Research, 76,* 273–286.

Schimmelmann, B.G., Huber, C.G., Lambert, M., Cotton, S., McGorry, P.D., & Conus, P. (2008). Impact of duration of untreated psychosis on pre-treatment, baseline, and outcome characteristics in an epidemiological first-episode psychosis cohort. *Journal Of Psychiatric Research, 42,* 982–990.

Schmidt, S.J., Mueller, D.R., & Roder, V. (2009). Untersuchung der Beziehung zwischen Neurokognition, sozialer Kognition und psychosozialem Funktionsniveau bei schizophren Erkrankten mittels Strukturgleichungsmodellen. In F. Schneider & M. Grözinger (Eds.), *Psychische Erkrankungen in der Lebensspanne – Abstractband zum DGPPN Kongress 2009, Berlin* (DOI 10.3287/dgppn.2009.1, 85). Berlin, Germany: Deutsche Gesellschaft für Psychiatrie, Psychotherapie und Nervenheilkunde.

Schüttler, R., Bell, V., Blumenthal, S., Neumann, N.U., & Vogen, R. (1990). Haben 2 kognitive Therapieprogramme messbaren Einfluss auf Basissymptome bei Schizophrenien? In G. Huber (Ed.), *Idiopathische Psychosen. Psychopathologie, Neurobiologie, Therapie* (S. 219–240). Stuttgart: Schattauer.

Semkovska, M., Bedard, M.A., Godbout, L., Limoge, F., & Stip, E. (2004). Assessment of executive dysfunction during activities of daily living in schizophrenia. *Schizophrenia Research, 69,* 289–300.

Sergi, M.J., Green, M.F., Widmark, C., Reist, C., Erhart, S., Braff, D.L., ... Mintz, J. (2007). Social cognition and neurocognition: Effects of risperidone, olanzapine, and haloperidol. *American Journal of Psychiatry, 164,* 1585–1592.

Sergi, M.J., Rassovsky, Y., Nuechterlein, K.H., & Green, M.F. (2006). Social perception as a mediator of the influence of early visual processing on functional status in schizophrenia. *American Journal of Psychiatry, 163,* 448–454.

Sergi, M.J., Rassovsky, Y., Widmark, C., Reist, C., Erhart, S., Braff, D.L., ... Green, M.F. (2007). Social cognition in schizophrenia: Relationships with neurocognition and negative symptoms. *Schizophrenia Research, 90,* 316–324.

Sharma, T., Lancaster, E., Lee, D., Lewis, S., Sigmundsson, T., Takei, N., ... Murray, R.M. (1998). Brain changes in schizophrenia. Volumetric MRI study of families multiply affected with schizophrenia: The Maudsley Family Study 5. *British Journal of Psychiatry, 173,* 132–138.

Silver, H., Goodman, C., Knoll, G., & Isakov, V. (2004). Brief emotion training improves recognition of facial emotions in chronic schizophrenia. A pilot study. *Psychiatry Research, 128,* 147–154.

Silverstein, M.L., Harrow, M., & Bryson, G.J. (1994). Neuropsychological prognosis and clinical recovery. *Psychiatry Research, 52,* 265–272.

Silverstein, M. L., Mavrolefteros, G., & Close, D. (2002). Premorbid adjustment and neuropsychological performance in schizophrenia. *Schizophrenia Bulletin, 28*, 157–165.

Silverstein, S. M., & Bellack, A. S. (2008). A scientific agenda for the concept of recovery as it applies to schizophrenia. *Clinical Psychology Review, 28*, 1108–1124.

Silverstein, S. M., Hatashita-Wong, M., Solak, B. A., Uhlhaas, P., Landa, Y., Wilkniss, S. M., . . . Smith, T. E. (2005). Effectiveness of a two-phase cognitive rehabilitation intervention for severely impaired schizophrenia patients. *Psychological Medicine, 35*, 829–837.

Silverstein, S. M., Menditto, A. A., & Stuve, P. (2001). Shaping attention span: An operant conditioning procedure to improve neurocognition and functioning in schizophrenia. *Schizophrenia Bulletin, 27*, 247–257.

Silverstein, S. M., Valone, C., Jewell, T. C., Corry, R., Nghiem, K., Saytes, M., & Portrude, S. (1999). Integrating shaping and skills training techniques in the treatment of chronic treatment refractory individuals with schizophrenia. *Psychiatric Rehabilitation Skills, 3*, 41–58.

Sitskoorn, M. M., Aleman, A., Ebich, S. J. H., Appels, M. C. M., & Kahn, R. S. (2004). Cognitive deficits in relatives of patients with schizophrenia: A meta-analysis. *Schizophrenia Research, 71*, 285–295.

Smith, E. T., Bellack, A. S., & Lieberman, R. P. (1996). Social skills training for schizophrenia: Review and future directions. *Clinical Psychology Review, 16*, 599–617.

Smith, G. N., Boydell, J., Murray, R. M., Flynn, S., McKay, K., Sherwood, M., & Honer, W. G. (2006). The incidence of schizophrenia in European immigrants to Canada. *Schizophrenia Research, 87*, 205–211.

Smith, T. E., Hull, J. W., Goodman, M., Hedayat-Harris, A., Wilson, D. F., Israel, L. M., & Munich, R. L. (1999). The relative influences of symptoms, insight, and neurocognition on social adjustment in schizophrenia and schizoaffective disorder. *Journal of Nervous and Mental Disorders, 187*, 102–108.

Sohlberg, M. M., & Mateer, C. A. (1987). Effectiveness of an attention-training program. *Journal of Clinical and Experimental Neuropsychology, 9*, 117–130.

Spaulding, W. (1986). Assessment of adult-onset pervasive behavior disorders. In H. Adams & K. Calhoun (Eds.), *Handbook of behavior assessment* (2nd ed., pp. 631–669). New York: Wiley.

Spaulding, W. (1994). *Cognitive technology in psychiatric rehabilitation*. Lincoln, NE: University of Nebraska Press.

Spaulding, W., & Nolting, J. (2006). Psychotherapy for schizophrenia in the year 2030: Prognosis and prognostication. *Schizophrenia Bulletin, 32*(Suppl. 1), 94–105.

Spaulding, W., Sullivan, M., & Poland, J. (2003). *Treatment and rehabilitation of severe mental illness*. New York: Guilford.

Spaulding, W. D., Reed, D., Sullivan, M., Richardson, C., & Weiler, M. (1999). Effects of cognitive treatment in psychiatric rehabilitation. *Schizophrenia Bulletin, 25*, 657–676.

Spauwen, J., Krabbendam, L., Lieb, R., Wittchen, H. U., & van Os, J. (2006). Impact of psychological trauma on the development of psychotic symptoms: Relationship with psychosis proneness. *British Journal of Psychiatry, 188*, 527–533.

Sprong, M., Schothorst, P., Vos, E., Hox, J., & van Engeland, H. (2007). Theory of mind in schizophrenia. *British Journal of Psychiatry, 191*, 5–13.

Stern, R. A., & White, T. (2003). *Neuropsychological Assessment Battery*. Lutz, FL: Psychological Assessment Resources, Inc.

Stevens, J. R. (1997). Anatomy of schizophrenia revisited. *Schizophrenia Bulletin, 23*, 373–383.

Stramke, W. G., & Brenner, H. D. (1983). Psychologische Trainingsprogramme zur Minderung defizitärer kognitiver Störungen in der Rehabilitation chronisch schizophrener Patienten. In H. D. Brenner, E. R. Rey, & W. G. Stramke (Eds.), *Empirische Schizophrenieforschung* (pp. 182–199). Bern, Switzerland: Huber.

Stramke, W. G., Hodel, B., & Brauchli, B. (1983). Untersuchungen zur Wirksamkeit psychologischer Therapieprogramme in der Rehabilitation chronisch schizophrener Patienten. In H. D. Brenner, E. R. Rey, & W. G. Stramke (Eds.), *Empirische Schizophrenieforschung* (pp. 216–234). Bern, Switzerland: Huber.

Straube, E. (1993). The heterogeneous prognosis of schizophrenia: Possible determinants of the short-term and five-year outcome. In R. L. Cromwell & C. R. Snyder (Eds.), *Schizophrenia: Origins, processes, treatment and outcome* (pp. 258–274). New York: Oxford Press.

Suddath, R. L., Christison, G. W., Torrey, E. F., Casanova, M. F., & Weinberger, D. R. (1990). Anatomical abnormalities in the brains of monozygotic twins discordant for schizophrenia. *The New England Journal of Medicine, 322*, 789–794.

Sullivan, P. F., Kendler, K. S., & Neale, M. C. (2003). Schizophrenia as a complex trait: Evidence form a meta-analysis of twin studies. *Archives of General Psychiatry, 60*, 1187–1192.

Süllwold, L. (1977). *Symptome schizophrener Erkrankungen.* Berlin, Germany: Springer.

Süllwold, L. (1991). *Frankfurter Beschwerde-Fragebogen (FBF).* Berlin, Germany: Springer.

Swartz, M. S., Perkins, D. O., Stroup, T. S., Davis, S. M., Capuano, G., Rosenheck, R. A., . . . Lieberman, J. (2007). Effects of antipsychotic medications on psychosocial functioning in patients with chronic schizophrenia: Findings from the NIMH CATIE study. *American Journal of Psychiatry, 164*, 428–436.

Takai, A., Uematsu, M., Kadama, Y., Ueki, H., & Sones, K. (1993). Kognitives Therapieprogramm bei chronisch schizophrenen Japanern. Eine kontrollierte Therapiestudie über die Auswirkungen auf Symptomatik und Bewältigungsmechanismen. *Schizophrenie, 8*(1), 29–34.

Tandon, R., Keshavan, M. S., & Nasrallah, H. A. (2008). Schizophrenia, "just the facts" what we know in 2008. Epidemiology and etiology. *Schizophrenia Research, 102*, 1–18.

Tarrier, N. (1992). Management and modification of residual psychotic symptoms. In M. Birchwood & N. Tarrier (Eds.), *Innovation in the psychological management of schizophrenia* (pp. 109–131). Chichester, UK: Wiley.

Tarrier, N., Barrowclough, C., Vaughn, C., Bamrah, J. S., Porceddu, K., Watts, S., & Freeman, H. (1988). The community management of schizophrenia: A controlled trial of a behavioural intervention with families to reduce relapse. *British Journal of Psychiatry, 153*, 532–542.

Tarrier, N., Wells, A., & Haddock, G. (Eds.). (1998). *Treating complex cases: The cognitive behavioral therapy approach.* Chichester, UK: Wiley.

Tennant, C. (1985). Stress and schizophrenia: A review. *Integrative Psychiatry, 3*, 248–255.

Theilemann, S. (1993). Beeinflussung kognitiver Störungen bei schizophrenen und schizoaffektiven Psychosen mit Hilfe kognitiver Therapie im Vergleich zur Soziotherapie. *Nervenarzt, 64*, 587–593.

Thornicroft, G., Tansella, M., Becker, T., Knapp, M., Leese, M., Schene, A., . . . EPSILON Study Group. (2004). The personal impact of schizophrenia in Europe. *Schizophrenia Research, 69*, 125–132.

Thorup, A., Petersen, L., Jeppesen, P., Ohlenschlaeger, J., Christensen, T., Krarup, G., . . . Nordentoft, M. (2007). Gender differences in young adults with first-episode schizophrenia spectrum disorders at baseline in the Danish OPUS study. *Journal of Nervous and Mental Disease, 195*, 396–405.

Tomas, P. (2009). *Entrenamiento cognitivo en la esquizofrenia.* Unpublished Tesis Doctoral. Valencia, Spain: Universitat de Valencia.

Toomey, R., Wallace, C. J., Corrigan, P. W., Schuldberg, D., & Green, M. F. (1997). Social processing correlates of nonverbal social perception in schizophrenia. *Psychiatry, 60*, 292–300.

Twamley, E. W., Doshi, R. R., Nayak, G. V., Palmer, B. W., Golshan, S., Heaton, R. K., . . . Jeste, D. V. (2002). Generalized cognitive impairments, ability to perform everyday tasks, and level of independence in community living situations of older patients with psychosis. *American Journal of Psychiatry, 159*, 2013–2020.

Twamley, E. W., Jeste, D. V., & Bellack, A. S. (2003). A review of cognitive training in schizophrenia. *Schizophrenia Bulletin, 29*, 359–382.

Twamley, E. W., Savla, G. N., Zurhellen, C. H., & Heaton, R. H. (2008). Development and pilot testing of a novel compensatory cognitive training intervention for people with psychosis. *American Journal of Psychiatric Rehabilitation, 11*, 144–163.

Twamley, E. W., Woods, S. P., Zurhellen, C. H., Vertinski, M., Narvaez, J. M., Mausbach, B. T., . . . Jeste, D. V. (2008). Neuropsychological substrates and everyday functioning implications of prospective memory impairments in schizophrenia. *Schizophrenia Research, 106*, 42–49.

Ueland, T., & Rund, B. R. (2004). A controlled randomized treatment study: The effects of a cognitive remediation program on adolescents with early onset psychosis. *Acta Psychiatrica Scandinavica, 109*, 70–74.

Ullman, L., & Krasner, L. (1965). *Case studies in behavior modification.* New York: Holt, Rinehart & Winston.

Usall, J., Haro, J. M., Araya, S., Moreno, B., Munoz, P. E., Martinez, A., & Salvador, L. (2007). Social functioning in schizophrenia: What is the influence of gender? *European Journal of Psychiatry, 21*, 199–205.

Usall, J., Haro, J. M., Ochosa, S., Marquez, M., & Araya, S. (2002). Influence of gender on social outcome in schizophrenia. *Acta Psychiatrica Scandinavica, 106*, 337–342.

Vallina-Fernandez, O., Lemos-Giraldez, S., Roder, V., Garcia-Saiz, A., Otero-Garzia, A., Alonso-Sanchez, M., & Gutiérrez-Pérez, A. M. (2001). An integrated psychological therapy program for schizophrenia. *Psychiatric Services, 52*, 1165–1167.

Van der Gaag, M. (1992). *The results of cognitive training in schizophrenic patients.* Delft, The Netherlands: Eburon.

Van der Gaag, M., Kern, R. S., van den Bosch, R. J., & Liberman, R. P. (2002). A controlled trial of cognitive remediation in schizophrenia. *Schizophrenia Bulletin, 28*, 167–176.

Van Horn, J. D., & McManus, I. C. (1992). Ventricular enlargement in schizophrenia. A meta-analysis of studies of the ventricle: brain ratio. *British Journal of Psychiatry, 160*, 687–697.

Van Os, J., Burns, T., Cavallaro, R., Leucht, S., Peuskens, J., Helldin, L., . . . Kane, J. M. (2006). Standardized remission criteria in schizophrenie. *Acta Psychiatrica Scandinavica, 113*, 91–95.

Van Os, J., Krabbendam, L., Myin-Germeys, I., & Delespaul, P. (2005). The schizophrenia evironment. *Current Opinion in Psychiatry, 58*, 141–145.

Van Os, J., & Selten, J. P. (1998). Prenatal exposure to maternal stress and subsequent schizophrenia. The May 1940 invasion of The Netherlands. *British Journal of Psychiatry, 172*, 324–326.

Vauth, R., Corrigan, P. W., Clauss, M., Dietl, M., Dreher-Rudolph, M., Stieglitz, R. D., & Vater, R. (2005). Cognitive strategies versus self-management skills as adjunct to vocational rehabilitation. *Schizophrenia Bulletin, 33*, 55–66.

Vauth, R., Dietl, M., Stieglitz, R.-D., & Olbrich, H. M. (2000). Kognitive Remediation: Eine neue Chance in der Rehabilitation schizophrener Störungen? *Nervenarzt, 71*, 19–29.

Vauth, R., Joe, A., Seitz, M., Dreher-Rudolph, M., Olbrich, H., & Stieglitz, R. D. (2001). Differenzielle Kurz- und Langzeitwirkung eines "Trainings Emotionaler Intelligenz" und des "Integrierten Psychologischen Therapieprogramms" für schizophrene Patienten. *Fortschritte in Neurologie und Psychiatrie, 69*, 518–525.

Vauth, R., Rüsch, N., Wirtz, M., & Corrigan, P. W. (2004). Does social cognition influence the relation between neurocognitive deficits and vocational functioning in schizophrenia? *Psychiatry Research, 128*, 155–165.

Vauth R., & Stieglitz, R. D. (2007). *Chronisches Stimmenhören und persistierender Wahn. Fortschritte der Psychotherapie.* Göttingen: Hogrefe.

Vauth, R., & Stieglitz, R. D. (2008). *Training Emotionaler Intelligenz bei schizophrenen Störungen. Ein Therapiemanual.* Göttingen: Hogrefe.

Velligan, D.I., & Bow-Thomas, C.C. (2000). Two case studies of cognitive adaption training for outpatients with schizophrenia. *Psychiatric Services, 51*, 25–29.

Velligan, D.I., Bow-Thomas, C.C., Huntzinger, C., Ritch, J., Ledbetter, N., Prihoda, T.J., & Miller, A.L. (2000). Randomized controlled trial of the use of compensatory strategies to enhance adaptive functioning in outpatients with schizophrenia. *American Journal of Psychiatry, 157*, 1317–1323.

Velligan, D.I., Kern, R.S., & Gold, J.M. (2006). Cognitive rehabilitation for schizophrenia and the putative role of motivation and expectancies. *Schizophrenia Bulletin, 32*, 474–485.

Velligan, D.I., Mueller, J., Wang, M., Dicocco, M., Diamond, P.M., Maples, N.J., & Davis, B. (2006). Use of environmental supports among people with schizophrenia. *Psychiatric Services, 57*, 219–224.

Velligan, D.I., Prihoda, T.J., Ritch, J.L., Maples, N., Bow-Thomas, C.C., & Dassori, A. (2002). A randomized single-blind pilot study of compensatory strategies in schizophrenia outpatients. *Schizophrenia Bulletin, 28*, 283–292.

Ventura, J., Bilder, S., Seise, S., & Keefe, R.S.E. (2008). *CAI Cognitive Assessment Interview* (Version 2). Los Angeles, CA: University of California.

Ventura, J., Cienfuegos, A., Boxer, O., & Bilder, R. (2008). Clinical global impression of cognition in schizophrenia (CGI-CogS): Reliability and validity of a co-primary measure of cognition. *Schizophrenia Research, 106*, 59–69.

Vita, A., Cocchi, A., Contini, A., Giannelli, A., Guerrini, A., Invernizzi, G., . . . Petrovich, L. (2002). Applicazione multicentrica del metodo riabilitativo strutturato IPT (Terapia Psicologica Integrata) per pazienti schizofrenici. *Psichiatria Oggi, 15*, 11–18.

Vogeley, K., & Falkai, P. (1998). The dysconnectivity hypothesis of schizophrenia. *Neurology-Psychiatry-and-Brain-Research, 6*(3), 113–122.

Walker, E.F., & Diforio, D. (1997). Schizophrenia: A neural diathesis-stress model. *Psychological Review, 104*, 667–685.

Wallace, C.J., Liberman, R.P., Tauber, R., & Wallace, J. (2000). The independent living skills survey: A comprehensive measure of the community functioning of severely and persistently mentally ill individuals. *Schizophrenia Bulletin, 26*, 631–658.

Wang, Y., Chan, R.C.K., Yu, X., Shi, J., & Deng, Y. (2008). Prospective memory deficits in subjects with schizophrenia spectrum disorders: A comparison study with schizophrenic subjects, psychometrically defined schizotypical subjects, and healthy controls. *Schizophrenia Research, 106*, 70–80.

White, C., Stirling, J., Hopkins, R., Morris, J., Montague, L., Tantam, D., & Lewis, S. (2009). Predictors of 10-year outcome of first-episode psychosis. *Psychological Medicine, 39*, 1447–1456.

WHO World Health Organization. (1988). *Psychiatric Disability Assessment Schedule (WHO/DAS)*. Geneva, Switzerland: Author.

WHO World Health Organization. (1999). *Schedules for Clinical Assessment in Neuropsychiatry (SCAN)* (Version 2.1). Geneva, Switzerland: Author.

Wilk, C.M., Gold, J.M., Humber, K., Dickerson, F., Fenton, W., & Buchanan, R. (2004). Brief cognitive assessment in schizophrenia: Normative data for the Assessment of Neuropsychological Status. *Schizophrenia Research, 70*, 175–186.

Wittorf, A., Wiedemann, G., Buchkremer, G., & Klingberg, S. (2008). Prediction of community outcome in schizophrenia 1 year after discharge from inpatient treatment. *European Archives of Psychiatry and Clinical Neuroscience, 258*, 48–58.

Wobrock, T., Schneider, M., Kadovic, D., Schneider-Axmann, T., Ecker, U.K.H., Retz, W., . . . Falkai, P. (2008). Reduced cortical inhibition in first-episode schizophrenia. *Schizophrenia Research, 105*, 252–261.

Wölwer, W., Frommann, N., Halfmann, S., Piaszek, A., Streit, M., & Gaebel, W. (2005). Remediation of impairments in facial affect recognition in schizophrenia: Efficacy and specificity of a new training program. *Schizophrenia Research, 80,* 295–303.

Woodruff, P. W., Wright, I. C., Shuriquie, N., Russouw, H., Rushe, T., Howard, R. J., . . . Murray, R. M. (1997). Structural brain abnormalities in male schizophrenics reflect fronto-temporal dissociation. *Psychological Medicine, 27,* 1257–1266.

Woods, S. P., Twamley, E. W., Dawson, M. S., Narvaez, J. M., & Jeste, D. V. (2007). Deficits in cue detection and intention retrieval underlie prospective memory impairment in schizophrenia. *Schizophrenia Research, 90,* 344–350.

Woodward, N. D., Purdon, S. E., Meltzer, H. Y., & Zald, D. H. (2007). A meta-analysis of cognitive change with haloperidol in clinical trials of atypical antipsychotics: Dose effects and comparison to practice effects. *Schizophrenia Research, 89,* 211–224.

Wykes, T., & van der Gaag, M. (2001). Is it time to develop a new cognitive therapy for psychosis – cognitive remediation therapy (CRT)? *Clinical Psychology Review, 21,* 1227–1256.

Wykes, T., & Reeder, C. (2005). *Cognitive Remediation Therapy for schizophrenia.* London, UK: Routledge.

Wykes, T., Reeder, C., Corner, J., Williams, C., & Eyeritt, B. (1999). The effects of neurocognitive remediation on executive processing in patients with schizophrenia. *Schizophrenia Bulletin, 25,* 291–307.

Wykes, T., Reeder, C., Williams, C., Corner, J., Rice, C., & Everitt, B. (2003). Are the effects of cognitive remediation therapy (CRT) durable? Results from an exploratory trial in schizophrenia. *Schizophrenia Research, 61,* 163–174.

Wykes, T., Steel, C., Everitt, B., & Tarrier, N. (2008). Cognitive behavior therapy for schizophrenia: Effect sizes, clinical methods, and methodological rigor. *Schizophrenia Bulletin, 34,* 523–537.

Yager, J. A., & Ehmann, T. S. (2006). Untangling social function and social cognition: A review of concepts and measurement. *Psychiatry, 69*(1), 47–68.

Zanello, A., Perrig, L., & Huguelet, P. (2006). Cognitive functions related to interpersonal problem-solving skills in schizophrenic patients compared with healthy subjects. *Psychiatry Research, 142,* 67–78.

Zimmer, M., Dunsan, A. V., Laitano, D., Ferreira, E. E., & Belmonte-de-Abreu, P. (2007). A twelve-week randomized controlled study of the cognitive-behavioral Integrated Psychological Therapy program: Positive effect on the social functioning of schizophrenic patients. *Revista Brasileira de Psiquiatria, 29*(2), 140–147.

Zimmermann, G., Favrod, J., Trieu, V., & Pomini, V. (2005). The effect of cognitive behavioral treatment on the positive symptoms of schizophrenia spectrum disorders: A meta-analysis. *Schizophrenia Research, 77,* 1–9.

Zubin, J., & Spring, B. J. (1977). Vulnerability: A new view of schizophrenia. *Journal of Abnormal Psychology, 86,* 103–126.

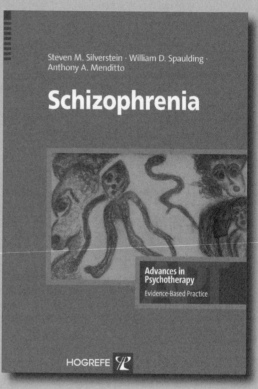
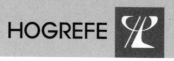

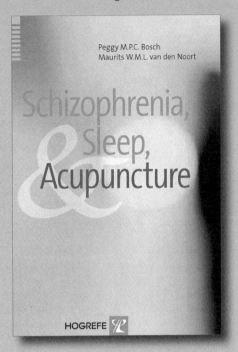
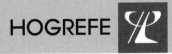